Recent Advances in Biomaterials and Dental Disease

Recent Advances in Biomaterials and Dental Disease

Editors

Naji Kharouf
Salvatore Sauro
Davide Mancino

MDPI • Basel • Beijing • Wuhan • Barcelona • Belgrade • Manchester • Tokyo • Cluj • Tianjin

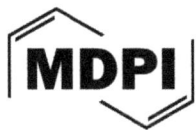

Editors

Naji Kharouf
Faculty of Dental Medicine,
Department of Biomaterials
and Bioengeneering
INSERM UMRS 1121
Strasbourg University
Strasbourg
France

Salvatore Sauro
Dental Biomaterials and
Minimally Invasive Dentistry,
Department of Dentistry
CEU Cardenal Herrera
University
CEU Universities
Valencia
Spain

Davide Mancino
Faculty of Dental Medicine,
Department of Biomaterials
and Bioengineering
INSERM UMRS 1121
Strasbourg University
Strasbourg
France

Editorial Office
MDPI
St. Alban-Anlage 66
4052 Basel, Switzerland

This is a reprint of articles from the Special Issue published online in the open access journal *Bioengineering* (ISSN 2306-5354) (available at: www.mdpi.com/journal/bioengineering/special_issues/biomaterials_root).

For citation purposes, cite each article independently as indicated on the article page online and as indicated below:

LastName, A.A.; LastName, B.B.; LastName, C.C. Article Title. *Journal Name* **Year**, *Volume Number*, Page Range.

ISBN 978-3-0365-6815-7 (Hbk)
ISBN 978-3-0365-6814-0 (PDF)

© 2023 by the authors. Articles in this book are Open Access and distributed under the Creative Commons Attribution (CC BY) license, which allows users to download, copy and build upon published articles, as long as the author and publisher are properly credited, which ensures maximum dissemination and a wider impact of our publications.

The book as a whole is distributed by MDPI under the terms and conditions of the Creative Commons license CC BY-NC-ND.

Contents

About the Editors . . . . **vii**

Preface to "Recent Advances in Biomaterials and Dental Disease" . . . . **ix**

Naji Kharouf, Salvatore Sauro, Louis Hardan, Youssef Haikel and Davide Mancino
Special Issue "Recent Advances in Biomaterials and Dental Disease" Part I
Reprinted from: *Bioengineering* **2023**, *10*, 55, doi:10.3390/bioengineering10010055 . . . . **1**

Naji Kharouf, Salvatore Sauro, Louis Hardan, Amr Fawzi, Ilona Eveline Suhanda and Jihed Zghal et al.
Impacts of Resveratrol and Pyrogallol on Physicochemical, Mechanical and Biological Properties of Epoxy-Resin Sealers
Reprinted from: *Bioengineering* **2022**, *9*, 85, doi:10.3390/bioengineering9030085 . . . . **7**

Calogero Bugea, Denise Irene Karin Pontoriero, Gaia Rosenberg, Giacomo Mario Gerardo Suardi, Gianmarco Calabria and Eugenio Pedullà et al.
Maxillary Premolars with Four Canals: Case Series
Reprinted from: *Bioengineering* **2022**, *9*, 757, doi:10.3390/bioengineering9120757 . . . . **25**

Victor Pinheiro Feitosa, Mara Natiere Mota, Roseane Savoldi, Tainah Rifane, Diego de Paula and Livia Borges et al.
The Allogenic Dental Pulp Transplantation from Son/Daughter to Mother/Father: A Follow-Up of Three Clinical Cases
Reprinted from: *Bioengineering* **2022**, *9*, 699, doi:10.3390/bioengineering9110699 . . . . **35**

Mateusz Radwanski, Corrado Caporossi, Monika Lukomska-Szymanska, Arlinda Luzi and Salvatore Sauro
Complicated Crown Fracture of Permanent Incisors: A Conservative Treatment Case Report and a Narrative Review
Reprinted from: *Bioengineering* **2022**, *9*, 481, doi:10.3390/bioengineering9090481 . . . . **45**

Krystyna Pietrzycka, Mateusz Radwanski, Louis Hardan, Rim Bourgi, Davide Mancino and Youssef Haikel et al.
The Assessment of Quality of the Root Canal Filling and the Number of Visits Needed for Completing Primary Root Canal Treatment by Operators with Different Experience
Reprinted from: *Bioengineering* **2022**, *9*, 468, doi:10.3390/bioengineering9090468 . . . . **59**

Hakjun Lee, Keunbada Son, Du-Hyeong Lee, So-Yeun Kim and Kyu-Bok Lee
Comparison of Wear of Interim Crowns in Accordance with the Build Angle of Digital Light Processing 3D Printing: A Preliminary In Vivo Study
Reprinted from: *Bioengineering* **2022**, *9*, 417, doi:10.3390/bioengineering9090417 . . . . **75**

Alejandro Elizalde-Hernández, Louis Hardan, Rim Bourgi, Cristina Pereira Isolan, Andressa Goicochea Moreira and J. Eliezer Zamarripa-Calderón et al.
Effect of Different Desensitizers on Shear Bond Strength of Self-Adhesive Resin Cements to Dentin
Reprinted from: *Bioengineering* **2022**, *9*, 372, doi:10.3390/bioengineering9080372 . . . . **89**

Louis Hardan, Davide Mancino, Rim Bourgi, Carlos Enrique Cuevas-Suárez, Monika Lukomska-Szymanska and Maciej Zarow et al.
Treatment of Tooth Wear Using Direct or Indirect Restorations: A Systematic Review of Clinical Studies
Reprinted from: *Bioengineering* **2022**, *9*, 346, doi:10.3390/bioengineering9080346 . . . . **101**

Ryan Harouny, Louis Hardan, Elie Harouny, Cynthia Kassis, Rim Bourgi and Monika Lukomska-Szymanska et al.
Adhesion of Resin to Lithium Disilicate with Different Surface Treatments before and after Salivary Contamination—An In-Vitro Study
Reprinted from: *Bioengineering* **2022**, *9*, 286, doi:10.3390/bioengineering9070286 . . . . **115**

Marc Krikor Kaloustian, Claire El Hachem, Carla Zogheib, Walid Nehme, Louis Hardan and Pamela Rached et al.
Effectiveness of the REvision System and Sonic Irrigation in the Removal of Root Canal Filling Material from Oval Canals: An In Vitro Study
Reprinted from: *Bioengineering* **2022**, *9*, 260, doi:10.3390/bioengineering9060260 . . . . **125**

Roberto Luongo, Fabio Faustini, Alessandro Vantaggiato, Giuseppe Bianco, Tonino Traini and Antonio Scarano et al.
Implant Periapical Lesion: Clinical and Histological Analysis of Two Case Reports Carried Out with Two Different Approaches
Reprinted from: *Bioengineering* **2022**, *9*, 145, doi:10.3390/bioengineering9040145 . . . . **137**

Louis Hardan, Rim Bourgi, Carlos Enrique Cuevas-Suárez, Monika Lukomska-Szymanska, Elizabeth Cornejo-Ríos and Vincenzo Tosco et al.
Disinfection Procedures and Their Effect on the Microorganism Colonization of Dental Impression Materials: A Systematic Review and Meta-Analysis of In Vitro Studies
Reprinted from: *Bioengineering* **2022**, *9*, 123, doi:10.3390/bioengineering9030123 . . . . **149**

Calogero Bugea, Federico Berton, Antonio Rapani, Roberto Di Lenarda, Giuseppe Perinetti and Eugenio Pedullà et al.
In Vitro Qualitative Evaluation of Root-End Preparation Performed by Piezoelectric Instruments
Reprinted from: *Bioengineering* **2022**, *9*, 103, doi:10.3390/bioengineering9030103 . . . . **165**

Inês Francisco, Raquel Travassos, Catarina Nunes, Madalena Ribeiro, Filipa Marques and Flávia Pereira et al.
What Is the Most Effective Technique for Bonding Brackets on Ceramic—A Systematic Review and Meta-Analysis
Reprinted from: *Bioengineering* **2022**, *9*, 14, doi:10.3390/bioengineering9010014 . . . . **175**

Inês Francisco, Anabela Baptista Paula, Madalena Ribeiro, Filipa Marques, Raquel Travassos and Catarina Nunes et al.
The Biological Effects of 3D Resins Used in Orthodontics: A Systematic Review
Reprinted from: *Bioengineering* **2022**, *9*, 15, doi:10.3390/bioengineering9010015 . . . . **219**

About the Editors

Naji Kharouf

Dr. Naji Kharouf currently works at the Laboratory INSERM UMRS 1121 and Faculty of Dental Medicine, University of Strasbourg, France. Naji carries out research on dental biomaterials, root canal anatomy, endodontic treatment, and restorative dentistry. Lecturer in: Microsurgical techniques Diploma, "Micro-endodontie Clinique et chirurgical" Diploma & Master of Biomaterials for health. Naji has a diploma in Microsurgical techniques, a Master in Biomaterials and Bioengineering, a certificate in endodontics, a certificate in oral implantology, a diploma in Esthetic smile and a PhD in Endodontics.

Salvatore Sauro

Prof. Dr. Salvatore Sauro is a Dental Research Coordinator and Professor in Dental Biomaterials and Minimally Invasive Dentistry Departamento de Odontologia, Facultad de Ciencias de la Salud, Universidad CEU-Cardenal Herrera Valencia, Spain. He is a Visiting Lecturer Centre of Oral Clinical & Translational Sciences Faculty of Dentistry, Oral & Craniofacial Sciences, King's College London (UK). Furthermore, he is Honorary Professor Faculty of Dentistry, The University of Hong Kong, Hong Kong, P.R. China. He is a Visiting Professor, Dipartimento Interdisciplinare, Università di Bari "Aldo Moro", Bari, Italia. He is a Visiting Professor, Department of Therapeutic Dentistry, I. M. Sechenov First Moscow State Medical University, Moscow, Russia.

Davide Mancino

Dr. Mancino Davide currently works at the Department of conservative and endodontic at the faculty of dental medicine, Strasbourg, France. Dr. Mancino carries out research in the field of dentistry. He is the director of "Micro-endodontie Clinique et chirurgical" diploma at Faculty of Dental Medicine.

Preface to "Recent Advances in Biomaterials and Dental Disease"

The researchers involved in this reprint will continue their studies to improve the existent dental biomaterials in order to achieve optimal dental treatment with biocompatible, bioactive, and stable properties. As the Guest Editors, we sincerely value and thank the reviewers for their insightful comments and the support of the team at Bioengineering. Finally, we express our gratitude to all contributing authors for their valuable research. Altogether, the 16 research papers/reviews in this Special Issue entitled "Recent Advances in Biomaterials and Dental Disease" reflect the importance of in vitro and in vivo studies for improving the efficacy of using biomaterials in dental treatment.

Naji Kharouf, Salvatore Sauro, and Davide Mancino
Editors

Editorial

Special Issue "Recent Advances in Biomaterials and Dental Disease" Part I

Naji Kharouf [1,2,*], Salvatore Sauro [3,4], Louis Hardan [5], Youssef Haikel [1,2,6] and Davide Mancino [1,2,6]

1. Department of Biomaterials and Bioengeneering, INSERM UMR_S, Strasbourg University, 67000 Strasbourg, France
2. Department of Endodontics, Faculty of Dental Medicine, Strasbourg University, 67000 Strasbourg, France
3. Dental Biomaterials and Minimally Invasive Dentistry, Department of Dentistry, CEU Cardenal Herrera University, CEU Universities, C/Santiago Ramón y Cajal, s/n., Alfara del Patriarca, 46115 Valencia, Spain
4. Department of Therapeutic Dentistry, I. M. Sechenov First Moscow State Medical University, 119146 Moscow, Russia
5. Department of Restorative Dentistry, School of Dentistry, Saint-Joseph University, Beirut 1107 2180, Lebanon
6. Pôle de Médecine et Chirurgie Bucco-Dentaire, Hôpital Civil, Hôpitaux Universitaire de Strasbourg, 67000 Strasbourg, France

* Correspondence: dentistenajikharouf@gmail.com; Tel.: +33-667522841

1. Introduction

Oral cavities provide an entry point for food and nutrients. Teeth consist of various hard and soft tissues, such as enamel, dentin, cementum, dental pulp, and the root canal system. Adsorbed macromolecules which are delivered by bacteria, blood, saliva, gingival fluids, particles, and molecules from the diet comprise the salivary pellicles [1]. Oral bacteria can adhere to the enamel surfaces (Figure 1) and demineralize dental hard tissues, resulting in the development of dental caries.

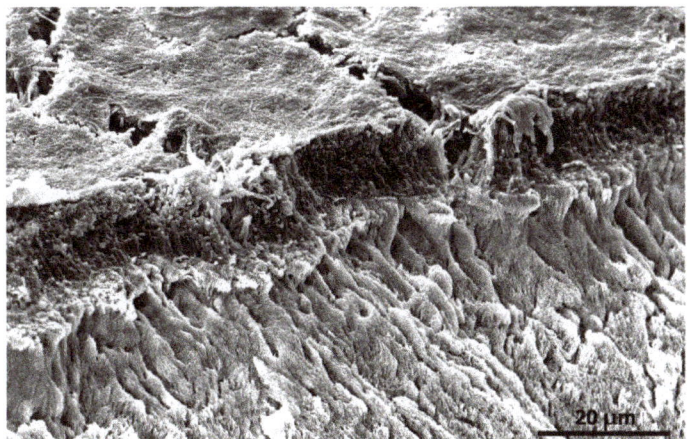

Figure 1. Scanning electron microscopy (SEM) shows the adhesion of oral biofilm to the enamel surface.

2. Individual Contribution

2.1. Enamel and Dentin Restoration

Once caries are established in the enamel and dentin structures, they can be eliminated with burs; then, the enamel and dentin structures can be restored with direct or indirect dental restorations [2–5]. These restorative biomaterials bond effectively to dental tissues, providing both durability and aesthetically satisfactory results [2,4,6,7]. Different desensitizers can produce chemical interactions with dentinal structures; these can be used in luting cements and may impact their bonding and sealing properties [8].

2.2. Modifications of Coronal Restorative Materials

Researchers have been working to improve the biological properties of coronal restorative biomaterials through adding bioactive molecules to their composition in order to ensure antibacterial and antioxidant properties [2,9]. Kharouf et al. [2] used pyrogallol to modify a dental adhesive. They reported that pyrogallol, a polyphenol–vegetable tannin, may preserve the polymer–dentin bonding interface and provide a certain degree of antibacterial activity.

2.3. Root Canal Treatment

Once bacteria arrive in the root pulp system, an endodontic treatment should be performed. The choice of endodontic treatment depends on the clinical situation [10].

Vital pulp therapy could be performed using pulp capping, partial pulpotomy, of full pulpotomy therapy [11–13]. Successful endodontic treatment consists of an appropriate access cavity [14], good shaping [15], proper cleaning using irrigants [16], and an optimal 3D obturation for the root canal system using sealer and gutta-percha [10,17,18]. Endodontic sealers must be used with gutta-percha to entomb the bacteria and ensure optimal sealing for the root canal system [19]. Several endodontic materials with different chemical compositions, such as zinc oxide eugenol, gutta-percha flow, epoxy–resin, and calcium silicate, have been introduced in the dental market. In addition, different studies have modified endodontic sealers with different polyphenols to enhance their properties [20]. Various endodontic treatments, such as pulpotomy, pulp capping, perforation, open apex, and the retrograde endodontic procedure, should be performed with materials that are more viscous than endodontic sealers, for example, endodontic cements (putty) [21].

2.4. Calcium Silicate Materials in Endodontic Treatment

Recently, calcium silicate (CS) materials were introduced to the dental market. The advantageous antibacterial activity, biocompatibility, filling ability, and physicochemical properties of CS materials have led this product to be the primary choice in modern clinical endodontics [11,21,22]. Moreover, these materials can be used in both permanent and primary teeth [23]. Despite the advantages of the evolution which has occurred in the endodontic field, some cases should be retreated with mechanical and chemical procedures to eliminate root canal materials which are no longer in use, clean the root canal system, and retreat re-infected teeth [24,25]. When orthograde endodontic treatment cannot be performed correctly, surgical endodontic treatment must be performed to improve the effectiveness of root canal debridement, and the quality of the retro-preparation and the retro-obturation of the apical part of the dental root [26,27]. Moreover, different regenerative endodontic techniques could offer good alternatives for pulp revitalization in some endodontic situations [28].

2.5. Final Restoration Materials and Preparation Steps

Today, a major challenge for dentists is in restoring the functionality of endodontically treated teeth. Several materials and techniques have been proposed to have a good restoration ability; these also ensure the durability of a restoration. Until now, there is no specific restoration for endodontically treated teeth which could avoid the restorative complications that lead to failure and tooth extraction [29–31]. Recently, Kharouf et al. [32] studied a new material—a bidirectional, spiral-winding, fiber-reinforced composite—which demonstrated a high compressive strength resistance; this material could be a promising solution for restoring endodontically treated teeth. In addition, different techniques could be used to fabricate the final restoration, such as the digital light-processing 3D-printing technique [7]. Several materials can be used in the final restoration, such as composite resin, zirconia, and lithium disilicate. Cleaning and disinfection procedures of these restorations, including impression materials, are recommended to ensure the quality of dental treatment. Hardan et al. reported that several disinfection agents could be used to disinfect dental impression materials [33]. Harouny et al. demonstrated that the use of phosphoric acid on the lithium disilicate surface provide efficient cleaning [34]. Therefore, the main aim of studies in the dental restoration field is to ameliorate the mechanical properties, bond strength, and durability of direct and indirect restoration approaches, as well as to improve the techniques used to bond brackets to teeth with different restorative materials in orthodontic treatments [35,36].

2.6. Dental Implant

Dental implants have been a solution for replacing lost teeth and for supporting fixed or removable prostheses for over 40 years. However, during the implantation planning stage, any sources of infection in the edentulous area should be carefully identified in advance to avoid complications with the dental implants [37].

3. Conclusions

Finally, the researchers involved in this Special Issue will continue their studies to improve the existent dental biomaterials in order to have an optimal dental treatment with biocompatible, bioactive, and stable properties.

As the Guest Editors, we sincerely value and thank the reviewers for their insightful comments and the support of the team at *Bioengineering*. Finally, we express our gratitude to all contributing authors for their valuable research. Altogether, the 15 research papers/reviews in this Special Issue—entitled Recent Advances in Biomaterials and Dental Disease—reflect the importance of in vitro and in vivo studies for improving the efficacy of using biomaterials in dental treatment.

Author Contributions: Conceptualization, N.K., Y.H., D.M., L.H. and S.S.; validation, N.K., Y.H., D.M., L.H. and S.S.; formal analysis, N.K., Y.H., D.M., L.H. and S.S.; investigation, N.K., Y.H., D.M., L.H. and S.S.; writing—original draft preparation, N.K.; writing—review and editing, N.K., Y.H., D.M., L.H. and S.S.; visualization, N.K., Y.H., D.M., L.H. and S.S.; supervision, N.K.; project administration, N.K., Y.H., D.M., L.H. and S.S. All authors have read and agreed to the published version of the manuscript.

Funding: This editorial received no external funding.

Conflicts of Interest: The editors declare no conflicts of interest.

References

1. Kharouf, N.; Haikel, Y.; Ball, V. Polyphenols in Dental Applications. *Bioengineering* **2020**, *7*, 72. [CrossRef]
2. Kharouf, N.; Eid, A.; Hardan, L.; Bourgi, R.; Arntz, Y.; Jmal, H.; Foschi, F.; Sauro, S.; Ball, V.; Haikel, Y.; et al. Antibacterial and Bonding Properties of Universal Adhesive Dental Polymers Doped with Pyrogallol. *Polymers* **2021**, *13*, 1538. [CrossRef]
3. Hardan, L.; Mancino, D.; Bourgi, R.; Cuevas-Suárez, C.E.; Lukomska-Szymanska, M.; Zarow, M.; Jakubowicz, N.; Zamarripa-Calderón, J.E.; Kafa, L.; Etienne, O.; et al. Treatment of Tooth Wear Using Direct or Indirect Restorations: A Systematic Review of Clinical Studies. *Bioengineering* **2022**, *9*, 346. [CrossRef] [PubMed]
4. Kharouf, N.; Ashi, T.; Eid, A.; Maguina, L.; Zghal, J.; Sekayan, N.; Bourgi, R.; Hardan, L.; Sauro, S.; Haikel, Y.; et al. Does Adhesive Layer Thickness and Tag Length Influence Short/Long-Term Bond Strength of Universal Adhesive Systems? An In-Vitro Study. *Appl. Sci.* **2021**, *11*, 2635. [CrossRef]
5. Kharouf, N.; Mancino, D.; Rapp, G.; Zghal, J.; Arntz, Y.; Haikel, Y.; Reitzer, F. Does Etching of the Enamel with the Rubbing Technique Promote the Bond Strength of a Universal Adhesive System. *J. Contemp. Dent. Pract.* **2020**, *21*, 1117–1121. [CrossRef] [PubMed]
6. Hardan, L.; Bourgi, R.; Cuevas-Suárez, C.E.; Lukomska-Szymanska, M.; Monjarás-Ávila, A.J.; Zarow, M.; Jakubowicz, N.; Jorquera, G.; Ashi, T.; Mancino, D.; et al. Novel Trends in Dental Color Match Using Different Shade Selection Methods: A Systematic Review and Meta-Analysis. *Materials* **2022**, *15*, 468. [CrossRef]
7. Lee, H.; Son, K.; Lee, D.-H.; Kim, S.-Y.; Lee, K.-B. Comparison of Wear of Interim Crowns in Accordance with the Build Angle of Digital Light Processing 3D Printing: A Preliminary In Vivo Study. *Bioengineering* **2022**, *9*, 417. [CrossRef]

8. Elizalde-Hernández, A.; Hardan, L.; Bourgi, R.; Isolan, C.P.; Moreira, A.G.; Zamarripa-Calderón, J.E.; Piva, E.; Cuevas-Suárez, C.E.; Devoto, W.; Saad, A.; et al. Effect of Different Desensitizers on Shear Bond Strength of Self-Adhesive Resin Cements to Dentin. *Bioengineering* **2022**, *9*, 372. [CrossRef]
9. Toledano, M.; Osorio; Vallecillo-Rivas, M.; Osorio, E.; Lynch, C.D.; Aguilera, F.S.; Toledano, R.; Sauro, S. Zn-doping of silicate and hydroxyapatite-based cements: Dentin mechanobiology and bioactivity. *J. Mech. Behav. Biomed. Mater.* **2021**, *114*, 104232. [CrossRef]
10. Bugea, C.; Pontoriero, D.I.K.; Rosenberg, G.; Suardi, G.M.G.; Calabria, G.; Pedullà, E.; La Rosa, G.R.M.; Sforza, F.; Scarano, A.; Luongo, R.; et al. Maxillary Premolars with Four Canals: Case Series. *Bioengineering* **2022**, *9*, 757. [CrossRef]
11. Eid, A.; Mancino, D.; Rekab, M.S.; Haikel, Y.; Kharouf, N. Effectiveness of Three Agents in Pulpotomy Treatment of Permanent Molars with Incomplete Root Development: A Randomized Controlled Trial. *Healthcare* **2022**, *10*, 431. [CrossRef]
12. Richman, J.A. Properties of Pulp Capping Materials. *Pediatr. Dent.* **2022**, *44*, 319.
13. Marinčák, D.; Doležel, V.; Přibyl, M.; Voborná, I.; Marek, I.; Šedý, J.; Žižka, R. Conservative Treatment of Complicated Crown Fracture and Crown-Root Fracture of Young Permanent Incisor—A Case Report with 24-Month Follow-Up. *Children* **2021**, *8*, 725. [CrossRef]
14. Jamleh, A.; Aljohani, S.M.; Alzamil, F.F.; Aljuhayyim, S.M.; Alsubaei, M.N.; Alali, S.R.; Alotaibi, N.M.; Nassar, M. Assessment of the educational value of endodontic access cavity preparation YouTube video as a learning resource for students. *PLoS ONE* **2022**, *17*, e0272765. [CrossRef]
15. Pedullà, E.; Kharouf, N.; Caruso, S.; La Rosa, G.R.M.; Jmal, H.; Haikel, Y.; Mancino, D. Torsional, Static, and Dynamic Cyclic Fatigue Resistance of Reciprocating and Continuous Rotating Nickel-Titanium Instruments. *J. Endod.* **2022**, *48*, 1421–1427. [CrossRef] [PubMed]
16. Kharouf, N.; Pedullà, E.; La Rosa, G.R.M.; Bukiet, F.; Sauro, S.; Haikel, Y.; Mancino, D. In Vitro Evaluation of Different Irrigation Protocols on Intracanal Smear Layer Removal in Teeth with or without Pre-Endodontic Proximal Wall Restoration. *J. Clin. Med.* **2020**, *9*, 3325. [CrossRef]
17. Mancino, D.; Kharouf, N.; Cabiddu, M.; Bukiet, F.; Haïkel, Y. Microscopic and chemical evaluation of the filling quality of five obturation techniques in oval-shaped root canals. *Clin. Oral. Investig.* **2021**, *25*, 3757–3765. [CrossRef] [PubMed]
18. Pietrzycka, K.; Radwanski, M.; Hardan, L.; Bourgi, R.; Mancino, D.; Haikel, Y.; Lukomska-Szymanska, M. The Assessment of Quality of the Root Canal Filling and the Number of Visits Needed for Completing Primary Root Canal Treatment by Operators with Different Experience. *Bioengineering* **2022**, *9*, 468. [CrossRef] [PubMed]
19. Mancino, D.; Kharouf, N.; Hemmerlé, J.; Haïkel, Y. Microscopic and Chemical Assessments of the Filling Ability in Oval-Shaped Root Canals Using Two Different Carrier-Based Filling Techniques. *Eur. J. Dent.* **2019**, *13*, 166–171. [CrossRef] [PubMed]
20. Kharouf, N.; Sauro, S.; Hardan, L.; Fawzi, A.; Suhanda, I.E.; Zghal, J.; Addiego, F.; Affolter-Zbaraszczuk, C.; Arntz, Y.; Ball, V.; et al. Impacts of Resveratrol and Pyrogallol on Physicochemical, Mechanical and Biological Properties of Epoxy-Resin Sealers. *Bioengineering* **2022**, *9*, 85. [CrossRef]
21. Kharouf, N.; Zghal, J.; Addiego, F.; Gabelout, M.; Jmal, H.; Haikel, Y.; Bahlouli, N.; Ball, V. Tannic acid speeds up the setting of mineral trioxide aggregate cements and improves its surface and bulk properties. *J. Colloid Interface Sci.* **2021**, *589*, 318–326. [CrossRef]
22. Kharouf, N.; Sauro, S.; Eid, A.; Zghal, J.; Jmal, H.; Seck, A.; Macaluso, V.; Addiego, F.; Inchingolo, F.; Affolter-Zbaraszczuk, C.; et al. Physicochemical and Mechanical Properties of Premixed Calcium Silicate and Resin Sealers. *J. Funct. Biomater.* **2023**, *14*, 9. [CrossRef]
23. Hachem, C.E.; Chedid, J.C.A.; Nehme, W.; Kaloustian, M.K.; Ghosn, N.; Sahnouni, H.; Mancino, D.; Haikel, Y.; Kharouf, N. Physicochemical and Antibacterial Properties of Conventional and Two Premixed Root Canal Filling Materials in Primary Teeth. *J. Funct. Biomater.* **2022**, *13*, 177. [CrossRef]
24. Kaloustian, M.K.; Hachem, C.E.; Zogheib, C.; Nehme, W.; Hardan, L.; Rached, P.; Kharouf, N.; Haikel, Y.; Mancino, D. Effectiveness of the REvision System and Sonic Irrigation in the Removal of Root Canal Filling Material from Oval Canals: An In Vitro Study. *Bioengineering* **2022**, *9*, 260. [CrossRef] [PubMed]
25. Garrib, M.; Camilleri, J. Retreatment efficacy of hydraulic calcium silicate sealers used in single cone obturation. *J. Dent.* **2020**, *98*, 103370. [CrossRef] [PubMed]
26. Bugea, C.; Berton, F.; Rapani, A.; Di Lenarda, R.; Perinetti, G.; Pedullà, E.; Scarano, A.; Stacchi, C. In Vitro Qualitative Evaluation of Root-End Preparation Performed by Piezoelectric Instruments. *Bioengineering* **2022**, *9*, 103. [CrossRef]
27. Ashi, T.; Mancino, D.; Hardan, L.; Bourgi, R.; Zghal, J.; Macaluso, V.; Al-Ashkar, S.; Alkhouri, S.; Haikel, Y.; Kharouf, N. Physicochemical and Antibacterial Properties of Bioactive Retrograde Filling Materials. *Bioengineering* **2022**, *9*, 624. [CrossRef]
28. Feitosa, V.P.; Mota, M.N.; Savoldi, R.; Rifane, T.; de Paula, D.; Borges, L.; Solheiro, L.K.; Aguiar Neto, M.; Vieira, L.; Moreira, A.C.; et al. The Allogenic Dental Pulp Transplantation from Son/Daughter to Mother/Father: A Follow-Up of Three Clinical Cases. *Bioengineering* **2022**, *9*, 699. [CrossRef]
29. Zarow, M.; Dominiak, M.; Szczeklik, K.; Hardan, L.; Bourgi, R.; Cuevas-Suárez, C.E.; Zamarripa-Calderón, J.E.; Kharouf, N.; Filtchev, D. Effect of Composite Core Materials on Fracture Resistance of Endodontically Treated Teeth: A Systematic Review and Meta-Analysis of In Vitro Studies. *Polymers* **2021**, *13*, 2251. [CrossRef]
30. Kharouf, N.; Sauro, S.; Jmal, H.; Eid, A.; Karrout, M.; Bahlouli, N.; Haikel, Y.; Mancino, D. Does Multi-Fiber-Reinforced Composite-Post Influence the Filling Ability and the Bond Strength in Root Canal? *Bioengineering* **2021**, *8*, 195. [CrossRef]

31. Radwanski, M.; Caporossi, C.; Lukomska-Szymanska, M.; Luzi, A.; Sauro, S. Complicated Crown Fracture of Permanent Incisors: A Conservative Treatment Case Report and a Narrative Review. *Bioengineering* **2022**, *9*, 481. [CrossRef]
32. Kharouf, N.; Sauro, S.; Hardan, L.; Jmal, H.; Bachagha, G.; Macaluso, V.; Addiego, F.; Inchingolo, F.; Haikel, Y.; Mancino, D. Compressive Strength and Porosity Evaluation of Innovative Bidirectional Spiral Winding Fiber Reinforced Composites. *J. Clin. Med.* **2022**, *11*, 6754. [CrossRef] [PubMed]
33. Hardan, L.; Bourgi, R.; Cuevas-Suárez, C.E.; Lukomska-Szymanska, M.; Cornejo-Ríos, E.; Tosco, V.; Monterubbianesi, R.; Mancino, S.; Eid, A.; Mancino, D.; et al. Disinfection Procedures and Their Effect on the Microorganism Colonization of Dental Impression Materials: A Systematic Review and Meta-Analysis of In Vitro Studies. *Bioengineering* **2022**, *9*, 123. [CrossRef]
34. Harouny, R.; Hardan, L.; Harouny, E.; Kassis, C.; Bourgi, R.; Lukomska-Szymanska, M.; Kharouf, N.; Ball, V.; Khairallah, C. Adhesion of Resin to Lithium Disilicate with Different Surface Treatments before and after Salivary Contamination—An In-Vitro Study. *Bioengineering* **2022**, *9*, 286. [CrossRef]
35. Francisco, I.; Travassos, R.; Nunes, C.; Ribeiro, M.; Marques, F.; Pereira, F.; Marto, C.M.; Carrilho, E.; Oliveiros, B.; Paula, A.B.; et al. What Is the Most Effective Technique for Bonding Brackets on Ceramic—A Systematic Review and Meta-Analysis. *Bioengineering* **2022**, *9*, 14. [CrossRef]
36. Francisco, I.; Paula, A.B.; Ribeiro, M.; Marques, F.; Travassos, R.; Nunes, C.; Pereira, F.; Marto, C.M.; Carrilho, E.; Vale, F. The Biological Effects of 3D Resins Used in Orthodontics: A Systematic Review. *Bioengineering* **2022**, *9*, 15. [CrossRef] [PubMed]
37. Luongo, R.; Faustini, F.; Vantaggiato, A.; Bianco, G.; Traini, T.; Scarano, A.; Pedullà, E.; Bugea, C. Implant Periapical Lesion: Clinical and Histological Analysis of Two Case Reports Carried Out with Two Different Approaches. *Bioengineering* **2022**, *9*, 145. [CrossRef] [PubMed]

Disclaimer/Publisher's Note: The statements, opinions and data contained in all publications are solely those of the individual author(s) and contributor(s) and not of MDPI and/or the editor(s). MDPI and/or the editor(s) disclaim responsibility for any injury to people or property resulting from any ideas, methods, instructions or products referred to in the content.

Article

Impacts of Resveratrol and Pyrogallol on Physicochemical, Mechanical and Biological Properties of Epoxy-Resin Sealers

Naji Kharouf [1,2,*], Salvatore Sauro [3,4], Louis Hardan [5], Amr Fawzi [6], Ilona Eveline Suhanda [1], Jihed Zghal [7,8], Frédéric Addiego [9], Christine Affolter-Zbaraszczuk [2], Youri Arntz [1,2], Vincent Ball [1,2], Florent Meyer [1,2,10], Youssef Haikel [1,2,10] and Davide Mancino [1,2,10]

1. Department of Endodontics and Conservative Dentistry, Faculty of Dental Medicine, Université de Strasbourg, 67000 Strasbourg, France; ilona-eveline.suhanda@etu.unistra.fr (I.E.S.); youri.arntz@unistra.fr (Y.A.); vball@unistra.fr (V.B.); fmeyer@unistra.fr (F.M.); youssef.haikel@unistra.fr (Y.H.); mancino@unistra.fr (D.M.)
2. Institut National de la Santé et de la Recherche Médicale, INSERM UMR_S 1121 Biomaterials and Bioengineering, 67085 Strasbourg, France; c.affolter-zbaraszczuk@unistra.fr
3. Dental Biomaterials and Minimally Invasive Dentistry, Department of Dentistry, Cardenal Herrera-CEU University, CEU Universities, C/Santiago Ramón y Cajal, s/n., Alfara del Patriarca, 46115 Valencia, Spain; salvatore.sauro@uchceu.es
4. Department of Therapeutic Dentistry, I. M. Sechenov First Moscow State Medical University, 119146 Moscow, Russia
5. Department of Restorative Dentistry, Saint-Joseph University, Beirut 11072180, Lebanon; louis.hardan@usj.edu.lb
6. UWA Dental School, University of Western Australia, Nedlands, WA 6009, Australia; amr.fawzy@uwa.edu.au
7. ICube Laboratory, UMR 7357 CNRS, Mechanics Department, University of Strasbourg, 67000 Strasbourg, France; zghal@unistra.fr
8. Laboratoire Energetique Mecanique Electromagnetisme, University of Paris Ouest, 50 rue de Sèvres, 92410 Ville d'Avray, France
9. Luxembourg Institute of Science and Technology (LIST), Department Materials Research and Technology (MRT), ZAE Robert Steichen, 5 rue Bommel, L-4940 Hautcharage, Luxembourg; frederic.addiego@list.lu
10. Pôle de Médecine et Chirurgie Bucco-Dentaire, Hôpital Civil, Hôpitaux Universitaires de Strasbourg, 67000 Strasbourg, France
* Correspondence: dentistenajikharouf@gmail.com; Tel.: +33-(0)66-752-2841

Abstract: This study aimed at evaluating the physicochemical and biological properties of experimental epoxy-resin sealers containing polyphenols such as resveratrol and pyrogallol. A conventional epoxy resin (OB) was modified by adding different concentrations of resveratrol (RS) or pyrogallol (PY) to its composition. Antibacterial and antioxidant activities, mechanical properties, along with wettability and morphological changes were investigated. The results were statistically analyzed using ANOVA and multiple comparison tests ($\alpha = 0.05$). The incorporation of the tested polyphenols into the epoxy resin enhanced its mechanical properties. PY demonstrated much better antioxidant and antibacterial activities than RS, which were associated with a higher release of PY. In contrast, PY showed a higher cytotoxicity than OB and OB doped with RS. OB containing PY presented a rougher surface and higher water absorption than OB doped with RS. Both tested polyphenols caused no notable changes to the overall porosity of OB. Resveratrol and pyrogallol may not only influence the morphology and mechanical properties of epoxy-resin sealers, but could also enhance antioxidant activity and antibacterial effects against *Enterococcus faecalis*. Most epoxy-resin sealers currently available in the market can be considered as "passive" materials. Thus, doping their composition with specific polyphenols may be a suitable strategy to confer some antibacterial properties, antioxidant potential, along with improvement of some mechanical properties.

Keywords: endodontic sealer; polyphenols; resveratrol; pyrogallol; biological activity

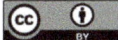

1. Introduction

For appropriate preparation of a cavity access, good shaping, proper cleaning and well-sealed tridimensional filling of the root canal space are essential factors in order to achieve a successful endodontic treatment [1,2]. Since it does not seem possible to entirely eliminate bacteria in an infected root canal system, a clinician should try to entomb such residual bacteria during obturation procedures, along with their byproducts, as much as possible. Indeed, to provide a hermetic tridimensional seal of the root canal system, gutta-percha is used in combination with root canal sealers during endodontics procedures [2,3].

Nevertheless, the incidence of voids formation during such procedures is still very high and proliferation of residual bacteria in such circumstances is inevitable; the risk for failure in the long-term outcome of root canal treatments is highly plausible [1–3]. A root canal sealer should be characterized as having good sealing ability, exhibiting low solubility, along with having high biocompatibility and antibacterial activity [3,4]. Depending on their chemical compositions, several types of root canal sealers are currently available in clinics, such as glass ionomer cements, silicone-based sealers, epoxy resins, calcium silicate-based sealers and zinc oxide-eugenol [3,5]. Calcium silicate-based sealers demonstrate good filling ability and antibacterial activity [3,6] but they are still overly expensive [7]. Conversely, epoxy resin-based sealers are relatively inexpensive, but they are characterized by limited or no antibacterial activity [8–10] especially against *Enterococcus faecalis* (*E. faecalis*), a predominant bacteria found in persistent endodontic infections and root canal re-treatment cases [3,8].

Polyphenols have been used to modify various dental materials in order to enhance their mechanical properties, biological activity and bonding strength to tooth tissues [11]. For instance, Hu et al. [12] used epigallocatechin-3-gallate (EGCG) in glass ionomer cements to improve their antibacterial ability, along with flexural strength and surface microhardness. In a further study [4] a cement with a mineral trioxide aggregate (MTA) base was doped with tannic acid (TA); there was an increase in compressive stiffness at higher concentrations of TA. Resveratrol (RS) (3,4,5-trihydroxystylbene), a polyphenol from the stilbene family characterized by a phytoalexin phenolic compound, was incorporated into dentin bonding agents in order to improve their biocompatibility [13]. RS has been used to treat dentin before the application of dental adhesives in order to preserve the dentin-resin bond over time [14]. Moreover, pyrogallol (PY) (1,2,3-trihydroxybenzene) is a well-known organic compound produced in plants [15] that is often used for its potent antibacterial activity against *Staphylococcus aureus* [16]. PY has been used in endosseous implant applications as a nanocoating; the release of PY can reduce significantly the growth of planktonic bacteria [17]. Moreover, the presence of pyrogallol groups in tannic acid have been demonstrated to play a role in the treatment of dentin hypersensitivity [18]. Several studies reported that resveratrol and pyrogallol exhibit antibacterial activity against Gram- and Gram+ bacteria [16,19–21].

Since epoxy-resin sealers have no evident antibacterial activity, the main idea of the present study was to incorporate some specific polyphenols with antibacterial properties into a conventional sealer currently available in the market. Thus, the purpose of the present study was to evaluate morphological changes, antibacterial activity, cytotoxicity and chemical-mechanical properties of an epoxy-resin endodontic sealer doped with different polyphenols, such as pyrogallol and resveratrol. The null hypothesis was that the addition of the different polyphenols (RS or PY) would have no impact on physicochemical and biological properties of tested epoxy-resin sealers.

2. Materials and Methods

2.1. Experimental and Control Materials

A conventional epoxy-resin dental sealer currently available in the market (OB) (Obturys, ITENA Clinical, Paris, France) was used in this study and labelled as the control group (Table 1). It was also used to generate several experimental cements by mixing different concentrations (0.5 wt%, 1 wt% and 5 wt%) of pyrogallol "PY" (Sigma Aldrich,

Saint-Quentin-Fallavier, France, ref. P0381) or resveratrol "RS" (Sigma Aldrich, Saint-Quentin-Fallavier, France, ref. R5010). It was not possible to incorporate more than 5% of RS or PY to prepare such experimental materials as a result of issues related to mixing, which caused inhomogeneous blends on a visual basis.

Table 1. Endodontic sealer and polyphenols: chemical compositions and references.

Materials	Reference	Chemical Composition
Obturys (OB)	OBAX1-5	Base: DGEBA, zirconium oxide, bismuth oxychloride, ytterbium oxide, fumed silica Catalyst: diamine, zirconium oxide, bismuth oxychloride, ytterbium oxide, fumed silica, silane quaternary ammonium salt
Pyrogallol (PY)	P0381-250G	$C_6H_3(OH)_3$ 1,2,3-Trihydroxybenzene
Resveratrol (RS)	R5010-500MG	$C_{14}H_{12}O_3$ 3,5,4'-trihydroxy-*trans*-stilbene

2.2. Specimen Preparations

The epoxy-resin dental sealer (OB) used in this study has two components (base and catalyst), but the polyphenols (RS or PY) were only added to the base part of the sealer and mixed using a mixing spatula for approximately 1 min until a homogenous paste was obtained on a visual basis. Subsequently, the complex (powder + base) was added to the catalyst paste and mixed for 1 min in order to obtain the experimental PY@OB or RS@OB sealers. All groups of specimens were labelled as OB (control group, epoxy resin without the addition of polyphenols), OB@RS (epoxy-resin modified with resveratrol) and OB@PY (epoxy-resin modified with pyrogallol). Stainless steel ring molds (internal diameter 20 ± 0.1 mm and height 1.6 ± 0.1 mm) were used to prepare the specimens for solubility, contact angle and roughness tests. Meanwhile, discs of 10 mm in diameter and 2 mm in height were prepared to test the release kinetic of the polyphenols and to perform surface ultra-morphology analysis via scanning electron microscopy. Finally, cylindrical specimens (internal diameter 3 mm and height 3.8 mm) were prepared for evaluation of their compressive strength, porosity, cytotoxicity and antioxidant properties. All specimens were stored in the dark in a container at 37 °C for 48 h in order to achieve a proper setting time.

2.3. Antimicrobial Activity

2.3.1. Bacterial Strain

Enterococcus faecalis (*E. faecalis*, ATCC 29212) was cultured in Brain Heart Infusion medium (BHI) (Darmstadt, Germany). In all tests, the turbidity of BHI containing *E. faecalis* was adjusted to $OD_{600\ (nm)} = 0.3$.

2.3.2. Agar Diffusion Tests (ADT)

The ADT tests were performed as described in previous studies [3]. In brief, six agar-filled petri dishes each containing 25 mL of BHI agar were used to evaluate antibacterial activity of the experimental materials OB@RS and/or OB@PY at different concentrations of PY and RS (0.5 wt%, 1 wt% and 5 wt%). A precise amount of the bacterial medium (100 µL) was spread homogeneously onto the petri dishes. Four wells in each petri dish, 3.0 mm in diameter and 3.0 mm in depth, were made with an adapted whack (3 mm, PFM medical, Köln, Germany) by removing the agar. The first three wells were filled with 0.5, 1 and 5 wt% of OB@PY or OB@RS, while the fourth well was filled with the control group (OB). All the agar petri dishes were incubated at 37 °C for 24 h. The inhibition zone in each group was assessed after 24 h of incubation [3].

2.3.3. Direct Contact Tests (DCT)

Immediately after mixing, for each tested group (in triplicate), each composite was placed (0.06 g per well) in the center of each well (24-well culture plates) (Trefflab, Degersheim, Switzerland). A specific amount of *E. faecalis* (1 mL) was added to each well and incubated for 24 h anaerobically at 37 °C under constant stirring (450 rpm). Positive control was set as *E. faecalis* culture without material. At each time step, the *E. faecalis* concentration was measured by manual counting. Briefly, 10-fold serial dilutions up to 10^5 in BHI were performed on each specimen of *E. faecalis* solution. Onto a BHI agar plate was homogeneously spread 100 µL of each dilution, and then incubated at 37 °C. After 24 h of incubation, colonies on the plate were counted and their CFU/mL (colony forming units/mL) were determined from the dilution plate.

2.4. Cytotoxicity Test

NIH3T3 cell line (mouse fibroblast ATCC CRL-1658) was cultivated in high-glucose content Dulbecco's Modified Eagle Medium (DMEM) with 10% fetal bovine serum and 1% of penicillin-streptomycin (Dominique Dutscher, Bernolsheim, France). Activated media were prepared by incubating OB, OB@5%RS and OB@5%PY specimens (in triplicate) in 500 µL of complete medium for 24 h at 37 °C. Prior to the experiment, NIH3T3 were seeded in a 96-well plate at a concentration of 8000 cells per well, in complete medium and incubated overnight. After the incubation period, the cell medium was removed and replaced with 100 µL of activated medium and incubated for a further 24 h at 37 °C, 5% CO_2. The medium was then removed and 100 µL of complete medium containing 3–(4,5-dimethylthiazol-2-yl)–2,5-diphenyltetrazolium bromide (MTT) at 0.5 mg/mL was added to each well. Cells were incubated for 2 h at 37 °C. The medium was carefully discarded and 100 µL of dimethyl sulfoxide (DMSO) was added per well. The plate was then incubated at room temperature for 15 min under gentle stirring in order to dissolve MTT crystals. The absorbance of the solution was measured at 570 nm using a spectrophotometer (Safas, Monaco, Monaco). Cell viability was then calculated from a standard curve, generated under the same conditions, with control medium (w/o material) as 100%.

2.5. Antioxidant Activity

One specimen from each group (OB, OB@5%RS and OB@5%PY) was immersed in 10 mL of 2,2-diphenyl-1-picrylhydrazyl (DPPH) (10^{-4} mol/L in 70% ethanol). After 30 min and 2 h, 0.5 mL of each supernatant solution above the specimens was taken (after vigorous shaking) using a calibrated pipette. The absorption spectrum of each solution was measured at a wavelength range between 300 and 600 nm. The solution that was in contact with OB was used in the reference cell. Digital pictures of all DPPH solutions above the specimens were also captured after 5 min and 2 h of contact.

2.6. Release Kinetics of RS and of PY in Water and pH Measurement

Stock solutions of RS (0.1 mg/mL) and PY (0.1 mg/mL) were prepared and diluted gradually between 2 and 100 times with distilled water. Absorption spectra from each group were acquired using a double beam mc^2 spectrophotometer (SAFAS, 98000 Monaco, Monaco) in order to establish a calibration curve allowing for the quantification of RS and PY release from the OB@RS and OB@PY sealers. The measurement cuvette was filled with a solution containing RS or PY, whereas the reference cuvette was filled with distilled water. One specimen from each material (OB, OB@RS and OB@PY) (containing 250 mg of each composite) was immersed in 15 mL of distilled water using a glass bottle. After 1, 3, 6, 24, 48 and 72 h, 0.5 mL of each supernatant solution was taken (after vigorous shaking). Subsequently, the absorption spectrum was measured (wavelength range between 200 and 700 nm). An absorption peak was observed at λ = 306 nm for the RS solutions and at λ = 267 nm for the PY solutions. The solution in contact with OB (control group) was used as reference. After each measurement, 0.5 mL of distilled water was added into each glass bottle in order to maintain a constant volume. pH measurements were performed at

24 ± 2 °C after incubation of the specimens in distilled water, under the same conditions as for the release experiment (3 h, 24 h and 72 h).

2.7. Solubility Evaluation

Three specimens from each tested material were prepared as reported in a previous study [3] and analyzed in accordance with the ISO standards 6876:2001. The specimens were weighed three times using a digital system (accuracy ± 0.0001 g) before different aging immersion periods (24 h and 7 days). After two immersion periods in 50 mL of distilled water at 37 °C, the specimens were removed from distilled water, gently washed with distilled water and dried at 37 °C for 24 h. Subsequently, the weight of each specimen was assessed three times and averaged to obtain the final weight. The solubility percentage of each tested material was determined from the difference in mass between the initial weight (before the immersion period in water) and the final weight [3].

2.8. Scanning Electron Microscopy (SEM) and Energy Dispersive X-ray (EDX) Analysis

Three specimens from each material group (OB, OB@5%RS and OB@5%PY) were created as described in Section 2.2 and immersed in phosphate-buffered saline (PBS10×, Dominique Dutscher, Bernolsheim, France) at 37 °C for 72 h and 7 days. After storage, all specimens were sputter-coated with gold-palladium (20/80) using a Hummer JR sputtering device (Technics, California, USA) and analyzed at a magnification of ×5000 for their chemical, mineral and morphological changes using an SEM-EDX (Quanta 250 FEG scanning electron microscope "FEI Company, Eindhoven, The Netherlands"; 10 kV acceleration voltage of the electrons). The weight percentages of the chemical elements were acquired from the outer surfaces of the specimens.

2.9. Water Sorption Tests, Roughness and Porosity Measurements

Five measurements were performed for each of the tested materials (OB, OB@5%PY and OB@5%RS), which were prepared as described in Section 2.2. A contact angle measurement device (Attention Theta, Biolin Scientific, Götenborg, Sweden) was used to measure the time of adsorption of an 8-microliter droplet of distilled water onto the surface of the tested materials. A video was recorded (10 frames per second) by a digital camera in order to track the profile of the water droplet and to calculate the contact angle of the water droplet at interval times.

The internal structures of OB, OB@5%RS and OB@5%PY were inspected in 3D by means of micro-computed X-ray tomography (µCT) (EasyTom 160 from RX Solutions, Chavanod, France). Imaging was conducted at a voltage of 45 kV and a current of 160 mA, using a micro-focused tube equipped with a tungsten filament. The source-to-detector distance (SDD) and the source-to-object distance (SOD) were adjusted in such ways to obtain a voxel size of around 2.3 µm. Volume reconstruction was performed with the software Xact64 (RX Solutions) after applying treatments such as geometrical corrections and ring artefact attenuation. Image treatment was performed with the Avizo software (ThermoFisher, Waltham, MA, USA) that enabled us to (i) de-noise the images with a median filter; (ii) segmentate the image intensity to reveal the objects of interest (here the pores); (iii) remove insignificant small objects (below a size of 10 pixels from the segmented 3D data); and (iv) determine the 3D geometrical aspects of the objects of interest (volume and equivalent diameter).

Atomic force microscopy (AFM) imaging was carried out in contact mode using the Bioscope Catalyst (Bruker Inc., Santa Barbara, CA, USA) equipped with MLCT cantilevers (0.7 N/m) (Bruker Inc., Santa Barbara, CA, USA). Images were obtained at a specific resolution (256 × 256 pixels) with a scan rate of 1 Hz (field of view of 10 × 10 µm). The roughness (Ra) was measured on three different representative regions of interest using the shareware software GWYDION.

2.10. Compressive Strength

Sixteen specimens were prepared from each test material and observed with an optical microscope at 10× magnification (Zumax medical, Suzhou New District, China) for the presence of voids or fractures. All specimens that presented such defects were discarded from the mechanical analysis. Half of the specimens were kept dry, while the other half were stored in water for 72 h. After storage, the specimens were tested using the uni-axial compression test in order to determine the stiffness of the cement and the maximum load before rupture. Such tests were performed using a universal electromechanical tensile Instron 3345 (Norwood, MA, USA) device instrumented with a 1 kN cell force (Class 0.5 following ISO 7500-1) and with a displacement sensor. The tests were performed at a constant crosshead speed of 0.5 mm/min. The compressive strength was calculated in megapascals (MPa) according to the following formula:

$$\sigma c = 4P/\pi D^2$$

where P is the recorded load during the test and D is the initial sample diameter.

2.11. Statistical Analysis

Statistical analysis was performed using SigmaPlot (release 11.2, Systat Software, Inc., San Jose, CA, USA). The Shapiro–Wilk test was used to verify the normality of the data in all groups. Analysis of the Variance (ANOVA) including a multiple comparison procedure (Holm-Sidak method) were used in order to determine whether significant differences existed in the compressive strength values, antibacterial activity, water sorption tests, roughness measurements and solubility evaluations between the different composites. In all tests, a statistical significance level of $\alpha = 0.05$ was adopted.

3. Results

3.1. Antibacterial Activity

Generally speaking, the incorporation of PY into the sealer materials increased antibacterial activity against *Enterococcus faecalis*, whilst RS caused bacterial growth similar to the positive control.

3.1.1. Agar Diffusion Tests

The OB sealer (control group) produced no inhibition zone on agar plates (Figure 1a,b). Conversely, OB@5%PY presented a large inhibition zone (5 ± 1 mm) (Figure 1b). OB@1%RS and OB@5%RS created only very small inhibition zones (1–1.5 mm). Note that the inhibition zones as well as part of the gel appeared brown in the presence of OB@5%PY as a result of the release of PY from the specimens (Figure 1b).

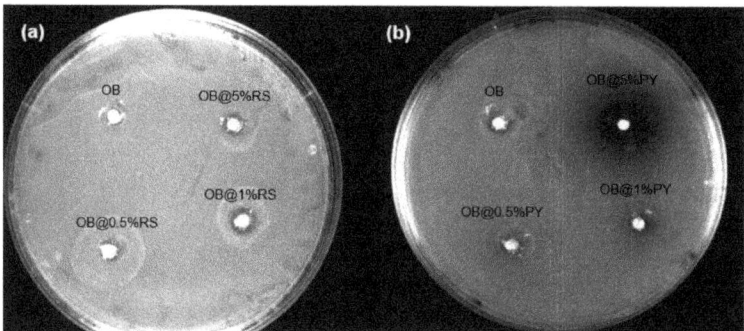

Figure 1. Agar diffusion tests with the different materials. (**a**) Control group (Obturys "OB") and the sealer modified with different concentrations of resveratrol (OB@RS); (**b**) control group (OB) and the sealer modified with different concentrations of pyrogallol (OB@PY).

3.1.2. Direct Contact Tests

The sealer (OB) caused significantly less bacterial growth than the control group (bacterial medium) ($p < 0.05$). The experimental OB@5%PY killed about 94% of *E. faecalis* bacteria after 24 h compared to the bacterial medium (Figure 2). In addition, OB@5%PY presented greater antibacterial activity than OB (<0.05). However, no differences were found between OB and OB@0.5%RS/PY, OB@1%RS/PY and OB@5%RS at 24 h; they all killed between 70% and 78% of the bacteria (Figure 2). However, it was evident that 5%PY was by far much more efficient than 5%RS against *E. faecalis*.

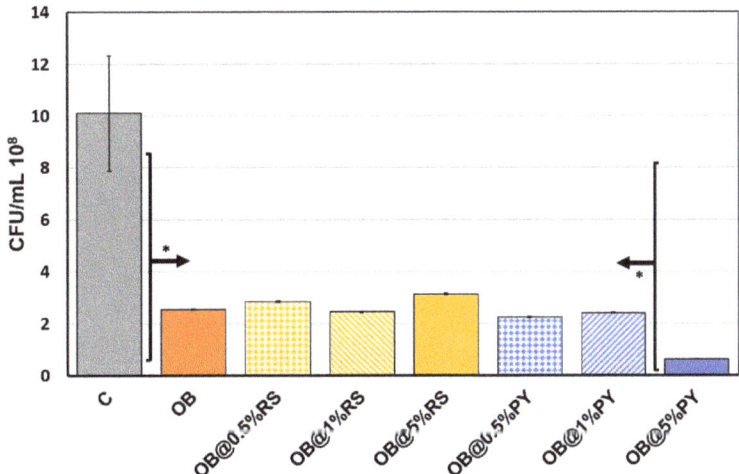

Figure 2. Number of colony forming units/mL of *E. faecalis* in the presence of sealer (OB) and sealer + different concentrations of RS/PY after 24 h of culture. C represents the control CFU experiment, without any material in each case. * $p < 0.05$.

3.2. Antioxidant Activity

As expected, the control group (OB) had no effect on the color of the DPPH solution, hence there was no antioxidant activity (Figure 3). However, incorporation of either PY or RS provided this additional property to the experimental sealers tested in this study (Figure 3). After 5 min and 2 h of contact between the DPPH solution and tested materials, the solution in contact with the PY group appeared much clearer than the solution in contact with the RS group (Figure 3, Table 2). Using an extinction coefficient of 1.09×10^4 L·mol^{-1}·cm^{-1} for DPPH at $\lambda = 525$ nm [22], we calculate from the absorbance decrease values provided in Table 2 that 53% and 43% of DPPH are quenched after 30 min of contact with OB@5%PY and with OB@5%RS, respectively. One PY and one RS molecule are equivalent to three TROLOX molecules from an antioxidant point of view [22].

Table 2. Antioxidant activity, as measured by a reduction in absorbance at 525 nm corresponding to a discoloration of 2,2-diphenyl-1-picrylhydrazyl (DPPH) solutions in contact with OB, OB@5%RS and OB@5%PY composites.

	30 min	2 h
PY (525 nm)	−0.58 ± 0.02	−0.54 ± 0.01
RS (525 nm)	−0.47 ± 0.01	−0.45 ± 0.004

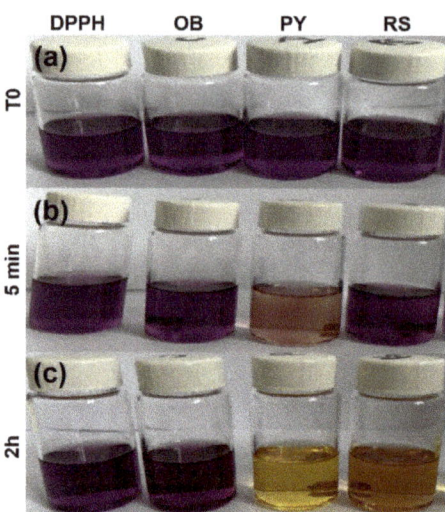

Figure 3. Digital pictures of color changes undergone by a 2,2-diphenyl-1-picrylhydrazyl (DPPH) solution (10^{-4} mol/L in 70% ethanol); (**a**) before (upper row, T0); (**b**) after 5 min; and (**c**) after 2 h of contact with the different composites.

3.3. Cytotoxicity

Cytotoxicities of leachable components from OB, OB@5%RS and OB@5%PY were evaluated at 24 h and it was observed that OB and OB@5%RS have good cell viabilities, (92.79 ± 6.18)% and (87.93 ± 4.89)%, respectively. In contrast, at 24 h it was observed that activated media from OB@5%PY showed acute toxicity with 0% cell viability.

3.4. Release Kinetics of RS and of PY in Water and pH Measurement of Water in Contact with the Composites

A maximum of 22.5% of the initial PY was released after 72 h (Figure 4) for OB@5%PY. In contrast, the maximum release of OB@RS was 0.2%, which was reached in the case of the addition of 5% RS (Figure 4a). These results showed that the higher the PY concentration, the higher the concentration of PY released in water (Figure 4). The release of PY and RS induced a slight decrease in the pH of water in contact with the different materials. After 72 h, such a reduction in pH was more pronounced in the case of OB@5%PY compared to the other tested materials (Figure 4b).

3.5. Solubility Evaluation

The results of solubility percentages (wt.%) of the tested composites after 1 and 7 days are presented in Figure 5. None of the solubility percentages exceeded 1.1% after 7 days. OB@5%PY demonstrated significantly higher solubility percentages for both testing periods compared to all the other tested materials ($p < 0.05$).

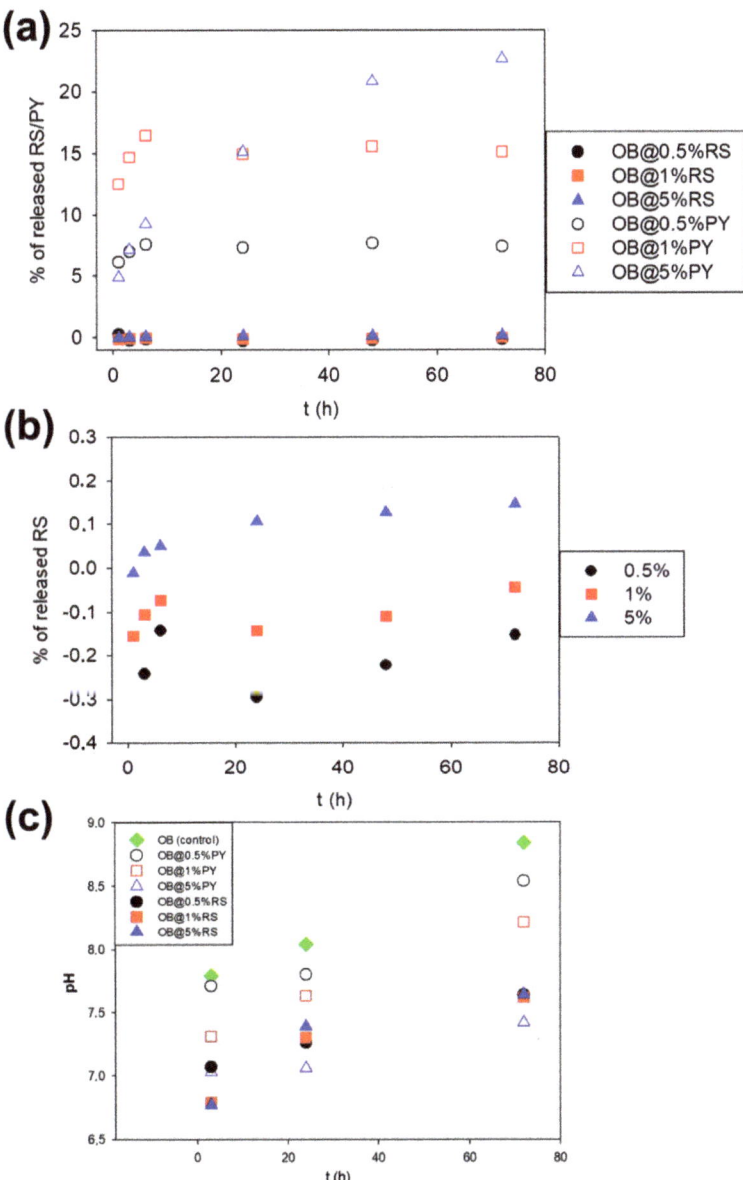

Figure 4. (a) Percentages of RS and PY released from the different composites versus time with respect to different initial mass fractions in the composites; (b) percentages of RS released from the different composites versus time with respect to the different initial mass fractions in the composites; (c) pH changes with time of water put in contact with sealer sample (control) and sealer modified with different concentrations of PY and/or RS as shown in the inset.

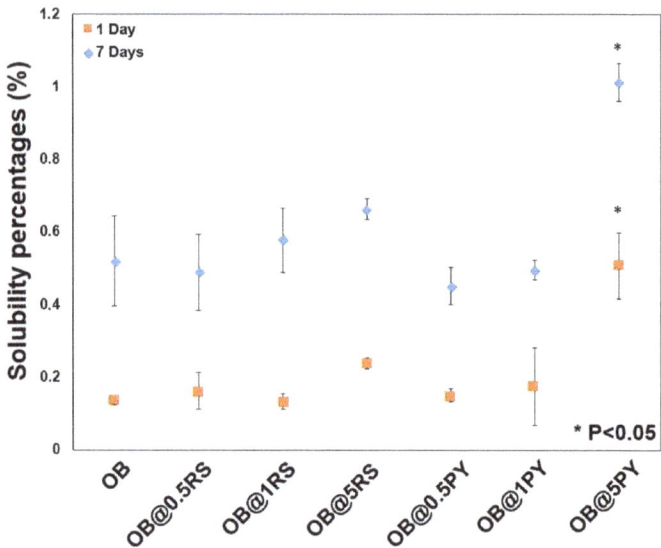

Figure 5. Solubility percentages (wt.%) ($n = 3$) of OB and OB modified with different concentrations of RS and PY in distilled water at 37 °C after 1 and 7 days. * $p < 0.05$.

3.6. Scanning Electron Microscopy (SEM) and Energy Dispersive X-ray (EDX) Analysis

The results of the tested materials' surfaces after immersion in PBS are depicted in Figure 6 and Table 3. Larger crystallites were observed on OB@PY/RS surfaces after 7 d compared to those on the OB surface. The chemical analyses of these surfaces determined by EDX analysis showed a remarkable decrease in the carbon content of the large crystallites in the RS and PY specimens after 7 d. The different chemical compositions are provided in Table 3.

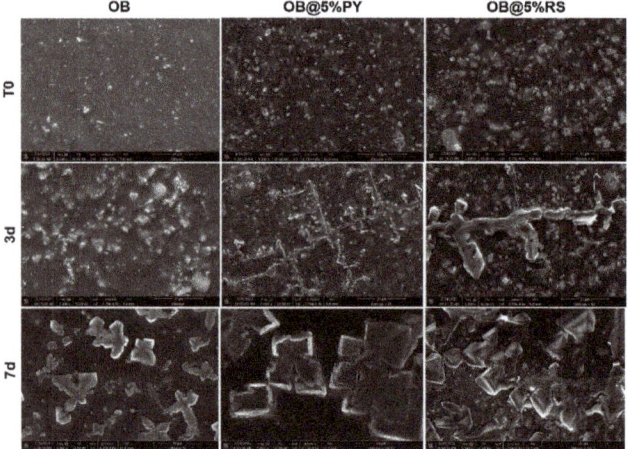

Figure 6. Representative scanning electron microscopy images at 5000× magnification. The morphologies of OB, OB@5%RS and OB@5%PY surfaces were analyzed in dry condition (T0); and after 3 and 7 days in PBS at 37 °C.

Table 3. Relative compositions of the experimental sealers as measured by means of EDX at T0 and after 7 days of immersion in PBS.

	Elements	T0	T7 Days
	C (%)	70 ± 2	66 ± 4.5
	O (%)	19 ± 1	17 ± 1.6
Obturys (OB)	Zr (%)	7.5 ± 2	5 ± 2.3
	Si (%)	1.5 ± 0.2	1 ± 0.4
	Cl (%)	1 ± 0.1	6 ± 2
	Na (%)	0	5 ± 1.8
	C (%)	63 ± 1.5	53 ± 4
	O (%)	18 ± 0.8	15 ± 2
OB@5%RS	Zr (%)	14 ± 1	11 ± 2
	Si (%)	2.2 ± 0.3	1.6 ± 0.4
	Cl (%)	1.6 ± 0.8	10 ± 4
	Na (%)	0	8.5 ± 3.6
	C (%)	62 ± 2.5	48 ± 11
	O (%)	20 ± 0.2	12 ± 2.2
OB@5%PY	Zr (%)	13 ± 3	7 ± 3
	Si (%)	2.5 ± 0.4	1 ± 0.5
	Cl (%)	1.7 ± 0.8	17 ± 7
	Na (%)	0	14 ± 5

3.7. Water Sorption Tests and Roughness

A further significant influence of the addition of PY (5%) into the epoxy-resin structure was a resulting increase in its hydrophilicity (Figure 7). Contact angles of $(58 \pm 1)°$ and $(46 \pm 2)°$ for OB@5%PY were detected after 20 s and 100 s, respectively. These were significantly lower than the respective contact angles observed in OB $(74 \pm 4°, 66 \pm 5°)$ and OB@5%RS $(68 \pm 5°, 62 \pm 5°)$, $p < 0.05$. No significant differences were found between OB and OB@5%RS ($p > 0.05$). All tested materials analyzed using AFM displayed rough surfaces (Figure 7a–c). However, a rougher surface was observed in OB@5%PY $(69.45 \pm 17.3$ nm$)$ compared to OB control $(11.11 \pm 5.9$ nm, $p < 0.001)$ and OB@5%RS $(30.27 \pm 10.27$ nm, $p = 0.003)$.

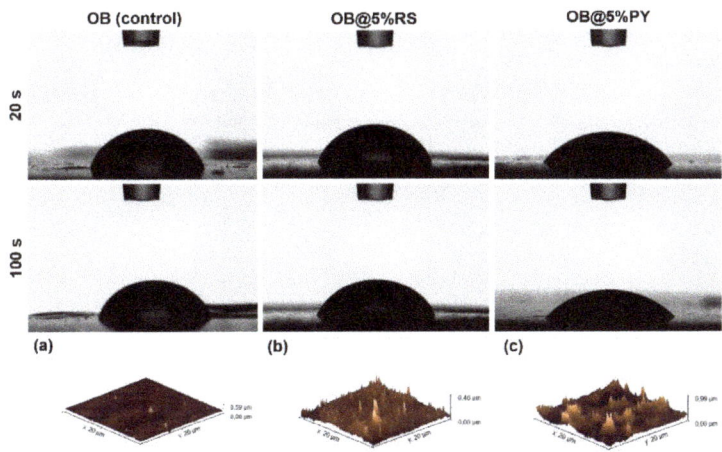

Figure 7. Contact angles of a water droplet (initial volume of 8 µL) deposited onto different composite surfaces (OB, OB@5%RS and OB@5%PY) after 20 and 100 s post deposition. AFM micrographs (20 µm × 20 µm) of the different composite surfaces (**a**) OB, (**b**) OB@5%RS and (**c**) OB@5%PY.

3.8. Compressive Strength and Porosity

In Figure 8 it is possible to compare the compressive strength values of the tested materials. There were significant differences between OB (18.78 ± 2.91 MPa) and both OB@5%RS (34.30 ± 5.71 MPa) and OB@5%PY (33.34 ± 2.98) in dry conditions ($p < 0.05$). However, all compressive strength values decreased after 72 h of storage in water at 37 °C (Figure 8). No significant differences were found among the compression values of all tested composites in wet conditions ($p > 0.05$).

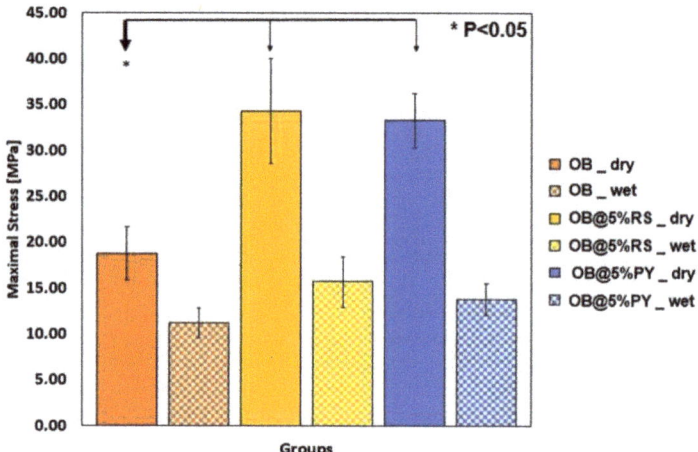

Figure 8. Evolution of maximal stress under compression for OB, OB@5%RS and OB@5%PY in dry conditions; and after immersion in water for 72 h. * $p < 0.05$ bold arrow.

The pore average equivalent diameters and volume percentages were evaluated for the different materials using μCT. No notable differences were found between the unmodified sealer when compared to the sealer doped with RS or PY (Figure 9, Table 4). Therefore, the three cases exhibited quite similar pore characteristics.

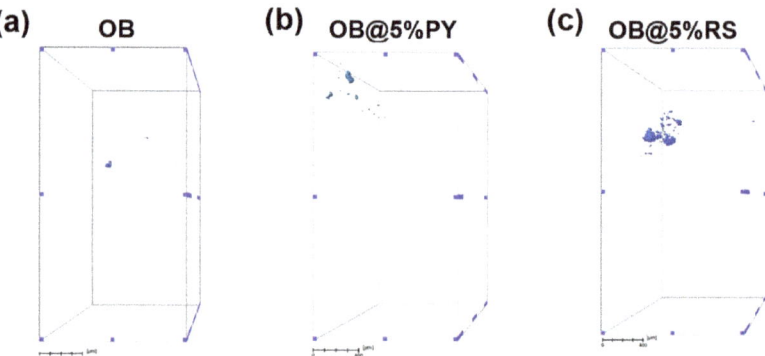

Figure 9. Micro-computed X-ray tomography analysis (scale bar of 400 μm). Volume rendering of the segmented pores in (**a**) OB (unmodified sealer); (**b**) OB@5%PY (sealer doped with 5%PY); and (**c**) OB@5%RS (sealer doped with 5%RS).

Table 4. Pore characteristics of OB, OB@5%RS and OB@5%PY as calculated from μCT imaging.

Group	Pore Average Equivalent Diameter (μm)	Pore Volume Density (%)
OB	15.1	1.2×10^{-3}
OB@5%PY	14.0	5.1×10^{-3}
OB@5%RS	19.0	2.6×10^{-2}

4. Discussion

To the best of our knowledge, this is the first study to incorporate pyrogallol and/or resveratrol into an epoxy-resin endodontic sealer in order to modify its biological, mechanical and physicochemical properties. Indeed, the general hypothesis of this study was that the addition of such polyphenols into epoxy resin-based sealers would have provided an enhancement to some biological and mechanical qualities. In the current study, incorporation of the tested polyphenols was performed into the base part (Table 1) of the epoxy resin-based sealer. We believe that since the catalyst part of the epoxy resin contains amines, oxidation of PY could have activated the polymerization and/or reduced beneficial effects of the phenolic compounds via formation of covalent bonds with the amines [23]. One of the first outcomes obtained in this study was that the control (free of polyphenols) sealer had some antibacterial effects against *E. faecalis* after 24 h. Ruiz-Linares et al. [24] analyzed an epoxy resin-based sealer (AH-Plus, Dentsply Sirona, Konstanz, Germany) against *E. faecalis* and they showed that such material could induce some antibacterial effects as a result of the release of formaldehyde and/or other toxic non-polymerized components, such as amines or epoxy monomers.

However, the incorporation of 5 wt%PY into the epoxy-resin sealer promoted greater antibacterial effects against *E. faecalis* compared to other experimental sealers doped with different percentages of RS. Both antibacterial tests (DCT and ADT) showed great antibacterial efficacy for the sealer doped with 5%PY as well as a peculiar brown-colored zone in the agar (Figure 1b). The brown color observed during the study with the experimental material was probably induced by oxidation of the pyrogallol in the bacterial medium [16,21]. In accordance with such a hypothesis, increased and more rapid antioxidant activity were observed for the OB@5%PY sealer when compared to specimens in the OB@5%RS group. Our hypothesis is that such findings may be principally associated with a relatively significant release of PY from the experimental materials, in comparison to release of RS (Figure 4a). Moreover, the significant release of PY may be a consequence of its smaller molecular weight compared to that of RS. From a chemical point of view, PY has three hydroxyl groups on the benzene ring, whilst the RS molecule has two benzene rings with three hydroxyl groups. It is possible that the different positions of the hydroxyl groups may have affected antibacterial activity of the experimental materials, exactly the same as that described by Cueva et al. [25]. Indeed, those authors reported that the numbers and positions of substitutions in the benzene rings of the phenolic acids, along with the saturated side-chain lengths, influenced antimicrobial properties of the phenolic acids against different microorganisms. The antibacterial effects of PY incorporated into dental adhesive (adhesive-resin with acidic function monomers) against *Streptococcus mutans* and its effects against Staphylococcus aureus when incorporated into plaster of Paris were previously reported [16,21]. Moreover, the antibacterial properties of resveratrol against various *bacteria*, including *E. faecalis*, were also reported in a previous study [26].

The antioxidant activity of OB doped with the tested polyphenols was evaluated using the DPPH discoloration method [16]. OB@5%PY presented increased and more rapid antioxidant activity than OB@5%RS. As stated before, these findings could be related also to the greater release of PY from the tested materials. Atalayin et al. [13], reported that RS reduced DNA damage and reactive oxygen species (ROS) produced by different dental resin-adhesive systems. Platzer et al. [27] reported significant antioxidant activity of PY associated with its structure and number of OH groups. Our study showed that resveratrol has good biocompatibility when it is incorporated into an epoxy-resin endodontic sealer, whilst PY can exert a cytotoxic effect on fibroblasts (NIH3T3). However, the protective effects of RS against ROS production and the decrease in cell viability were previously reported [13]. In contrast, the significant PY release from tested materials induced a negative effect on cell viability (Figure 3). This is in accordance with the observations of Park [28], who reported that PY was relatively toxic for human pulmonary fibroblasts (HPF), and induced cell death and a dose-dependent decrease in cell growth. Our study has also shown that the liberation of PY in water induced a slight decrease in pH (Figure 4b). Similar observations were reported in previous studies [16,21]. Subsequent to the evaluation of the biological properties of the experimental epoxy-resin sealer doped with PY or RS, their solubilities were also analyzed in accordance with the ISO standards 6876:2012; the solubility of dental sealer should not exceed 3% mass after 24 h in water [3]. It is known that high solubility may create pathways for microorganism infiltration into the root canal system [3]. The epoxy resin doped with 5%PY demonstrated the highest solubility compared to other tested materials. However, this solubility did not exceed 3% mass after 24 h and 7 d. Such findings may be correlated to the significant release of PY from the experimental sealers tested in this study. SEM was used to observe morphological changes induced by the incorporation of PY or RS into the experimental sealers. Larger crystallites were observed on the surfaces of OB@5%PY and of OB@5%RS rather than OB (unmodified epoxy-resin) after an immersion period of 7 days in PBS (at 37 °C).

Different polyphenols have been used in dental applications in order to evoke mineral precipitation and remineralization [10]. For instance, grape seed extracts were used in order to induce mineral precipitation in dentin [29]. Liu et al. [30] demonstrated that resveratrol could reduce tooth movement and root resorption during orthodontic therapy. Furthermore, gallic acid facilitated the participation of hydroxyapatite crystallites with specific particle size [31]. The sorption test applied with the different experimental materials was performed using a contact angle method. The profile of an 8-microliter droplet of distilled water on each composite surface was analyzed and the OB@5%PY sealer demonstrated greater wettability (lower contact angle) compared to OB and OB@5%RS. These findings suggest that OB@5%PY may have a greater surface energy [32,33]. Moreover, OB@5%PY presented a rougher surface during AFM analysis compared to OB and OB@5%RS. The greater surface roughness may in part explain the wettability results obtained with some specific experimental materials tested in this study. Indeed, one of the main factors that may assign the contact angle measurements and wettability evaluations is the surface roughness [33]. In accordance with Wenzel or Cassie-Baxter [33], chemical composition of the surface can also play an important role in contact angle measurements. Therefore, we can affirm that the OB@5%PY sealer had both a rougher and more hydrophilic surface than other composites. Zuo et al. [34] reported that PY could be applied in polymer materials in order to fabricate hydrophilic coatings. The mechanical properties of endodontic sealers are very important to strengthen treated root canals as well as to increase resistance to displacement of the gutta-percha cone during and after its placement [3,35]. The results of this study showed that the addition of both polyphenols in an epoxy-resin sealer significantly increased its compression stress values in dry conditions compared to the unmodified control sealer. However, no notable differences were observed for the pore size/volume between different materials tested in this study. The higher compressive strength of OB@PY/RS compared to the control group may be explained by the hypothesis that these polyphenols play the role as a sort of bonding agent between sealer elements. Moreover, it has been demonstrated that the presence of a polyphenol, TA, in mineral trioxide aggregate could increase a sealer's compressive strength [4]. Such an outcome may be related to the ability of such molecules to adsorb on all kinds of surfaces [36] and to ultimately favor interparticular interactions. After immersion in water, both experimental materials showed lower compressive strength values compared to the same materials tested in dry conditions. It is hypothesized that such outcomes may be a result of the liberation of polyphenols in water; this may have degraded bonding links that were probably present in dry conditions. However, no statistical differences were found between the unmodified sealers in dry or wet conditions when compared to OB@PY/RS in wet conditions. Therefore, the compressive strengths of sealers modified with the tested polyphenol, after immersion in water, yielded similar results to the unmodified sealer. In accordance, Kharouf et al. [4] reported an increase in compressive strength of mineral trioxide aggregate (MTA) doped with tannic acid in dry conditions. However, they also found that MTA doped with tannic acid presented weaker mechanical properties in wet conditions. The current study showed both positive and negative outcomes when pyrogallol or resveratrol were incorporated into epoxy-resin sealers. For instance, mechanical properties and antioxidant activity of the epoxy-resin dental sealer were enhanced by incorporating RS and PY into its compositions. The material doped with pyrogallol was more efficient in terms of antibacterial activity against *E. faecalis* than the experimental sealer doped with resveratrol or the control unmodified resin. However, pyrogallol displayed high toxicity towards fibroblasts, and such cytotoxicity marred other favorable qualities (antibacterial and mechanical properties) produced from pyrogallol incorporation into endodontic sealers. In contrast, resveratrol presented better biocompatibility despite its limited antibacterial activity when compared to the pyrogallol group. For this reason, resveratrol may be considered as a suitable choice for incorporation into endodontic sealers with its important mechanical and antioxidant effects compared to unmodified sealers. Antioxidant activity introduced into an endodontic sealer could be useful in preventing harmful effects of oxidative stress and in stabilizing free radicals, thereby protecting cells from damage [37]. As mentioned in Section 2.2, the addition of both polyphenols was limited to 5% (wt.%) to avoid inhomogeneity within the materials resulting from phase separation. Therefore, our future studies will be focused on alternative strategies to incorporate more RS into an epoxy-resin sealer in order to enhance its antibacterial properties without affecting its cellular viability rate. However, the concentration of microorganisms found in root canal systems may be lower compared to those used in our DCT test. Hence, lower concentrations of PY or RS than those used in this in vitro study may be also suitable for real clinical scenarios. In addition, further investigations are required to analyze chemical interactions between the epoxy-resin sealer and polyphenols, and their effects on bond strength to root canal dentin.

5. Conclusions

Within the limitations of the present study, the addition of pyrogallol and resveratrol to an epoxy-resin dental sealer improved mechanical and biological properties. However, pyrogallol seems to have greater antibacterial and antioxidant activities than resveratrol, whereas the latter has fewer cytotoxic effects.

Author Contributions: Conceptualization, N.K. and D.M.; methodology, F.A., J.Z., I.E.S., C.A.-Z. and Y.A.; software, J.Z.; validation, F.M., A.F., L.H., S.S. and D.M. formal analysis, J.Z.; investigation, F.A., J.Z., I.E.S., C.A.-Z. and Y.A.; resources, F.A., J.Z., I.E.S., C.A.-Z. and Y.A.; data curation, N.K.; writing—original draft preparation, N.K., F.M., V.B. and D.M.; writing—review and editing, F.M., L.H., S.S., V.B., N.K., D.M. and A.F.; visualization, N.K.; supervision, D.M.; project administration, Y.H., V.B., N.K. and D.M.; funding acquisition, N.K. and Y.H. All authors have read and agreed to the published version of the manuscript.

Funding: This project was performed using the funds from grant Conectus 19- INSERM-108.

Institutional Review Board Statement: Not applicable.

Informed Consent Statement: Not applicable.

Data Availability Statement: The data presented in this study are available on request from the corresponding author. The data are not publicly available due to the reason that a small part of these data are shared with a private company.

Acknowledgments: We acknowledge Nadia Bahlouli, M. Hamdi Jmal and Platform IRIS and Mechanics ICube, UMR 7357, FMTS, Université de Strasbourg, for providing the experimental setups for the mechanical characterizations. This study was in part supported by the grant "Ministerio de Ciencia, Innovación y Universidades (PID2020-120346GB-I00) to PI: Salvatore Sauro.

Conflicts of Interest: The authors declare no conflict of interest.

References

1. Mancino, D.; Kharouf, N.; Cabiddu, M.; Bukiet, F.; Haïkel, Y. Microscopic and Chemical Evaluation of the Filling Quality of Five Obturation Techniques in Oval-Shaped Root Canals. *Clin. Oral Investig.* **2020**, *25*, 3757–3765. [CrossRef]
2. Mancino, D.; Kharouf, N.; Hemmerlé, J.; Haïkel, Y. Microscopic and Chemical Assessments of the Filling Ability in Oval-Shaped Root Canals Using Two Different Carrier-Based Filling Techniques. *Eur. J. Dent.* **2019**, *13*, 166–171. [CrossRef] [PubMed]
3. Kharouf, N.; Arntz, Y.; Eid, A.; Zghal, J.; Sauro, S.; Haikel, Y.; Mancino, D. Physicochemical and Antibacterial Properties of Novel, Premixed Calcium Silicate-Based Sealer Compared to Powder–Liquid Bioceramic Sealer. *J. Clin. Med.* **2020**, *9*, 3096. [CrossRef] [PubMed]
4. Kharouf, N.; Zghal, J.; Addiego, F.; Gabelout, M.; Jmal, H.; Haikel, Y.; Bahlouli, N.; Ball, V. Tannic acid speeds up the setting of mineral trioxide aggregate cements and improves its surface and bulk properties. *J. Colloid Interface Sci.* **2021**, *589*, 318–326. [CrossRef] [PubMed]
5. Nicholson, J.W.; Czarnecka, B. Materials for root canal filling. In *Materials for the Direct Restoration of Teeth, Woodhead Publishing Series in Biomaterials*; Woodhead Publishing: Amsterdam, The Netherlands, 2016; pp. 197–219.
6. Bose, K.; Ioannidis, K.; Foschi, F.; Bakhsh, A.; Kelly, R.D.; Deb, S.; Mannocci, F.; Niazi, S.A. Antimicrobial Effectiveness of Calcium Silicate Sealers against a Nutrient-Stressed Multispecies Biofilm. *J. Clin. Med.* **2020**, *9*, 2722. [CrossRef] [PubMed]
7. Komabayashi, T.; Colmenar, D.; Cvach, N.; Bhat, A.; Primus, C.; Imai, Y. Comprehensive Review of Current Endodontic Sealers. *Dent. Mater. J.* **2020**, *39*, 703–720. [CrossRef] [PubMed]
8. Mickel, A.; Nguyen, T.; Chogle, S. Antimicrobial Activity of Endodontic Sealers on Enterococcus Faecalis. *J. Endod.* **2003**, *29*, 257–258. [CrossRef]
9. Slutzky-Goldberg, I.; Slutzky, H.; Solomonov, M.; Moshonov, J.; Weiss, E.I.; Matalon, S. Antibacterial Properties of Four Endodontic Sealers. *J. Endod.* **2008**, *34*, 735–738. [CrossRef]
10. Singh, G.; Gupta, I.; Elshamy, F.M.M.; Boreak, N.; Homeida, H.E. In Vitro Comparison of Antibacterial Properties of Bioceramic-Based Sealer, Resin-Based Sealer and Zinc Oxide Eugenol Based Sealer and Two Mineral Trioxide Aggregates. *Eur. J. Dent.* **2016**, *10*, 366–369. [CrossRef]
11. Kharouf, N.; Haikel, Y.; Ball, V. Polyphenols in Dental Applications. *Bioengineering* **2020**, *7*, 72. [CrossRef]
12. Hu, J.; Du, X.; Huang, C.; Fu, D.; Ouyang, X.; Wang, Y. Antibacterial and Physical Properties of EGCG-Containing Glass Ionomer Cements. *J. Dent.* **2013**, *41*, 927–934. [CrossRef]
13. Atalayin, C.; Armagan, G.; Konyalioglu, S.; Kemaloglu, H.; Tezel, H.; Ergucu, Z.; Keser, A.; Dagci, T.; Onal, B. The Protective Effect of Resveratrol against Dentin Bonding Agents-Induced Cytotoxicity. *Dent. Mater. J.* **2015**, *34*, 766–773. [CrossRef]
14. Porto, I.C.C.M.; Nascimento, T.G.; Oliveira, J.M.S.; Freitas, P.H.; Haimeur, A.; França, R. Use of Polyphenols as a Strategy to Prevent Bond Degradation in the Dentin-Resin Interface. *Eur. J. Oral Sci.* **2018**, *126*, 146–158. [CrossRef] [PubMed]
15. Cynthia, I.F.; Sutanto, H.; Darmawan, A. Antibacterial and Antioxidant Activities of Pyrogallol and Synthetic Pyrogallol Dimer. *Res. J. Chem. Environ.* **2018**, *22*, 39–47.
16. Kharouf, N.; Mancino, D.; Zghal, J.; Helle, S.; Jmal, H.; Lenertz, M.; Viart, N.; Bahlouli, N.; Meyer, F.; Haikel, Y.; et al. Dual role of Tannic acid and pyrogallol incorporated in plaster of Paris: Morphology modification and release for antimicrobial properties. *Mater. Sci. Eng. C Mater. Biol. Appl.* **2021**, *127*, 112209. [CrossRef] [PubMed]
17. Geißler, S.; Gomez-Florit, M.; Wiedmer, D.; Barrantes, A.; Petersen, F.C.; Tiainen, H. In Vitro Performance of Bioinspired Phenolic Nanocoatings for Endosseous Implant Applications. *ACS Biomater. Sci. Eng.* **2019**, *5*, 3340–3351. [CrossRef]
18. Oh, D.X.; Prajatelistia, E.; Ju, S.-W.; Jeong Kim, H.; Baek, S.-J.; Joon Cha, H.; Ho Jun, S.; Ahn, J.-S.; Soo Hwang, D. A Rapid, Efficient and Facile Solution for Dental Hypersensitivity: The Tannin–Iron Complex. *Sci. Rep.* **2015**, *5*, 10884. [CrossRef]
19. Hu, Y.; Chen, D.; Zheng, P.; Yu, J.; He, J.; Mao, X.; Yu, B. The Bidirectional Interactions between Resveratrol and Gut Microbiota: An Insight into Oxidative Stress and Inflammatory Bowel Disease Therapy. *BioMed Res. Int.* **2019**, *2019*, 5403761. [CrossRef] [PubMed]
20. Alibi, S.; Crespo, D.; Navas, J. Plant-Derivatives Small Molecules with Antibacterial Activity. *Antibiotics* **2021**, *10*, 231. [CrossRef]
21. Kharouf, N.; Eid, A.; Hardan, L.; Bourgi, R.; Arntz, Y.; Jmal, H.; Foschi, F.; Sauro, S.; Ball, V.; Haikel, Y.; et al. Antibacterial and Bonding Properties of Universal Adhesive Dental Polymers Doped with Pyrogallol. *Polymers* **2021**, *13*, 1538. [CrossRef] [PubMed]
22. Villaño, D.; Fernández-Pachón, M.S.; Moyá, M.L.; Troncoso, A.M.; García-Parrilla, M.C. Radical scavenging ability of polyphenolic compounds towards DPPH free radical. *Talanta* **2007**, *71*, 230–235. [CrossRef]
23. Ball, V. Stabilization of [poly (allylamine)–tannic acid] multilayer films in acidic and basic conditions after crosslinking with NaIO4. *RSC. Adv.* **2015**, *5*, 55920–55925. [CrossRef]
24. Ruiz-Linares, M.; Baca, P.; Arias-Moliz, M.T.; Ternero, F.J.; Rodríguez, J.; Ferrer-Luque, C.M. Antibacterial and antibiofilm activity over time of GuttaFlow Bioseal and AH Plus. *Dent. Mater. J.* **2019**, *38*, 701–706. [CrossRef] [PubMed]

25. Cueva, C.; Moreno-Arribas, M.V.; Martín-Alvarez, P.J.; Bills, G.; Vicente, M.F.; Basilio, A.; Rivas, C.L.; Requena, T.; Rodríguez, J.M.; Bartolomé, B. Antimicrobial activity of phenolic acids against commensal, probiotic and pathogenic bacteria. *Res. Microbiol.* **2010**, *161*, 372–382. [CrossRef]
26. Paulo, L.; Ferreira, S.; Gallardo, E.; Queiroz, J.; Domingues, F. Antimicrobial activity and effects of resveratrol on human pathogenic bacteria. *World J. Microbiol. Biotechnol.* **2010**, *26*, 1533–1538. [CrossRef]
27. Platzer, M.; Kiese, S.; Herfellner, T.; Schweiggert-Weisz, U.; Miesbauer, O.; Eisner, P. Common Trends and Differences in Antioxidant Activity Analysis of Phenolic Substances Using Single Electron Transfer Based Assays. *Molecules* **2021**, *26*, 1244. [CrossRef] [PubMed]
28. Park, W.H. Pyrogallol induces the death of human pulmonary fibroblast cells through ROS increase and GSH depletion. *Int. J. Oncol.* **2016**, *49*, 785–792. [CrossRef]
29. Tang, C.; Fang, M.; Liu, R.; Dou, Q.; Chai, Z.; Xiao, Y.; Chen, J. The role of grape seed extract in the remineralization of demineralized dentine: Micromorphological and physical analyses. *Arch. Oral Biol.* **2013**, *58*, 1769–1776. [CrossRef]
30. Liu, X.-C.; Wang, X.-X.; Zhang, L.-N.; Yang, F.; Nie, F.-J.; Zhang, J. Inhibitory effects of resveratrol on orthodontic tooth movement and associated root resorption in rats. *Arch. Oral. Biol.* **2020**, *111*, 104642. [CrossRef]
31. Tang, B.; Yuan, H.; Cheng, L.; Zhou, X.; Huang, X.; Li, J. Effects of gallic acid on the morphology and growth of hydroxyapatite crystals. *Arch. Oral Biol.* **2015**, *60*, 167–173. [CrossRef]
32. Kontakiotis, E.G.; Tzanetakis, G.N.; Loizides, A.L. A comparative study of contact angles of four different root canal sealers. *J. Endod.* **2007**, *33*, 299–302. [CrossRef] [PubMed]
33. Ball, V. *Self-Assembly Processes at Interfaces*, 1st ed.; Akademic Press: London, UK, 2018; pp. 1–241.
34. Zuo, C.; Wang, L.; Tong, Y.; Shi, L.; Ding, W.; Li, W. Co-deposition of pyrogallol/polyethyleneimine on polymer membranes for highly efficient treatment of oil-in-water emulsion. *Sep. Purif. Technol.* **2021**, *267*, 118660. [CrossRef]
35. Branstetter, J.; von Fraunhofer, J.A. The physical properties and sealing action of endodontic sealer cements: A review of the literature. *J. Endod.* **1982**, *8*, 312–316. [CrossRef]
36. Sileika, T.S.; Barrett, D.G.; Zhang, R.; Lau, K.H.; Messersmith, P.B. Colorless multifunctional coatings inspired by polyphenols found in tea, chocolate, and wine. *Angew. Chem. Int. Ed. Engl.* **2013**, *52*, 10766–10770. [CrossRef] [PubMed]
37. Patel, S.; Hans, M.K.; Chander, S.; Ahluwalia, A.S. Antioxidants in Endodontics: A Strategic Review. *J. Clin. Diagn. Res.* **2015**, *9*, ZE12–ZE15. [CrossRef] [PubMed]

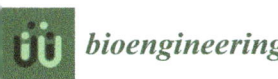

Case Report

Maxillary Premolars with Four Canals: Case Series

Calogero Bugea [1,*], Denise Irene Karin Pontoriero [2,3], Gaia Rosenberg [4], Giacomo Mario Gerardo Suardi [5], Gianmarco Calabria [6], Eugenio Pedullà [7], Giusy Rita Maria La Rosa [7], Francesco Sforza [8], Antonio Scarano [9], Roberto Luongo [10] and Giovanni Messina [11]

1. Private Practice, Lungomare G. Galilei, 73014 Gallipoli, Italy
2. Department of Prosthodontics, University of Siena, 53100 Siena, Italy
3. Department of Endodontics, University of Genoa, 16126 Genova, Italy
4. Private Practice, Via Ercole Ferrario, 1, 20144 Milano, Italy
5. Private Practice, Residenza Alberata 741 Via Salvo d'Acquisto 4/6, 20079 Basiglio, Italy
6. Private Practice, Via Alessandro Volta 21, 88046 Lamezia Terme, Italy
7. Department of General Surgery and Surgical-Medical Specialties, University of Catania, 95123 Catania, Italy
8. Private Practice, Corso Umberto I 115, 72012 Carovigno, Italy
9. Department of Medical, Oral and Biotechnological Sciences, University of Chieti-Pescara, 66100 Chieti, Italy
10. Private Practice, Via Melo da Bari 229, 70121 Bari, Italy
11. Private Practice, Piazza Primavera 17, 92100 Agrigento, Italy
* Correspondence: calogerobugea@yahoo.it

Abstract: The aim of this case series is to contribute to the better knowledge and management of the complex anatomical configurations of maxillary premolars with four canals. The paper explains the endodontic treatment of five maxillary premolars with four canals, with three buccal and one palatal orifices, in different patients. The cases report several approaches in the treatment of four canal maxillary premolars including a conservative canal preparation with a hybrid shaping technique, endodontic microsurgery and the application of biomaterials. The use of an operating dental microscope, different operating strategies and the critical evaluation of radiographs are all necessary steps for the correct and safe endodontic management of these teeth.

Keywords: root; maxillary premolars; upper premolars; canal; root canal anomalies; anatomical variations; root morphology; coneless; MEA technique

1. Introduction

Understanding the anatomy of the root canal system is a key factor for success in endodontics [1–3]. For this reason, clinicians must know all the possible anatomical variations and assess the root and canal configuration prior to, during, and after endodontic treatment. Although the vast majority of maxillary premolars have two root canals, the presence of three distinct root canals has been reported in 1–6% of cases [4–9]. Previous case reports have shown several canal and root configurations in three-canal maxillary premolars: three canals in a single root, two canals in the buccal root and one in the palatal root, three separate roots and canals [10–12]. Only two studies have described four separate canals in a three-rooted premolar [13,14].

2. Materials and Methods

Five patients were found with a rare anatomical variant of a four-canal upper premolar (three first premolars and two s premolar). Each patient agreed to participate and signed a consent form. Assessment of the presence of the number of canals was documented via X-ray examination and clinical photographic evidence.

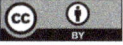

2.1. CASE 1

A 55-year-old male patient diagnosed with pulpitis with no swelling or fistulae. The pre-operative X-ray suggested tooth 14 had an unusual three-rooted anatomy, (Figure 1). After anesthesia and isolation, the whole endodontic procedure was carried out under microscope magnification (PROergo, Carl Zeiss Meditec AG, Munich, Germany) using ultrasonic instrumentation to access cavity refining (no. 3 Start-X, Maillefer Instruments Holding, Ballaigues, Switzerland). A lot of time and dedication was needed in order to identify and negotiate the two buccal canals, due to the closeness of the orifices and their deep location. An intra-operative X-ray was taken to evaluate the root canal system. A three-rooted system was confirmed. Canals were shaped using ProTaper Gold™ (Maillefer Instruments Holding Sàrl, Ballaigues, Switzerland) following the manufacturer's recommendations. Buccal canals were shaped up to the F1 instrument, while the palatal canal was shaped up to the F2 instrument. Passive ultrasonic irrigation was performed using 5.25% sodium hypochlorite, and a final 10% ethylene-diaminetetracetic acid rinse was carried out at the end. The canals were dried with sterile paper points, and obturated by injection of thermoplastic of gutta-percha using the Obtura III Max (Obtura Spartan Endodontics, Algonquin, IL, USA) in association with an endodontic sealant (Essenseal, Produits Dentaires Sa, Vevey, Switzerland). Upon closer examination, the final X-ray revealed an additional mesial root. After carefully re-examining the pulp chamber, another small orifice, was found very close to the others. This mesial canal was treated in the same session, following the same instrumentation (up to ProTaper Gold, F1), irrigation and obturation protocol used for the other canals. The obturation of the endodontic space was performed by a modification of the injection molding thermoplasticized gutta-percha by Yee [15]. The authors called this kind of obturation Coneless®. A final X-ray was taken, and the complete anatomy of this complex endodontic system is clearly shown in Figure 1. The access cavity was filled with a provisional filling material (3M ESPE™ CAVIT™, 3M Italia srl, Pioltello, Italy), and another appointment was scheduled one week later for the definitive restoration. The complete case is illustrated in Figure 1.

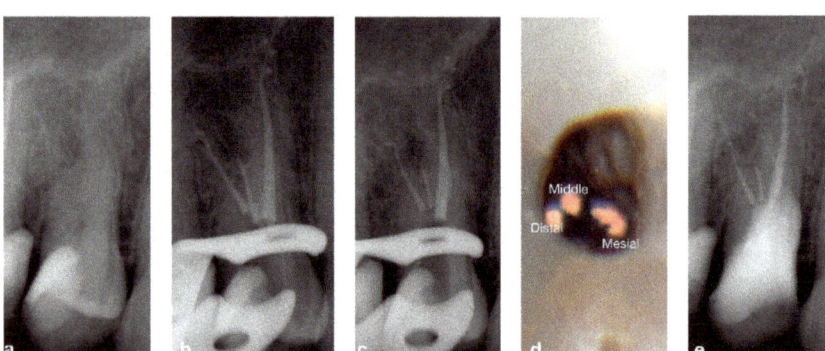

Figure 1. (a) Pre-operative X-ray showing the complex anatomy, (b) intra-operative X-ray after obturation of three canals, (c) intra-operative X-ray after obturation of the 4th canal, (d) intra-operative view of the three vestibular canals, (e) X-ray of 6-month follow-up.

2.2. CASE 2

A 47-year-old female patient presented to the practice because of swelling in the upper premolar area. Upon intra-oral radiographic examination, a periapical radiolucent area was found at tooth 14, so the patient was scheduled for an endodontic re-treatment. After anesthesia and isolation with a rubber dam, the pulp chamber was accessed, and three canal orifices (one buccal, two palatal) appeared immediately, so as to confirm the suspicion aroused by examination by the pre-operative X-ray. Considering the thickness of the roots, it was useful to prepare the untreated and treated roots of the 14 tooth with the "MEA and inverse taper technique" to keep the dentinal wall removal during the shaping phases under control [16]. The mixed endodontic alloy (MEA) inverse taper® is a hybrid shaping technique comprising the combination of different heat-treated instruments with austenitic files (i.e., Mtwo #10.04 and #15.05, Sweden Martina, Italy) employed in the initial phase of shaping followed by martensitic (i.e., Plex V #20.04 and 25.04, Orodeka, Shandong Province, China) in the second. The first instruments guarantee effective debris removal by means of the more rigid alloy and design; the second ensures improvement in the center ability with respect to the original anatomy. Moreover, the hybrid sequence, constituting the #10.04 and #15.05 files was followed by the #20.04, produced the first taper inversion at 5 mm from the apex while the second phase of #25.04 inverted the taper at 10 mm. It was impossible to completely dry the endodontic system on the first session, so calcium hydroxide was used as an intermediate medication, and the patient was prescribed antibiotic therapy with amoxicillin and clavulanic acid. On the second session, a fourth orifice was identified on the pulp chamber floor in the buccal–mesial root. The fourth canal was itself impossible to dry, so another calcium hydroxide dressing was carried out and the patient was scheduled for a third session, 30 days later, on which more difficulties were met because of the wetting of the apical third of all roots, so an apicoectomy was scheduled. The retrograde preparation was performed with an ultrasonic tip R1D (Piezomed, W&H, Bürmoos, Austria) [16] deep into the canal and obturated with Biodentine as the root-end filling. Seven days after the apicoectomy the patient was recalled for removing the suture and completing the root filling with a single cone and biomaterial (BioRoot™ RCS, Septodont, Saint-Maur-des-Fossés Cedex, France). Several follow-ups were scheduled at different months until the complete healing was obtained and visible by X-ray. The complete case is reported in Figures 2 and 3.

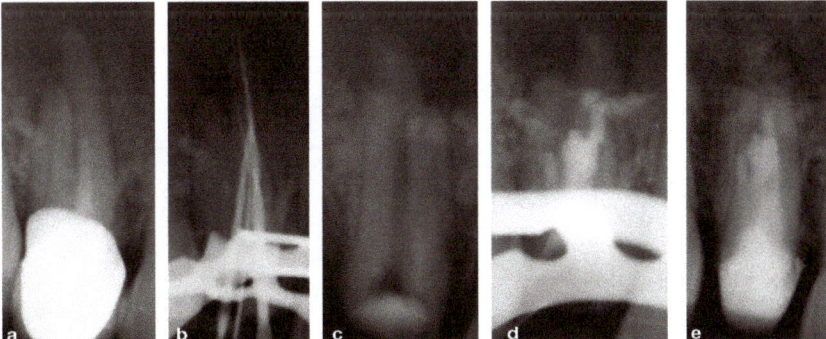

Figure 2. (**a**) Pre-operative X-rays showing the complex anatomy, (**b**) intra-operative X-ray with endodontic instruments to better understand the anatomy, (**c**) post-operative view of the endodontic surgery, (**d**) orthograde filling with gutta-percha, (**e**) 1-year follow-up.

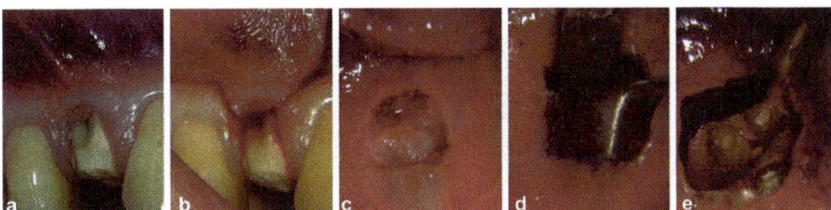

Figure 3. (**a**) Pre-operative view of the premolar, (**b**) flap design, (**c**) intra-operative view of the lesion, (**d**) ultrasonic tip in action, (**e**) intra-operative view of the retrograde obturation.

2.3. CASE 3

A 40-year-old male patient presented with pain and swelling located in the maxillary projection of tooth 24. An X-ray showed a previous inadequate endodontic treatment and a screw post. Analysis of the pre-operative X-ray suggested a missed canal. After administration with local anesthesia (articaine with 1:100,000 epinephrine) the field was isolated with a rubber dam. All the phases of the procedure, starting from the disassemble of the existing build-up, were performed under the magnification of an operative microscope (PROergo, Carl Zeiss Meditec AG, Germany). The screw post was removed from the palatal canal by means of ultrasound instrumentation (no. 3 Start-X, Maillefer Instruments Holding, Ballaigues, Switzerland).

Removal of the old canal filling began using M-Two Retreatment 25 (Sweden and Martina, Padova, Italy). Working length was determined by an apex locator (Apit Osada, Osada Electric co. Ltd., Tokyo, Japan) and the shaping was finished by Reciproc Blue 25 (Dentsply Sirona, Baden, Switzerland). Irrigation was performed with NaOCl 5.25% (NiClor, Ogna, Bologna, Italy) and activated using the Eddy VDW sonic tip (Dentsply Sirona, Switzerland).

As soon as the chamber and canals were clean, two additional canal orifices in-between were suspected and were easily identified with an endodontic probe DG 16 (Hu-Friedy, Chicago, IL, USA). The initial shaping was performed with M-two Retreatment 15 (Sweden e Martina, Italy) to enlarge the first 5–6 mm. After negotiation and measuring the working length with a manual k-file 10, the M-two 15 0.5 (Sweden e Martina, Padova, Italy) was used to shape up to the working length. All four canals were finished in terms of shaping with an M-two 35 0.4 (Sweden e Martina, Italy). Obturation of the canals was performed using a Bioceramic Cement TotalFill® BC SealerTM (Padova, La Chaux-de-Fonds, FKG Dentaire-Switzerland) with the single cone technique. After the treatment, a post-operative X-ray was taken, and the patient was scheduled for restorative treatment. The complete case is illustrated in Figure 4.

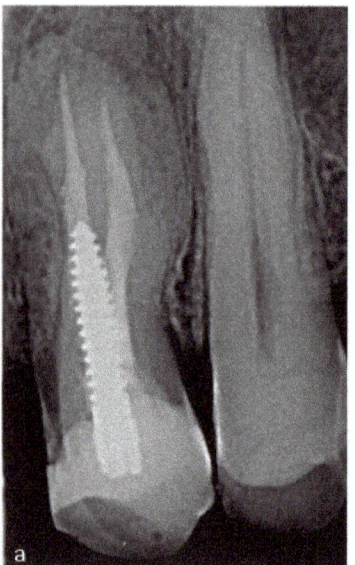
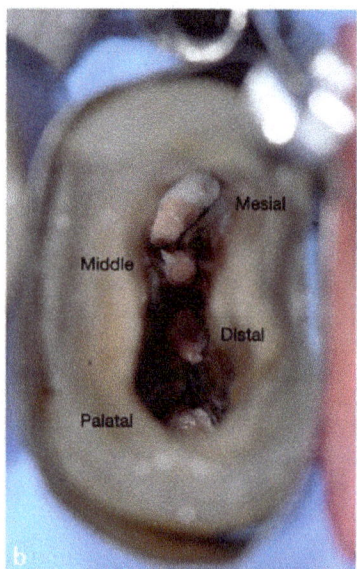
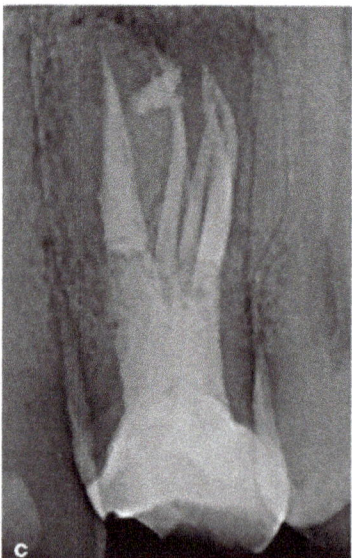

Figure 4. (a) Pre-operative view of the premolar, (b) post-operative X-ray of the four canals filled with gutta-percha (c) 1-year follow-up.

2.4. CASE 4

A 54-year-old male patient presented with a spontaneous crown fracture of tooth 25. The intra-oral examination revealed no swelling or sinus tracts, the tooth was vital. The tooth presented an old MOD amalgam restoration and an extended complicated crown fracture involving the palatal half of the crown. The pre-operative X-ray revealed an anatomy of a three-rooted premolar. The whole endodontic procedure was carried out under 4X loupes magnification and dedicated illumination (Carl Zeiss Meditec AG, Germany). After local anesthesia (2% lidocaine with 1:100,000 epinephrine), and rubber dam isolation, a conservative endodontic access cavity was performed using a long-shaft-rounded diamond bur, and dedicated endodontic ultrasonic tips Start X 3 (Maillefer Dentsply, Ballaigues, Switzerland). A careful inspection of the pulp chamber floor revealed an extremely unusual anatomy for a second maxillary premolar, four separate canal orifices were identified. After straight-line access preparation was obtained, root canals were negotiated with pre-curved stainless-steel K-files, sized 0.8 and 10 ISO (Maillefer-Dentsply, Ballaigues, Switzerland), and the WL was established with an apex locator (Root ZX Morita, Tokyo, Japan). A mixed shaping technique was adopted. Pre-flaring and glide path were performed to WL with a NiTi 10.04 and a 15.05 (Sweden e Martina, Padova, Italy) rotary file at 180 rpm and torque 2. All canals were finished with ProTaper Next X2 (Maillefer-Dentsply, Ballaigues, Switzerland). All shaping steps were carried out under 5.25% heated NaOCl irrigation (NiClor, Ogna, Bologna, Italy). After instrumentation, the root canals were irrigated with 17% EDTA solution Tubuliclean (Ogna, Bologna, Italy) for 3 min followed again by several 1-minute rinses with heated 5.25% sodium hypochlorite solution. A carrier-based obturation was performed using dedicated obturators Thermafil for ProTaper NEXT, X2, (Maillefer-Dentsply, Ballaigues, Switzerland) and a zinc oxide-based endodontic sealer. The intra-operative X-ray confirmed all four canals were independent throughout their entire length. A temporary restoration was performed using zinc oxide-based cement placed on the pulp chamber floor covered by a layer of glass ionomer cement (GCem, GC Co Tokyo, Japan). Follow-up after 1 year showed clinical and radiographic signs of healthy conditions. Figure 5 illustrates the complete case.

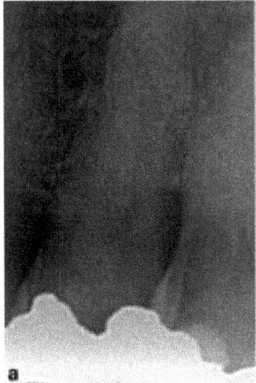 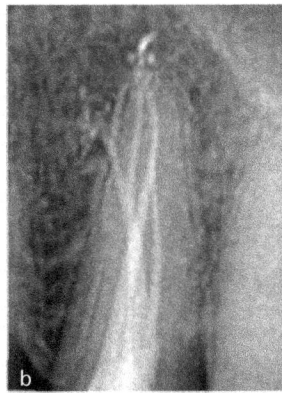 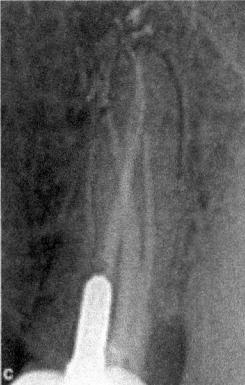

Figure 5. (a) Pre-operative view of the premolar, (b) post-operative X-ray of the four canals filled with gutta-percha, (c) 1-year follow-up.

2.5. CASE 5

A 54-year-old male patient was referred for treatment before prosthetic rehabilitation. The pre-operative X-ray revealed the presence of an accessory and an untreated canal of tooth 15, which presented an apical lesion. The whole treatment was conducted under magnification (Leica 525M, Leica Microsystems, Wetzlar, Germany). During disassemble of the cavity, access was refined by ultrasonic instrumentation (Start X no. 2 and 3, Maillefer,

Ballaigues, Switzerland) with the aim of locating the missed canal. The treated canals were shaped with a Komet EndoRestart 25/05 (Komet, Besigheim, Germany) and finished with a Protaper Next X2 (Maillefer-Dentsply, Ballaigues, Switzerland). Only the palatal canal was finished with the F3 instrument. The missed canal was then negotiated manually using a k-file 10/02 up to the working length and was then prepared mechanically with the following instrument sequence: M-two 10/04, (Sweden e Martina, Italy), Proglider and Protaper Next X1-X2 (Maillefer-Dentsply, Ballaigues, Switzerland). Warm vertical gutta-percha condensation with a Pulp Canal Sealer EWT (Kerr Dental, Orange, CA, USA) was used for canal obturation. The final X-ray showed unusual anatomy with four independent canals. The complete case is reported in Figure 6.

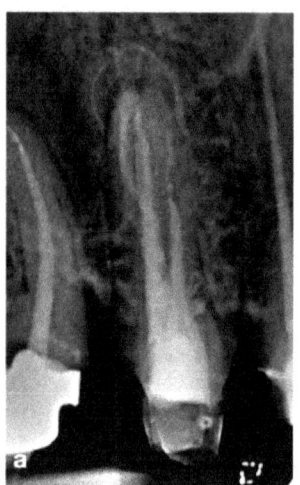 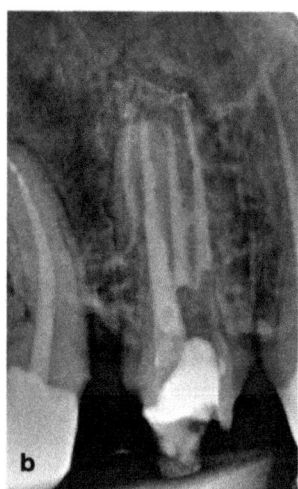 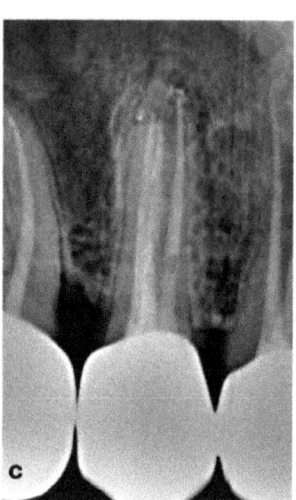

Figure 6. (**a**) Pre-operative view of the premolar, (**b**) post-operative X-ray of the four canals filled with gutta-percha, (**c**) 1-year follow-up.

3. Discussion

These cases are rare findings of maxillary premolars with four canals. Endodontic management in these complex anatomical configurations is challenging and depends on individual clinical skills as well as the procedural techniques applied [17].

Accurate radiographic examination using horizontal angle variation provides notable support for the endodontist to distinguish the roots and root canals and formulate a correct diagnosis, also in challenging anatomical configurations, as previously reported [12–14]. Furthermore, the detection of the pulp chamber anatomy during coronal access and adequate intracanal dentin removal contribute to the correct clinical location of the root canal orifices [12]. Cone beam-computed tomography (CBCT) is also a diagnostic imaging modality recommended for approaching the complex root canal anatomy [18,19]. Despite CBCT providing high-quality, accurate, three-dimensional (3D) representations of the anatomical dental structures, the presence of metallic restorations (e.g., amalgam restorations, metal posts and/or crowns) or even gutta-percha can determine significant radiographic artefacts which can impact the visualization of the root canal anatomy and pathological conditions, such as root resorption and root fractures [20]. Considering that cone beam-computed tomography implies an additional X-ray dose for the patient, the final decision to perform or not to perform a second-level radiologic exam should be based on the clinical and radiographic interpretation of each case. Within this context, the use of a CBCT exam was not considered pivotal for the management of the clinical cases described.

The microscopy is another essential tool in complex endodontic cases. It favors the localization of anatomical landmarks in the pulp chamber floor and thus the identification of eventual supplementary root canals or root canal aberrations [21]. In some selected cases, the operating microscope can help the clinician in identifying the point where the principal canal bi- or trifurcates and the orientation of the canal orifices [17].

Moreover, in such complex anatomical configurations the use of ultrasonic devices [22], dedicated file for re-treatment [23], and modified preparation techniques [16] could be useful in improving the procedural steps of endodontic treatment.

The mixed endodontic alloy (MEA) inverse taper® is a hybrid shaping technique proposed for the preparation of challenging anatomical configurations, such as double or abrupt curvatures and narrow canals. Inverting the taper during the treatment of a narrow, curved or double canal allows the treatment to be extremely safe. The 0.05% final taper ensures root cleaning until the apex maintaining open the eventual lateral canals. At the same time, the 0.05% taper allows for adequate final shaping for the filling phase. The hybrid sequence comprising the #10.04 and #15.05 austenitic files, followed by the martensitic #20.04 produce the first taper inversion at 5 mm from the apex, while the second phase of #25.04 invert the taper at 10 mm. Thus, the instrument does not engage the dentinal walls at D5 and D10 for #20.04 and #25.04, respectively, avoiding excessive file torsional stress and maintaining as much residual dentin as possible [16].

Finally, the use of straightforward and fast obturation techniques, such as the single cone technique combined with biosealers, which promote hydroxyapatite formation, are particularly useful in challenging root canal configurations [24,25].

These case series provide useful clinical information for performing root canal treatments in complex cases, while creating awareness about anatomical variations of maxillary premolars [26–28]. Of note, different clinical outcomes such as orthodontic movement and implant success depend on several factors [29,30], including root canal morphology [31,32]. Hence, a detailed knowledge of root canal morphology is useful in different clinical contexts.

4. Conclusions

The above clinical cases describe several approaches in the treatment of four-canal maxillary premolars, including a conservative canal preparation with a hybrid shaping technique, endodontic microsurgery and the application of biomaterials. The use of an operating dental microscope, different operating strategies and the critical evaluation of radiographs are all pivotal steps for the correct and predictable endodontic management of these teeth.

Author Contributions: Conceptualization, C.B. and G.M.; methodology, C.B.; software, G.R.M.L.R.; validation, E.P. and A.S.; investigation, C.B., D.I.K.P., G.R., G.M.G.S., G.C., F.S., A.S., R.L. and G.M.; resources, C.B., G.R., G.M.G.S., D.I.K.P., G.C., E.P., F.S., A.S., R.L. and G.M.; data curation, D.I.K.P.; writing—original draft preparation, C.B., D.I.K.P., G.R., G.M.G.S., G.C., E.P., F.S., A.S. and R.L.; writing—review and editing, G.R.M.L.R. and G.M.; visualization, G.R.M.L.R.; supervision, E.P. and A.S.; project administration, G.M. All authors have read and agreed to the published version of the manuscript.

Funding: This research received no external funding.

Institutional Review Board Statement: Not applicable.

Informed Consent Statement: Informed consent was obtained from all subjects involved in the study.

Data Availability Statement: Not applicable.

Conflicts of Interest: The authors deny any conflict of interest.

References

1. Ida, R.D.; Gutmann, J.L. Importance of anatomic variables in endodontic treatment outcomes: Case report. *Endod. Dent. Traumatol.* **1995**, *11*, 199–203. [CrossRef]
2. Lin, L.M.; Pascon, E.A.; Skribner, J.; Gängler, P.; Langeland, K. Clinical, radiographic and histologic study of endodontic treatment failures. *Oral Surg. Oral Med. Oral Pathol.* **1991**, *71*, 603–611. [CrossRef] [PubMed]
3. Ricucci, D.; Siqueira, J.F., Jr. Anatomic and microbiologic challenges to achieving success with endodontic treatment: A case report. *J. Endod.* **2008**, *34*, 1249–1254. [CrossRef] [PubMed]
4. Carns, E.J.; Skidmore, A.E. Configurations and deviations of root canals maxillary first premolars. *Oral Surg. Oral Med. Oral Pathol.* **1973**, *36*, 880–886. [CrossRef] [PubMed]
5. Pecora, J.D.; Sousa-Neto, M.D.; Saquy, P.C.; Woelfel, J.B. Root form and canal anatomy of maxillary first premolars. *Braz. Dent. J.* **1991**, *2*, 87–94.
6. Atieh, M.A. Root and canal morphology of maxillary first premolars in a Saudi population. *J. Contemp. Dent. Pract.* **2008**, *9*, 46–53. [CrossRef] [PubMed]
7. Neelakantan, P.; Subbarao, C.; Ahuja, R.; Subbarao, C.V. Root and canal morphology of Indian maxillary premolars by a modified root canal staining technique. *Odontology* **2011**, *99*, 18–21. [CrossRef] [PubMed]
8. Tian, Y.Y.; Guo, B.; Zhang, R.; Yu, X.; Wang, H.; Hu, T.; Dummer, P.M.H. Root and canal morphology of maxillary first pre-molars in a Chinese subpopulation evaluated using cone-beam computed tomography. *Int. Endod. J.* **2012**, *45*, 996–1003. [CrossRef]
9. Ahmad, I.A.; Alenezi, M.A. Root and Root Canal Morphology of Maxillary First Premolars: A Literature Review and Clinical Considerations. *J. Endod.* **2016**, *42*, 861–872. [CrossRef]
10. De Almeida-Gomes, F.; de Sousa, B.C.; de Souza, F.D.; Dos Santos, R.A.; Maniglia-Ferreira, C. Unusual anatomy of maxillary second premolars. *Eur. J. Dent.* **2009**, *3*, 145–149. [CrossRef]
11. De Almeida-Gomes, F.; De Sousa, B.C.; De Souza, F.D.; dos Santos, R.A.; Maniglia-Ferreira, C. Three root canals in the maxillary second premolar. *Indian J. Dent. Res.* **2009**, *20*, 241–242. [CrossRef] [PubMed]
12. Barros, D.B.; Guerreiro-Tanomaru, J.M.; Tanomaru-Filho, M. Root canal treatment of three-rooted maxillary second premolars: Report of four cases. *Aust. Endod. J.* **2009**, *35*, 73–77. [CrossRef] [PubMed]
13. Lea, C.; Deblinger, J.; Machado, R.; Nogueira Leal Silva, E.J.; Vansan, L.P. Maxillary premolar with 4 separate canals. *J. Endod.* **2014**, *40*, 591–593. [CrossRef] [PubMed]
14. Allahem, Z.; AlYami, S. Treatment of maxillary second premolar with 4 roots. *Case Rep. Dent.* **2020**, *2020*, 8634797. [CrossRef]
15. Yee, F.S.; Marlin, J.; Krakow, A.A.; Gron, P. Three-dimensional obturation of the root canal using injection-molded, thermoplasticized dental gutta-percha. *J. Endod.* **1977**, *3*, 168–174. [CrossRef]
16. Messina, G. Strumentazione mista e tecnica delle conicità invertite nei canali curvi. *Il Dent. Mod.* **2021**, *12*, 70–76.
17. Albuquerque, D.; Kottoor, J.; Hammo, M. Endodontic and clinical considerations in the management of variable anatomy in mandibular premolars: A literature review. *Biomed Res. Int.* **2014**, *2014*, 512574. [CrossRef]
18. Kottoor, J.; Velmurugan, N.; Surendran, S. Endodontic management of a maxillary first molar with eight root canal systems evaluated using cone-beam computed tomography scanning: A case report. *J. Endod.* **2011**, *37*, 715–719. [CrossRef]
19. Sberna, M.T.; Rizzo, G.; Zacchi, E.; Capparè, P.; Rubinacci, A. A preliminary study of the use of peripheral quantitative computed tomography for investigating root canal anatomy. *Int. Endod. J.* **2009**, *42*, 66–75. [CrossRef]
20. Patel, S.; Brown, J.; Pimentel, T.; Kelly, R.D.; Abella, F.; Durack, C. Cone beam computed tomography in Endodontics—A review of the literature. *Int. Endod. J.* **2019**, *52*, 1138–1152. [CrossRef]
21. Al-Fouzan, K.S. The microscopic diagnosis and treatment of a mandibular second premolar with four canals. *Int. Endod. J.* **2001**, *34*, 406–410. [CrossRef] [PubMed]
22. Plotino, G.; Pameijer, C.H.; Grande, N.M.; Somma, F. Ultrasonics in endodontics: A review of the literature. *J. Endod.* **2007**, *33*, 81–95. [CrossRef] [PubMed]
23. Das, S.; De Ida, A.; Das, S.; Nair, V.; Saha, N.; Chattopadhyay, S. Comparative evaluation of three different rotary instrumentation systems for removal of gutta-percha from root canal during endodontic retreatment: An in vitro study. *J. Conserv. Dent.* **2017**, *20*, 311–316. [PubMed]
24. Heran, J.; Khalid, S.; Albaaj, F.; Tomson, P.L.; Camilleri, J. The single cone obturation technique with a modified warm filler. *J. Dent.* **2019**, *89*, 103181. [CrossRef] [PubMed]
25. Sfeir, G.; Zogheib, C.; Patel, S.; Giraud, T.; Nagendrababu, V.; Bukiet, F. Calcium silicate- based root canal sealers: A narrative review and clinical perspectives. *Materials* **2021**, *14*, 3965. [CrossRef] [PubMed]
26. Bugea, C.; Berton, F.; Rapani, A.; Di Lenarda, R.; Perinetti, G.; Pedullà, E.; Scarano, A.; Stacchi, C. In Vitro Qualitative Evaluation of Root-End Preparation Performed by Piezoelectric Instruments. *Bioengineering* **2022**, *9*, 103. [CrossRef]
27. Ahmed, H.M.; Abbott, P.V. Accessory roots in maxillary molar teeth: A review and endodontic considerations. *Aust. Dent. J.* **2012**, *57*, 123–131. [CrossRef]
28. Silva, E.J.N.L.; Nejaim, Y.; Silva, A.V.; Haiter-Neto, F.; Cohenca, N. Evaluation of root canal configuration of mandibular molars in a Brazilian population using cone beam computed tomography: An in vivo study. *J. Endod.* **2013**, *39*, 849–852. [CrossRef]

29. Lucchese, A.; Gherlone, E.; Portelli, M.; Bertossi, D. Tooth Orthodontic Movement after Maxillofacial Surgery. *Eur. J. Inflamm.* **2012**, *10*, 227–232. [CrossRef]
30. Ferrari Cagidiaco, E.; Carboncini, F.; Parrini, S.; Doldo, T.; Nagni, M.; Uti, N.; Ferrari, M. Functional Implant Prosthodontic Score of a one-year prospective study on three different connections for single-implant restorations. *J. Osseointegr.* **2018**, *10*, 130–135.
31. Savignano, R.; Viecilli, R.F.; Oyoyo, U. Three-dimensional nonlinear prediction of tooth movement from the force system and root morphology. *Angle Orthod.* **2020**, *90*, 811–822. [CrossRef] [PubMed]
32. Juodzbalys, G.; Stumbras, A.; Goyushov, S.; Duruel, O.; Tözüm, T.F. Morphological Classification of Extraction Sockets and Clinical Decision Tree for Socket Preservation/Augmentation after Tooth Extraction: A Systematic Review. *J. Oral Maxillofac. Res.* **2019**, *10*, e3. [CrossRef] [PubMed]

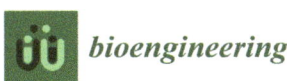

Case Report

The Allogenic Dental Pulp Transplantation from Son/Daughter to Mother/Father: A Follow-Up of Three Clinical Cases

Victor Pinheiro Feitosa [1,*], Mara Natiere Mota [1], Roseane Savoldi [1], Tainah Rifane [1], Diego de Paula [1], Livia Borges [1], Luzia Kelly Solheiro [1], Manoel Aguiar Neto [1], Lorena Vieira [1], Ana Carolina Moreira [1] and Salvatore Sauro [2]

[1] Research Division, Paulo Picanço School of Dentistry, 900 Joaquim Sá St., Fortaleza 60135-218, Ceará, Brazil
[2] Dental Biomaterials and Minimally Invasive Dentistry, Department of Dentistry, Cardenal Herrera-CEU University, CEU Universities, C/Santiago Ramón y Cajal, s/n., Alfara del Patriarca, 46115 Valencia, Spain
* Correspondence: victorpfeitosa@hotmail.com or victor.feitosa@facpp.edu.br; Tel.: +55-(85)-999164512

Abstract: The study investigated allogenic pulp transplantation as an innovative method of regenerative endodontic therapy. Three patients were selected for the endodontic treatment of single-root teeth, who also had a son/daughter with deciduous teeth or third molars scheduled for extraction. Receptor teeth were endodontically instrumented and irrigated using a tri-antibiotic solution. During the transplant procedures, the teeth from the son/daughter were extracted, sectioned, and the pulp was carefully removed. The harvested pulp from the donor was inserted into the root canal of the host tooth (father/mother), followed by direct pulp capping and resin composite restoration. The teeth were followed-up with for 2 years and were surveyed with computed tomography, the electric pulp vitality test, and Doppler ultrasound examination. At the 6-month follow-up, positive pulp vitality and the formation of periapical lesions were verified in cases 1 and 2. Case 3 showed remarkable periapical radiolucency before transplantation, but after 1 year, such lesions disappeared and there was positive vitality. All teeth were revascularized as determined by Doppler imaging after 2 years with no signs of endodontic/periodontal radiolucency. In conclusion, although this was a case series with only three patients and four teeth treated, it is possible to suppose that this allogenic pulp transplantation protocol could represent a potential strategy for pulp revitalization in specific endodontic cases.

Keywords: pulp; regeneration; revitalization; transplant

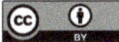

1. Introduction

The pulp–dentin complex may be repaired, and dental caries can be arrested by highly organized, vascularized, and cell-loaded pulpal tissue. Any injuries to such tissue may trigger an inflammatory response or necrosis, overturning its repair capacity. Such circumstances often require pulp removal, disinfection, instrumentation, and endodontic obturation with inert materials such as gutta-percha [1]. Regenerative endodontics are rapidly evolving thanks to the advent of innovative tissue-engineering protocols, treatments, and technologies [2]. Most of the strategies used to regenerate pulp tissue are based on the use of stem cells from periodontal ligament, bone, or dental pulp. These cells are usually seeded in scaffolds and later transferred into the in-root canal, where they can differentiate in specialized cells towards the formation of vessels, fibroblasts, odontoblasts, and further cells found in pulp [3].

The role of growth factors is also essential for cell differentiation and signaling to the accessibility of other cells. Nevertheless, most of the improvements in regenerative endodontics are found in in vitro or animal model studies [2–5]. In this regard, the uses of platelet-rich fibrin (PRF) and platelet-rich plasma (PRP) have demonstrated optimal potential to treat open apex situations, improving the revascularization procedure [6–9].

However, the actual formation of new pulp tissue is limited when using platelet concentrates. Only recently, the transplantation of all the pulp tissue [10] generated an optimal "scaffold" for regeneration. The auto-transplantation of dental pulp collected from a third molar requiring extraction to a host tooth in the same patient was demonstrated to be a clinically feasible procedure for true pulp regeneration without risks for body rejection and severe inflammation [11–13]. Nevertheless, to the best of our knowledge, dental pulp transplantation between two different people has never been investigated so far. Indeed, allogenic transplantation could be the next step to assess the clinical success of such a clinical procedure.

Therefore, this investigation aimed at describing the clinical procedures for dental pulp allogenic transplantation and conducted a clinical follow-up for at least 24 months for three patients treated with such a regenerative endodontic treatment.

2. Materials and Methods

Three patients requiring root canal treatment in single-root premolars with their sons/daughters in need of an extraction of deciduous teeth or the third molar were recruited in this study (Dental Clinics of School of Dentistry). The protocol and the treatment plan were evaluated and approved by the Local Ethics Committee of Paulo Picanço School of Dentistry (protocol 3585776), and all patients signed an informed consent form with the details of the aim of the study and potential complications and accepted the clinical/radiographic follow-up for a period of 1, 3, 6, 12, 18, and 24 months. The inclusion criteria were the following: patients were 18–60 years old with no gender predilection, undergoing irreversible pulpitis (case 2) or pulp necrosis (cases 1 and 3) signs with spontaneous pain (case 2) or periapical radiolucency (cases 1 and 3) in single-root teeth, thereby requiring root canal treatment, with a periodontal pocket depth < 3 mm. The presence of tooth discoloration was not an exclusion criterion. Furthermore, the patients' sons/daughters (donors) were aged between 9 and 21 years old and needed to have a deciduous tooth without root resorption or a third molar scheduled for extraction for reasons not related to this investigation. These donor teeth were tested for vitality with an electric pulp vitality test (Pulp Tester Digital, Odous de Deus, Belo Horizonte, Brazil).

First, panoramic radiography was performed on all patients in the three cases (Figures 1–3), as well as computed tomography (CT) scanning with a 0.25 mm voxel size in order to confirm the periapical status of each tooth requiring endodontic treatment. The extraction of teeth from the patients' children was performed without tooth sectioning and with extreme caution in order to avoid damaging the tooth and the apical structures. The extraction was carried out with local anesthesia using 1.8 mL of 2% lidocaine (1:80,000 epinephrine) through a nerve block technique. The extracted teeth were stored in a sterilized saline solution. At the same time and in the same dental office, the single-root teeth requiring root canal treatment were also anesthetized as aforementioned, isolated with a rubber dam, and pulp chamber access was executed with diamond burs with a high-speed handpiece under continuous and copious water irrigation. The canal instrumentation was performed using rotary files (Wave One Gold, Dentsply, Rio de Janeiro, Brazil) in combination with irrigation using a tri-antibiotic solution (ciprofloxacin, minocycline, and metronidazole at 500 µg/mL each) [14,15]. Prior to the rotary files, one #10 manual K-file (Dentsply) was used to perform the patency. No apical bleeding was performed because it was a different protocol than the revascularization strategy [15,16].

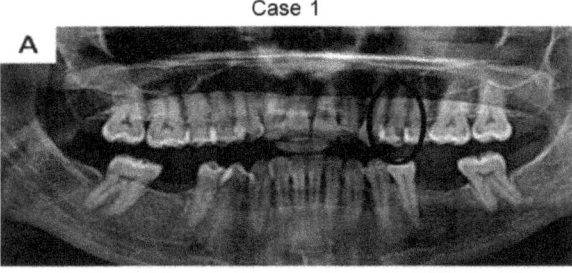
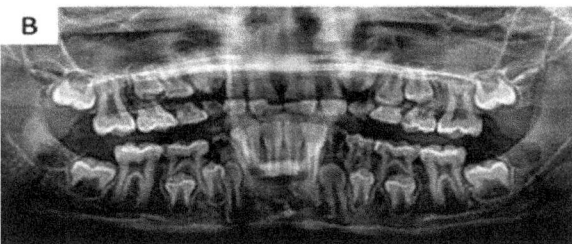

Figure 1. Panoramic radiographs of initial visit of the two patients from case 1. Black circle indicates the tooth requiring root canal treatment (receptor tooth) in the mother whilst the asterisks point to the primary canines in the son with planning for extraction (pulp donor tooth). The pulps from both canines were transplanted to the buccal and palatal canals from the first premolar of the mother.

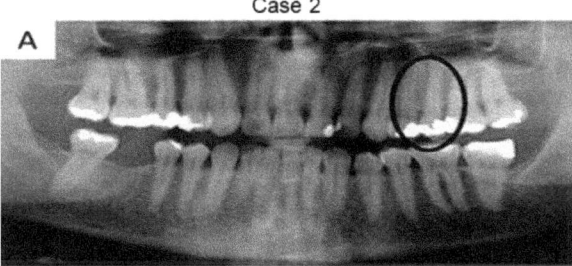
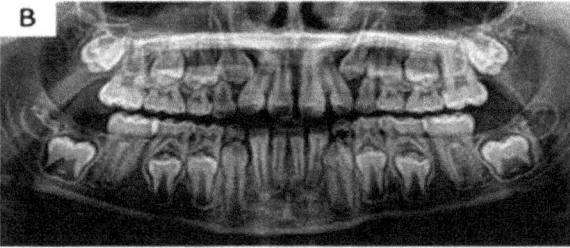

Figure 2. Panoramic radiographs of initial visit of the two patients in case 2. Black circle indicates the tooth requiring root canal treatment (receptor tooth) in the father whilst the asterisk points to the primary canine of the patient's daughter planned for extraction (pulp donor tooth).

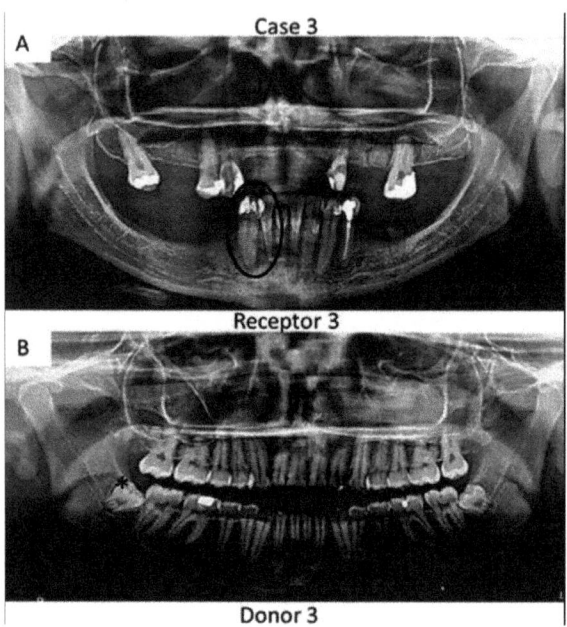

Figure 3. Panoramic radiographs of initial visit of the further two patients. Black circle indicates the teeth requiring root canal treatment (receptor teeth: lateral incisor and canine) in the mother whilst the asterisk highlights the third molar from the daughter demanding extraction (pulp donor tooth). The pulp from the donor tooth was sliced to obtain a mesial portion, which was transplanted to the lateral incisor of the mother; meanwhile, the distal part of the pulp was inserted into the mother's canine.

Sterile saline solution was used to remove the residues of the irrigating solution, while EDTA at 17% concentration was employed for 5 min for dentin conditioning and smear layer removal [17]. EDTA was rinsed twice using the saline solution, and the root canal was gently dried with an absorbent paper cone. The extracted teeth from the patients' children were first cut with a small diamond saw with a slow-speed handpiece [10] under a running sterilized saline solution. This first cut penetrated only 1–2 mm around the entire mesial and distal surfaces and 3–4 mm along the occlusal surface. This was performed to create a notch without touching the pulp tissue. The notch was pressed with a straight sharp syndesmotome to separate the tooth into two halves, which allowed for more careful pulp removal using small tweezers [10]. Pulp tissue (from the donor tooth) was inserted into the root canal of the receptor tooth (mother or father) with the aid of disinfected gutta-percha cones [10] to avoid damaging the pulp tissue.

Direct pulp capping was performed by means of Biodentine (Septodont, Paris, France) calcium silicate cement, which was manipulated according to the manufacturer's instructions and applied 2 mm below the bottom of the pulp chamber. After 10 min from the setting of the Biodentine, resin-modified glass ionomer cement (Riva Light-Cure, SDI, Bayswater, Australia) was applied as a liner and light-cured for 20 s with an LED Valo unit (1200 mW/cm^2, Ultradent, South Jordan, UT, USA) in order to avoid a negative reaction between the Biodentine and adhesive restoration [18]. A two-step self-etch adhesive (Clearfil SE Bond, Kuraray Medical, Kurashiki, Japan) was applied in the selective enamel etching mode by using 37% phosphoric acid gel only at enamel borders for 15 s, which was rinsed with distilled water for 30 s, and both the dentin and enamel were completely air-dried for 30 s prior to the application of the adhesive primer for 20 s. A slight air-blast was performed to evaporate the solvent, followed by an immediate application of the adhesive for 20 s. The adhesive system was light-cured for 40 s using a Valo LED unit, as previously described. Resin composite build-up was incrementally performed using 2 mm thick increments (Opallis, FGM, Joinville, Brazil), which were individually light-cured for 20 s. After occlusal check/adjustments, the patient was sent home with pharmacological support based on 600 mg of ibuprofen every 8 h for 3 days. No antibiotics were prescribed for any patient.

The receptor teeth were imaged by computed tomography in this first clinical visit (Figure 4(A1,B1,C1,C2)). Patients were scheduled for follow-up visits after 1 month and at every 3 months after the allogenic transplantation clinical procedure. At each recall visit, the treated teeth were evaluated via computed tomography (at 6, 12, and 24 months) and periapical radiography (at 3, 9, 15, and 18 months). Moreover, an electric pulp vitality test (Pulp Tester Digital, Odous de Deus, Belo Horizonte, Brazil) was performed on treated and further intact teeth from the same patient for control purposes, followed by occlusal check/adjustments of restorations and Doppler ultrasonic imaging at the 2-year follow-up. The device used was a Phillips HD11 ultrasonic device with color and spectral Doppler with a 1 cm/s rate by using a linear tip with 12–15 MHz frequency.

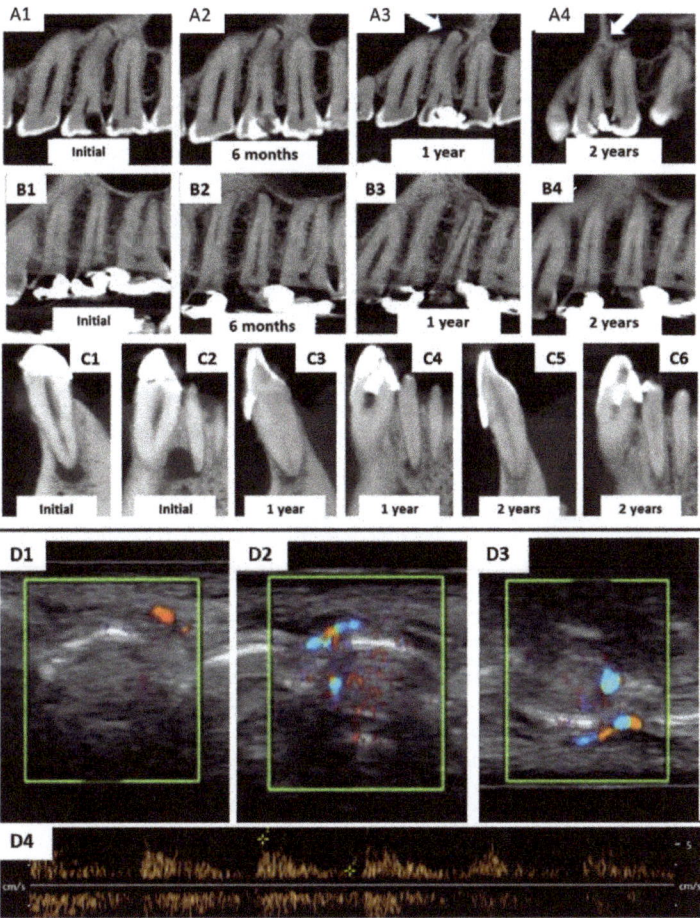

Figure 4. Computed tomography images of teeth receiving pulp allogenic transplantation. (**A1**–**A3**) are related to the patient's premolar in case 1, which showed small initial periapical radiolucency (**A1**) and

slightly increased in further follow-ups (**A2**,**A3**) but was entirely reduced at the 2-year follow-up (**A4**). The same trend occurred in the patient from case 2 (**B1,B2**) with a complete reduction of the periapical lesions at the 1-year follow-up (**B3**). This was confirmed by tomography at the 2-year stage (**B4**). In case 3, two teeth received allogenic pulp transplantation: the lateral incisor and mandibular canine. However, different tomographic slices were selected to show the treatment progression; (**C1,C3,C5**) depict lesion regression at the 1- and 2-year follow-ups. The same occurred with the lateral incisor, with a complete reduction of periapical radiolucency after 2 years. All four teeth from the 3 cases showed positive pulpal vitality with the electric test after 6–12 months. (**D1–D4**) depicts the Doppler ultrasonic assessment of the periapical revascularization in teeth from all three cases subjected to pulp allogenic transplantation. (**D1**) demonstrates high blood flux at the tooth receptor of the pulp of the patient from case 1. The blood flux of the teeth from case 2 (**D2**) was intense and similar to that of both teeth in case 3 (**D3**). The pulse intensity was normal in all four teeth (**D4**).

3. Results

During the 3-month follow-up, all patients reported slight pain at the periapical region of the receptor tooth, which started after 40 days and continued up to 2–3 months after the procedure. No response to the electrical pulp vitality test was detected until the 3-month follow-up. The patients in cases 1 and 2 showed a slight increase in periapical radiolucency as highlighted in the computed tomography at the 6-month follow-up period (Figure 4(A2,B2)) and at 1 year in case 1 (Figure 4(A3)). The details of patients from each case are presented in Table 1.

Table 1. Spreading of age and gender of donors and receptors in each case along with the teeth related.

	Age	Relationship	Teeth
Donor 1	11	Son	73
Receptor 1	25	Mother	24
Donor 2	10	Daughter	73
Receptor 2	49	Father	25
Donor 3	20	Daughter	38
Receptor 3	48	Mother	42 and 43

After one year from the allogenic transplantation, a complete regression of periapical lesions was verified for the patient in case 2 (Figure 4(B3)), and a remarkable reduction was verified for the patient in case 3 (Figure 4(C3,C4)). No signs of endodontic/periodontal complications/radiolucencies were observed for any patients at the 24-month follow-up stage (Figure 4(A4,B4,C5,C6)). Positive pulp vitality was confirmed, and revascularization was further proved for the three patients by Doppler imaging (Figure 4(D1–D4)) at the periapical region of each tooth.

4. Discussion

In modern dentistry, the auto-transplantation of teeth is a well-known and established procedure for the replacement of destroyed molars demanding immediate extraction. More recently, 3D-printing technology facilitated such a procedure by allowing the training of operators in a simulated clinical scenario [19]. Even the allogenic tooth transplantation of an entire tooth from the daughter to the mother was successfully demonstrated with the support of 3D-printing technology in order to achieve an optimal clinical outcome [20]. Such clinical procedures prompted the concept and idea of the present investigation, which was based on the use of the pulp tissue from an extracted primary tooth to replace the defective tissue in a different area of the oral environment in a third patient.

Several advantages are expected when performing a pulp tissue allogenic transplantation, such as the reduction of transplant rejection, similar DNA and RNA in all cells, completely mature connective tissue, formed neuronal network, as well as a properly formed vascularization network. Nevertheless, small inflammation would be expected at the initial time until the macrophages and lymphocytes recognize similar DNA fragments diminishing immunological reactions, thereby avoiding complete tissue rejection and the unsuccess of transplants [20]. Indeed, these factors may enhance the success of pulp regeneration treatments as in the strategy demonstrated by Liang et al. [13], which used minced pulp as a source of mesenchymal stem cells (MSCs) in order to provide odontogenic differentiation with high potential for protein and alkaline phosphatase expression. Furthermore, the in vivo clinical regeneration of pulp tissue would be faster than when using only conventional scaffolds, MSCs, and growth factors, especially once all the conjunctive tissue, blood vessels, and nerves are already constructed.

In a successful clinical procedure for pulp allogenic transplantation, the extraction of primary teeth or third molars from a relative, such as sons or daughters, must be performed with minimal damage of the tooth, avoiding tooth sectioning during extraction and excluding carious teeth or resorbed roots.

Indeed, when pulp tissue was removed from the donor teeth with tweezers, several odontoblasts were heavily damaged but were suitably replaced by stem cells after transplantation in order to achieve clinical success. Nevertheless, such a procedure is critical, as many cells could be damaged or killed, depending on how careful the pulp removal from the pulp chamber in the donor teeth was. A harsh procedure may inevitably cut the cellular processes from the odontoblast cell body, thereby increasing the failure rate of the entire transplantation procedure. In a therapeutic role, alkaline phosphatase may act as recovery mechanisms to heal the damaged tissue with odontoblast-like cells or with localized pulp mineralization [13].

Herein, the primary teeth extracted (asterisks in Figures 1 and 2) were scheduled to be extracted with minimal injury as they were vertically inclined, and permanent teeth were already formed/erupted in cases 1 and 2. Furthermore, the tooth must be stored as soon as possible in a sterilized saline solution; the complete disinfection prior to pulp removal and transplantation is mandatory [21]. The sectioning of the extracted tooth must be performed using a sterilized handpiece and diamond disks only after the root canal instrumentation of the receptor tooth [10]. Pulp should also be removed with sterilized tweezers (Figure 4B) and inserted into the roots of the acceptor teeth using disinfected gutta-percha cones. Indeed, all these procedures may promote minimal contamination during the clinical treatment, thereby increasing the probability to perform bacterial-free endodontic regeneration.

Moreover, root canal instrumentation and irrigation were performed by using rotary files and a tri-antibiotic solution [22], respectively. Although a recent report [23] suggested that clindamycin can replace minocycline to offer better angiogenic potential, we in the present case series employed the traditional solution used for revascularization procedures. A further feasible drug to replace minocycline would be doxycycline [24], which is approved by the US FDA and does not induce oxidative tooth staining over time [25]. However, doxycycline has been little investigated in pulp regeneration studies and the tri-antibiotic solution was used only as an irrigant, thereby diminishing the possibility of tooth staining. This is in contrast with the conventional procedure of revascularization performed by endodontic specialists, which requires keeping the tri-antibiotic solution for several days inside the root canals and pulp chamber. A further traditional procedure commonly performed in such a scenario is a final irrigation with 17% EDTA [17] prior to tissue transplantation [10]. It has been proposed that by opening dentinal tubules and conditioning the outer dentin, it would be possible to release several growth factors such as brain-derived neurotrophic factors and growth-differentiation factor 15 [8]. Particularly, these neuronal growth factors play an important role in the regeneration process of the transplanted pulp and obtain a faster recovery of the tooth vitality [26]. Furthermore, the intense blood flow in the bone surrounding the periapical apex may deliver vascular endothelial growth factors (VEGF) into root canals, likely reaching the two receptors (VEGFR-1 and VEGFR-2) in cells from mature blood vessels [26] within the transplanted pulp tissue. With entire vessels formed inside and outside the root canal in the apical region, a small vascular formation would restore blood to the transplanted pulp. All apexes from receptor teeth were kept without a high increase in diameter, but an open apex could help in revascularization and clinical success.

Concerning the few clinical studies available in the literature about pulp regeneration, the majority of them are focused on teeth diagnosed with irreversible pulpitis [8,9,12] with an absence of initial periapical radiolucency; this provides optimal vascularization and a lack of inflammatory mediators in the bone of the periapical region, which may facilitate the revascularization and reinnervation of transplanted tissue/cells. Conversely, in the current clinical cases, all patients presented periapical radiolucency either before or a few months after the allogenic transplantation. Such a feature may be a consequence of lower blood irrigation along with some inflammatory mediators due to the presence of allogenic cells, which may interfere with the success of the treatment. Nevertheless, successful outcomes were attained in the current study, along with a clear reduction of the periapical lesions in the treated teeth (Figure 4). Herein, we did not use prefabricated fibrin or collagen to avoid the contact of stem cells with different tissues, which could impair their differentiation and the success rate of transplantation. Stem cells replicate and differentiate more when in their natural tissue; this is the reason we did not use such materials.

Several protocols have been proposed for pulp transplantation to the root canal via endodontic regeneration, such as minced pulp [13], extracted/expanded DPSCs [12], platelet-rich fibrin [8], and leukocyte-platelet-rich fibrin [9]. Unfortunately, all these treatments require the support from a laboratory procedure to obtain platelet concentrates or stem cell expansion/replication [21]. In the present investigation, no laboratory intervention was demanded for pulp allogenic transplantation, which may represent a significant advance in comparison to previous clinical strategies. In fact, pulp allogenic transplantation as highlighted in the present report is entirely performed in a clinical dental office without the need for further external support.

In the clinical steps of the present case series, pulp capping after the allogenic transplantation was performed by using a gold standard procedure based on the use of calcium silicate cement (Biodentine, Septodont). This usually attains an optimal pulpal response, yielding a release of odontogenic growth factors, alkaline phosphatase release, and dentin bridge formation [9,27]. Afterwards, resin-modified glass ionomer cement was applied, followed by the application of [28] a two-step self-etch adhesive Clearfil SE Bond, which was employed in the selective enamel etching technique [29] in order to obtain the optimal sealing of the margins of the restored cavity. We believe that such pulp capping and restorative procedures may play an important role in the clinical long-term outcome of auto-transplanted pulps.

To confirm the apical revascularization, the three patients received a Doppler ultrasonic evaluation (Figure 4) of the four teeth that were treated for a pulp allogenic transplantation. This technique confirmed blood perfusion with characteristic pulse images (Figure 4(D4)), thereby demonstrating revascularization. Although such a method is not usual for the assessment of pulp vitality and periapical vascularization, an experienced M.D. radiologist trained with an obstetric ultrasound/Doppler device using his own teeth until it was calibrated prior to surveying the patients. Furthermore, electric pulp testing may vary from one device to another concerning the level of electric current and the tips employed, thereby jeopardizing the repeatability and reliability of the experiment.

This report is the very first attempt to demonstrate that the transplantation of pulp may be possible between close relatives such as parents and children, and perhaps between further family members. Indeed, future trends should focus on possible blood tests to survey the suitability for pulp transplants among distant family members and non-family-related donors/receptors. However, there are several limitations to the present treatment protocol related to the treatment of cases characterized by teeth presenting abscesses, purulency, or even when third molars are not well-positioned, which need to be extracted employing odonto-section procedures with a high risk for pulp damage and/or contamination. Furthermore, more improvements for the clinical procedure should focus on more suitable irrigation protocols and antibiotics, optimal root canal instrumentation, and the digitalization of the process in order to facilitate the current positioning of the pulp tissue into root canals with different shapes and sizes. Future trends may continue with the investigation of the health status of transplanted tissue by histochemical staining or cell culture studies, as well as the possible assessment of pulp transplantation between people from different families and a future feasible test to confirm gene compatibility tailored to such a novel sort of transplantation procedure.

5. Conclusions

Within the limitations of the present clinical report, the procedure of allogenic pulp transplantation may be feasible and provide revascularization, vitality restoration, and the reduction of periapical radiolucency. Further randomized clinical trials should be employed to study the actual success rate of such an innovative clinical treatment.

Author Contributions: V.P.F. and S.S., writing—original draft preparation; M.N.M. and L.V., clinical execution; T.R., writing—review and editing; D.d.P. and A.C.M., supervision and visualization; L.K.S., methodology and clinical execution; M.A.N., R.S. and L.B., methodology. All authors have read and agreed to the published version of the manuscript.

Funding: This research was supported by the Brazilian Ministry of Education (CAPES grant 23038.006958/2014-96, PI VPF).

Institutional Review Board Statement: The approval protocol of IRB was included in the manuscript.

Informed Consent Statement: Not applicable.

Data Availability Statement: No new data were created or analyzed in this study. Data sharing is not applicable to this article.

Acknowledgments: The authors thank David Araujo for the Doppler ultrasonic surveys.

Conflicts of Interest: The authors declare no conflict of interest.

References

1. Nakashima, M.; Iohara, K.; Bottino, M.C.; Fouad, A.F.; Nör, J.E.; Huang, G.T. Animal Models for Stem Cell-Based Pulp Regeneration: Foundation for Human Clinical Applications. *Tissue Eng. Part B Rev.* **2019**, *25*, 100–113. [CrossRef] [PubMed]
2. Li, X.; Ma, C.; Xie, X.; Sun, H.; Liu, X. Pulp regeneration in a full-length human tooth root using a hierarchical nanofibrous microsphere system. *Acta Biomater.* **2016**, *35*, 57–67. [CrossRef] [PubMed]
3. Athirasala, A.; Lins, F.; Tahayeri, A.; Hinds, M.; Smith, A.J.; Sedgley, C.; Ferracane, J.; Bertassoni, L.E. A Novel Strategy to Engineer Pre-Vascularized Full-Length Dental Pulp-like Tissue Constructs. *Sci. Rep.* **2017**, *7*, 3323. [CrossRef] [PubMed]
4. Nakashima, M.; Reddi, A.H. The application of bone morphogenetic proteins to dental tissue engineering. *Nat. Biotechnol.* **2003**, *21*, 1025–1032. [CrossRef]
5. Khayat, A.; Monteiro, N.; Smith, E.E.; Pagni, S.; Zhang, W.; Khademhosseini, A.; Yelick, P.C. GelMA-Encapsulated hDPSCs and HUVECs for Dental Pulp Regeneration. *J. Dent. Res.* **2017**, *96*, 192–199. [CrossRef]
6. Nagata, J.Y.; Gomes, B.P.; Rocha Lima, T.F.; Murakami, L.S.; de Faria, D.E.; Campos, G.R.; de Souza-Filho, F.J.; Soares, A. Traumatized immature teeth treated with 2 protocols of pulp revascularization. *J. Endod.* **2014**, *40*, 606–612. [CrossRef]
7. Shivashankar, V.Y.; Johns, D.A.; Maroli, R.K.; Sekar, M.; Chandrasekaran, R.; Karthikeyan, S.; Renganathan, S.K. Comparison of the Effect of PRP, PRF and Induced Bleeding in the Revascularization of Teeth with Necrotic Pulp and Open Apex: A Triple Blind Randomized Clinical Trial. *J. Clin. Diagn. Res. JCDR* **2017**, *11*, ZC34–ZC39. [CrossRef]
8. Nageh, M.; Ahmed, G.M.; El-Baz, A.A. Assessment of Regaining Pulp Sensibility in Mature Necrotic Teeth Using a Modified Revascularization Technique with Platelet-rich Fibrin: A Clinical Study. *J. Endod.* **2018**, *44*, 1526–1533. [CrossRef]
9. Meza, G.; Urrejola, D.; Saint Jean, N.; Inostroza, C.; López, V.; Khoury, M.; Brizuela, C. Personalized Cell Therapy for Pulpitis Using Autologous Dental Pulp Stem Cells and Leukocyte Platelet-rich Fibrin: A Case Report. *J. Endod.* **2019**, *45*, 144–149. [CrossRef]
10. Feitosa, V.P.; Mota, M.; Vieira, L.V.; de Paula, D.M.; Gomes, L.; Solheiro, L.; Aguiar Neto, M.A.; Carvalho, D.; Silvestre, F.A. Dental Pulp Autotransplantation: A New Modality of Endodontic Regenerative Therapy-Follow-Up of 3 Clinical Cases. *J. Endod.* **2021**, *47*, 1402–1408. [CrossRef]
11. Del Fabbro, M.; Lolato, A.; Bucchi, C.; Taschieri, S.; Weinstein, R.L. Autologous Platelet Concentrates for Pulp and Dentin Regeneration: A Literature Review of Animal Studies. *J. Endod.* **2016**, *42*, 250–257. [CrossRef] [PubMed]
12. Nakashima, M.; Iohara, K.; Murakami, M.; Nakamura, H.; Sato, Y.; Ariji, Y.; Matsushita, K. Pulp regeneration by transplantation of dental pulp stem cells in pulpitis: A pilot clinical study. *Stem Cell Res. Ther.* **2017**, *8*, 61. [CrossRef] [PubMed]

13. Liang, Z.; Kawano, S.; Chen, W.; Sadrkhani, M.S.; Lee, C.; Kim, E.; Moshaverinia, A.; Kim, R.H.; Kang, M.K. Minced Pulp as Source of Pulpal Mesenchymal Stem Cells with Odontogenic Differentiation Capacity. *J. Endod.* **2018**, *44*, 80–86. [CrossRef] [PubMed]
14. Miltiadous, M.E.; Floratos, S.G. Regenerative Endodontic Treatment as a Retreatment Option for a Tooth with Open Apex—A Case Report. *Braz. Dent. J.* **2015**, *26*, 552–556. [CrossRef]
15. Ruparel, N.B.; Teixeira, F.B.; Ferraz, C.C.; Diogenes, A. Direct effect of intracanal medicaments on survival of stem cells of the apical papilla. *J. Endod.* **2012**, *38*, 1372–1375. [CrossRef]
16. Estefan, B.S.; El Batouty, K.M.; Nagy, M.M.; Diogenes, A. Influence of Age and Apical Diameter on the Success of Endodontic Regeneration Procedures. *J. Endod.* **2016**, *42*, 1620–1625. [CrossRef]
17. Aksel, H.; Albanyan, H.; Bosaid, F.; Azim, A.A. Dentin Conditioning Protocol for Regenerative Endodontic Procedures. *J. Endod.* **2020**, *46*, 1099–1104. [CrossRef]
18. Palma, P.J.; Marques, J.A.; Antunes, M.; Falacho, R.I.; Sequeira, D.; Roseiro, L.; Santos, J.M.; Ramos, J.C. Effect of restorative timing on shear bond strength of composite resin/calcium silicate-based cements adhesive interfaces. *Clin. Oral Investig.* **2021**, *25*, 3131–3139. [CrossRef]
19. Kamio, T.; Kato, H. Autotransplantation of Impacted Third Molar Using 3D Printing Technology: A Case Report. *Bull. Tokyo Dent. Coll.* **2019**, *60*, 193–199. [CrossRef]
20. Xu, H.D.; Miron, R.J.; Zhang, X.X.; Zhang, Y.F. Allogenic tooth transplantation using 3D printing: A case report and review of the literature. *World J. Clin. Cases* **2019**, *7*, 2587–2596. [CrossRef]
21. Nakashima, M.; Iohara, K.; Zayed, M. Pulp Regeneration: Current Approaches, Challenges, and Novel Rejuvenating Strategies for an Aging Population. *J. Endod.* **2020**, *46*, S135–S142. [CrossRef] [PubMed]
22. Santiago, C.N.; Pinto, S.S.; Sassone, L.M.; Hirata, R., Jr.; Fidel, S.R. Revascularization Technique for the Treatment of External Inflammatory Root Resorption: A Report of 3 Cases. *J. Endod.* **2015**, *41*, 1560–1564. [CrossRef] [PubMed]
23. Dubey, N.; Xu, J.; Zhang, Z.; Nör, J.E.; Bottino, M.C. Comparative Evaluation of the Cytotoxic and Angiogenic Effects of Minocycline and Clindamycin: An In Vitro Study. *J. Endod.* **2019**, *45*, 882–889. [CrossRef] [PubMed]
24. Santos, L.; Chisini, L.A.; Springmann, C.G.; Souza, B.; Pappen, F.G.; Demarco, F.F.; Felippe, M.; Felippe, W.T. Alternative to Avoid Tooth Discoloration after Regenerative Endodontic Procedure: A Systematic Review. *Braz. Dent. J.* **2018**, *29*, 409–418. [CrossRef] [PubMed]
25. Palasuk, J.; Windsor, L.J.; Platt, J.A.; Lvov, Y.; Geraldeli, S.; Bottino, M.C. Doxycycline-loaded nanotube-modified adhesives inhibit MMP in a dose-dependent fashion. *Clin. Oral Investig.* **2018**, *22*, 1243–1252. [CrossRef]
26. Barta, P.; Kamaraj, R.; Kucharova, M.; Novy, Z.; Petrik, M.; Bendova, K.; Hajduch, M.; Pavek, P.; Trejtnar, F. Preparation, In Vitro Affinity, and In Vivo Biodistribution of Receptor-Specific ^{68}Ga-Labeled Peptides Targeting Vascular Endothelial Growth Factor Receptors. *Bioconj. Chem.* **2022**, *33*, 1825–1836. [CrossRef]
27. Pedano, M.S.; Li, X.; Yoshihara, K.; Landuyt, K.V.; Van Meerbeek, B. Cytotoxicity and Bioactivity of Dental Pulp-Capping Agents towards Human Tooth-Pulp Cells: A Systematic Review of In-Vitro Studies and Meta-Analysis of Randomized and Controlled Clinical Trials. *Materials* **2020**, *13*, 2670. [CrossRef]
28. Feitosa, V.P.; Sauro, S.; Zenobi, W.; Silva, J.C.; Abuna, G.; Van Meerbeek, B.; Sinhoreti, M.; Correr, A.B.; Yoshihara, K. Degradation of Adhesive-Dentin Interfaces Created Using Different Bonding Strategies after Five-year Simulated Pulpal Pressure. *J. Adhes. Dent.* **2019**, *21*, 199–207.
29. Van Meerbeek, B.; Yoshihara, K.; Van Landuyt, K.; Yoshida, Y.; Peumans, M. From Buonocore's Pioneering Acid-Etch Technique to Self-Adhering Restoratives. A Status Perspective of Rapidly Advancing Dental Adhesive Technology. *J. Adhes. Dent.* **2020**, *22*, 7–34.

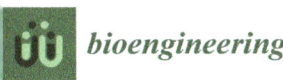

Case Report

Complicated Crown Fracture of Permanent Incisors: A Conservative Treatment Case Report and a Narrative Review

Mateusz Radwanski [1,†], Corrado Caporossi [2,†], Monika Lukomska-Szymanska [3,*,†], Arlinda Luzi [4] and Salvatore Sauro [4,5,*]

1. Department of Endodontics Chair, Conservative Dentistry, Endodontics Medical University of Lodz, 251 Pomorska Str., 92-213 Lodz, Poland
2. Independent Researcher, Roma, 65B, 00030 Labico, RM, Italy
3. Department of General Dentistry, Medical University of Lodz, 251 Pomorska Str., 92-213 Lodz, Poland
4. Group of Dental Biomaterials and Minimally Invasive Dentistry, Department of Dentistry, Cardenal Herrera-CEU Universities, C/Santiago Ramón y Cajal, s/n., Alfara del Patriarca, 46115 Valencia, Spain
5. Department of Therapeutic Dentistry, I. M. Sechenov First Moscow State Medical University, 119146 Moscow, Russia
* Correspondence: monika.lukomska-szymanska@umed.lodz.pl (M.L.-S.); salvatore.sauro@uchceu.es (S.S.); Tel.: +48-426-757461 (M.L.-S.)
† These authors contributed equally to this work.

Abstract: Dental trauma may have a severe impact on the social and psychological wellbeing of a patient. Most cases of dental injuries involve anterior teeth, especially the maxillary upper incisors. Crown fractures, with or without pulp exposure, are the most common trauma in permanent dentition. There are many methods of management, in which the initial state of the pulp, the time since the injury, and the presence of an accompanying injury play a key role. This case report aimed at showing a possible conservative treatment after complicated tooth fracture that consisted of partial pulpotomy followed by adhesive reattachment of the tooth fragment using a technique based on heated resin composite. Such a specific procedure represents a conservative approach to traumatic coronal lesions, providing a suitable opportunity to maintain the tooth vitality, aesthetics, and function. Indeed, reattachment of tooth fragment using a composite/adhesive is a simple technique to achieve excellent results in terms of aesthetic and function.

Keywords: traumatic dental injury; tooth fracture; adhesive reattachment

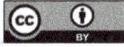

1. Introduction

Traumatic dental injuries (TDIs) concern mostly children and young adults [1]. TDIs may have a severe impact on the social and psychological wellbeing of a patient. Dental fractures are classified according to the fractured tissue and pulp involvement, and include enamel infractions, uncomplicated crown fractures (enamel fractures and enamel–dentin fractures), complicated crown fractures (enamel–dentin fractures with pulp exposure), and crown–root and root fractures [2]. Most of the cases of dental injuries involve anterior teeth, especially the maxillary upper incisors [3,4]. Conversely, lower central incisors and upper lateral incisors are less commonly involved [5,6]. Crown fractures, with or without pulp exposure, are the most common type of trauma in permanent dentition [3,7]. Complicated crown fractures involve enamel and dentin with pulp exposure; the occurrence of such trauma ranges between 2% and 13%, and the most common causes are falls, traffic accidents, domestic violence, fights, and sports [3,7].

The treatment of complicated crown fractures according to the International Association of Dental Traumatology (IADT, 2020) [1] includes conservative treatment of the pulp, such as partial pulpotomy, in both mature and immature roots. It is worth emphasizing that the condition of the pulp before starting treatment should be determined [1]. However, in the case of tooth injuries, it is possible to obtain false negative results, meaning no response despite vital pulp. After the trauma, the nervous response is temporarily lost, so the sensibility test (cold test and electric pulp test) may be negative [8]. Nevertheless, it is recommended that pulp vitality testing is performed after injury, as well as at follow-up visits, to assess any possible change over time [1,9]. In addition, tests for the evaluation of blood flow in the pulp, such as laser Doppler flowmetry (LDF), should be used [1].

During diagnosis, it is strongly recommended to take a parallel periapical radiograph. Additional radiographs are required if there are signs and symptoms of other potential injuries. For soft tissue injuries, X-rays of the lip and/or cheek are needed to look for tooth fragments or external debris. In the event of suspicion of other injuries, especially root fractures, crown–root fractures, or lateral luxations, the clinician should consider using cone beam computerized tomography (CBCT). This examination enables the determination of the location, extent, and direction of the injury [10]. The decision on additional patient exposure to radiation should be based on the fact that the obtained results will change the route of injury management.

When a tooth fragment is available, it should be reattached; if it is not available, it is recommended to cover the dentin with a glass-ionomer or a bonding agent and composite resin [1]. If a post is required to retain a crown in a mature tooth with complete root formation, root canal treatment is the preferred method.

The favorable outcomes include asymptomatic teeth with positive response to pulp sensibility testing, good quality restoration, and continued root development in immature teeth. Treatment outcome depends on the severity of the injury, quality, and timeliness of initial care, and recall protocol (after 14 days, 6–8 weeks, 3 and 6 months, and one year after the injury) [1]. The latter was performed via radiographic assessment and cold/hot vitality test. The present case report aimed at showing a possible conservative treatment after complicated tooth fracture that consisted of partial pulpotomy followed by adhesive reattachment of the tooth fragment.

2. Presentation of Cases

2.1. Diagnosis

A 15 year old male patient (case #1) experienced a blunt trauma during basketball game. The patient suffered from a complicated fracture of the crowns of 11 and 21 (Figure 1A,B). The fragments were recovered and kept immersed in milk until the appointment two days after the trauma.

Case #1   Case #2

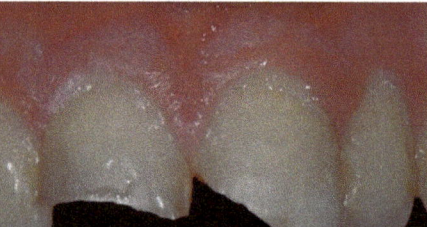
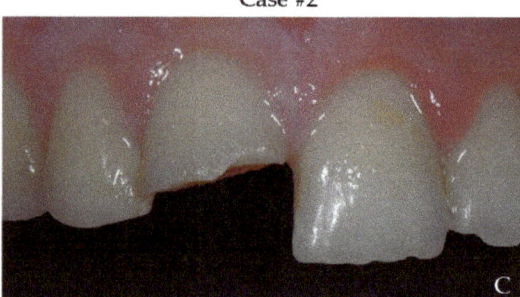

Figure 1. *Cont.*

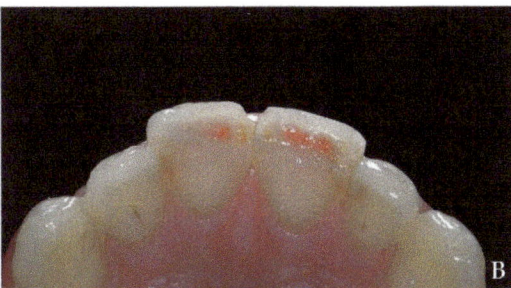 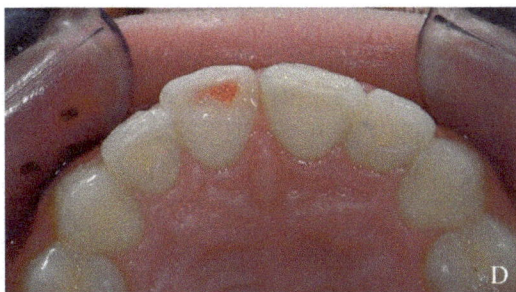

Figure 1. Intraoral photographs of both cases. (**A,C**)—buccal view; (**B,D**)—occlusal view.

In case #2, a 21 year old male patient reported to dental office immediately after a complicated crown fracture of the crowns of 11 during a tennis game (Figure 1C,D). The dental fragment was immediately stored in Hank's balanced saline solution.

In both cases, teeth were vital with thermal and electrical stimulus; no mobility and symptoms of other trauma were detected during clinical and X-ray examination (Figure 2A,B). The tooth fragments were not damaged, fit the tooth crowns, and did not interfere with the occlusion (Figure 3A,B).

Case #1   Case #2

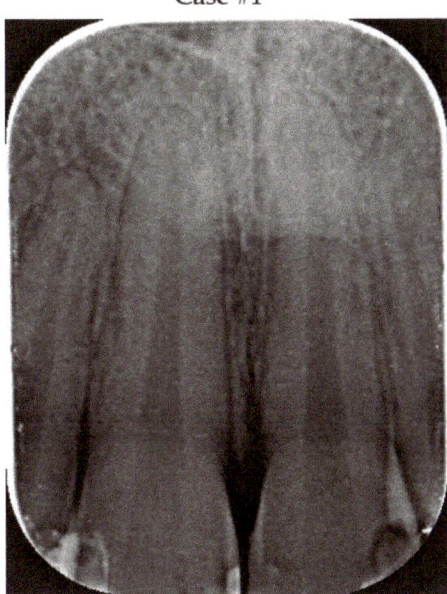 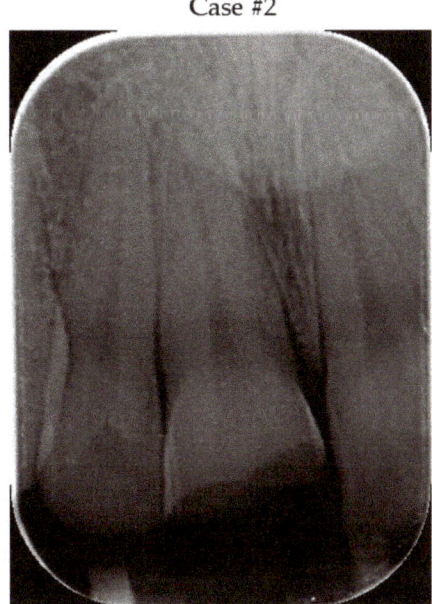

Figure 2. The preoperative X-rays.

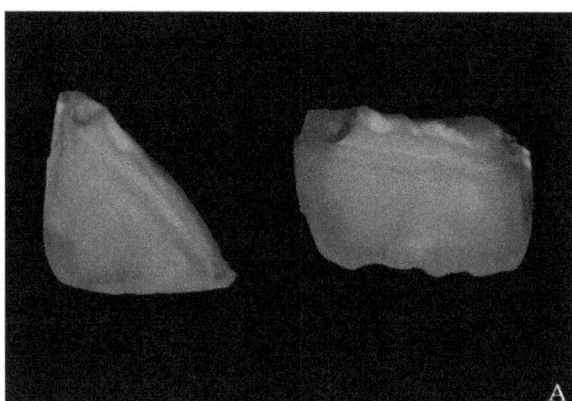
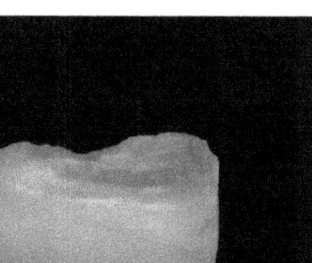

Figure 3. Fragments of teeth (**A**) 11 and 21, (**B**) 11.

2.2. Pulp Treatment Option

In case of complicated crown fractures, vital pulp therapy (VPT) interventions include direct pulp capping (DPC), partial pulpotomy (PP), and complete pulpotomy (CP) (Table 1).

Table 1. Treatment options of crown fractures with pulpal exposure.

Vital Pulp Therapy (VPT) Intervention	Description of the Method	Indication
Direct pulp capping (DPC)	(1) Placement of protective pulp capping material directly over the exposure	A recent and pinpoint-sized exposed vital pulp
Partial pulpotomy (PP)	(1) Partial removal of the coronal pulp; (2) Hemostasis; (3) Placement of a pulp capping material.	Pulp exposure treated within 14 days after trauma, caries-free, open apex or thin dentinal walls, and vital and asymptomatic pulp
Full (complete) pulpotomy (CP)	(1) Removal of the entire coronal pulp to the level of canal orifices; (2) Hemostasis; (3) Placement of a pulp capping material.	More than 2 week lapse between trauma and treatment, extensive pulp exposure

Based on the analysis of the clinical conditions and additional tests, it was decided to perform PP with adhesive/composite reattachment in case #1, as well as in case #2, maintaining the vitality of the treated teeth. PP was chosen as the treatment method following the admission of patients within 14 days after injury, no caries, and vital and asymptomatic pulp.

In general, VPT has a high success rate. However, clinical factors such as the vitality of the pulp, the time from exposure to intervention, age of the patient, other coexisting injuries, the cause of exposure, and the extent of exposure may influence the favorable outcome [11]. Additionally, PP has the advantage of preserving the cell-rich coronal pulp, which may provide greater healing potential, and so maintain the possibility of having physiological dentin deposition [12].

The diagnosis of injured tissue plays a key role, which can often be difficult in the case of trauma. Additionally, the tests used for sensitivity assessment (electric and/or thermal stimulation), which are dependent on neural response, may not be reliable in the first days after trauma [13]. In the case of difficulties, tests based on the measurement of actual blood flow, such as LDF or pulse oximetry, are recommended [13]. The increasing time between injury and intervention contributes to lower treatment success [11,14]. The age of the patient, and, thus, root development, does not influence the treatment prognosis [11]. It was believed that the pulp of the elderly contains more fibrous than cellular elements, which means that it has less repair capacity. Currently, it is thought that more important factor for treatment success is the complete removal of infected tissue, and, therefore, biological methods can be successfully applied to elderly individuals [15]. However, the presence of a further injury (e.g., luxation) associated with the crown fracture may adversely affect the outcome of the treatment [16]. The pulp exposed due to trauma, compared to carious exposure, has a greater chance of healing [11,17]. The extent of pulp exposure does not affect treatment prognosis, provided that it remains vital [11].

It is important to consider that the success of VPT is also influenced by factors such as proper infection control (rubber dam isolation), bleeding control, selection of the capping material providing a tight seal, and a final restoration.

2.3. Preparation of Operatory Field

In the presented cases, after administrating the anesthesia of 2% lidocaine with 1: 80,000 adrenalines not alkalinized (Dentsply, Konstanz, Germany), and performing a total rubber dam isolation to avoid cross-contamination, the partial pulpotomy was executed through high-speed bur under continuous saline irrigation.

Various local anesthetics and different vasoconstrictors concentration are used in VPT after trauma. Based on the available literature, the active substance and its concentration demonstrated no effect on the treatment results [18]. On the other hand, the vasoconstrictors may affect hemostasis, thus, making it difficult to assess the initial state of the pulp [18]. However, there are no clear guidelines for vasoconstrictor application in vital therapy.

The ability to control bleeding is an important factor determining the success of treatment, as prolonged bleeding is supposed to be a sign of an irreversible inflammatory process. The time needed to stop bleeding varies from 2 to 25 min, with no effect on the prognosis of pulpotomy [18]. Moreover, achieving hemostasis at the site of exposure does not provide an accurate assessment of pulp inflammation at the level of canal orifice [19]. Interestingly, immediate hemostasis does not determine the success of VPT [20]. Additionally, high blood flow may indicate good blood supply to the pulp, and high level of ability to repair and maintain vitality [20,21].

For bleeding control, the hemostatic agents are recommended. True hemostatic agents such as ferric sulphate or hydrogen peroxide are not recommended, due to the risk of masking the inflammation of the radicular pulp [21]. Several hemostatic products are available i.e., sodium hypochlorite, chlorhexidine, lidocaine with a vasoconstrictor, or saline, that show no adverse reaction to a pulp [22]. According to the guidelines (2021) of the American Association of Endodontists (AAE), the use of sodium hypochlorite is recommended, due to its bactericidal properties, and the ability to remove fibrin, clot, biofilm, and discolorations [23]. The sodium hypochlorite can be used safely in direct contact with pulp tissue (passive irrigation or soaked cotton pellet) at various concentrations, without adverse effect to the pulp and treatment prognosis [23]. Thereby, to control bleeding, cotton pellets soaked with 1% sodium hypochlorite were applied and the hemostasis was obtained after 2 min in both cases.

2.4. Choice of Materials

An ideal pulpotomy material should be biocompatible, non-toxic, induce hard tissue formation, and exhibit a disinfecting properties [24]. The materials used in pulpotomy are calcium hydroxide (CH) and calcium silicate materials (CSMs) [24,25].

CH exhibits bactericidal properties, high pH, and, therefore, it is characterized by the ability to neutralize acids and lipopolysaccharides [26]. These preparations contribute to the dentin bridge formation and healing of the pulp [25]. The most recommended form is an aqueous suspension of CH, which is applied to cover both the exposed pulp and the adjacent dentin. Aqueous solutions cause fewer hydroxyl ions to be released, and are less toxic due to the low content of additives [25]. However, the light-cured materials based on CH are not recommended, due to the cytotoxicity of the monomer [27]. The major disadvantage of CH products is instability and resorption over time. Numerous studies show that the formed dentin bridge is heterogeneous, with the presence of pores (tunnel defects) that can be the entry points for microorganisms. In addition, the high pH of CH has a negative effect on the pulp, which may contribute to its extensive necrosis [28–30].

Most CSMs, such as mineral trioxide aggregate (MTA), are based on Portland cement, consist mainly of dicalcium or tricalcium silicates, and are mixed with water [31,32]. They are called "hydraulic" because they can set in contact with water. MTA stimulates the pulp cells to produce a dentine deposition (e.g., dentin bridge) [33]. During setting, calcium hydroxide is released, providing the antimicrobial properties. MTA, compared with CH, exhibits a higher mechanical strength, is less toxic, and causes less pulpal inflammation [34]. The disadvantages of MTA include the difficulty of application, long setting time, and teeth discoloration [35].

One of the major aesthetic complications after pulpotomy with white and grey MTA can be the discoloration of the tooth [36,37]. It is caused mainly by the oxidation of heavy metal oxides (bismuth or iron), and by the interaction between erythrocytes and the unset cement in case of inadequate hemostasis [38–40]. To prevent the discoloration, different approaches are suggested, such as using cements with alternative radiopacifying agents such as zirconium oxide, sealing the surrounding dentinal tubules with dentin bonding agents before MTA application, or adding zinc oxide or aluminium fluoride to the powder [41–44]. Unfortunately, there is no consensus regarding that matter and, consequently, no guidelines for the prevention of discoloration were issued.

The powder of MTA is mixed with distilled water (3:1 ratio) to obtain a wet, gel-like consistency [45]. For mixing, a metal or plastic spatula and a glass plate or paper can be used. The working time with the material is about 5 min, and the setting time is long, from 3 to 4 h. Some substances may affect the setting time, causing it to shorten (sodium hypochlorite) or elongate (saline, lignocaine) [45]. However, the results for chlorhexidine are contradictory; some studies show no effect [46], while others show an alteration in the setting of the MTA [47]. The excavator, a retrograde amalgam that carries, can be used for the delivery of the prepared MTA, and paper points, pluggers, or ultrasounds for the condensation. The material should not be condensed with excessive force, due to the risk of reducing its strength and surface hardness [48]. The material should be applied excessively to cover pulp and all walls without the risk of creating voids. For the final condensation, it is recommended to use a cotton pellet moistened with sterile water to initiate the setting reaction and clean the excess of the material. Appropriate material thickness in the case of pulpotomy amounts up to 3–4 mm. The thickness and compaction of the MTA layer can be assessed with X-ray [49]. The coronal excess of material should be removed with use of cotton pellet or mechanically with burs. In the presented cases, MTA (ENDOPASS, DEI -Italia, Varese, Italy) was mixed with bi-distilled water using a plastic spatula on a glass pad, and condensed with paper points and moist cotton pellet (Figure 4A–D); the excess of material was removed with cotton pellet.

Many systematic review papers and meta-analyses report that there is no significant differences between MTA and CH regarding the survival rate of pulp, both for permanent immature teeth and teeth with closed apices [12,50–52]. On the other hand, some studies indicate the superiority of MTA-based materials due to lower solubility when compared with CH, greater biocompatibility, and the quicker formation of thicker and more homogenous dentin bridge, which may be a greater barrier to bacterial leakage [53,54]. Therefore, in the presented cases, MTA was applied.

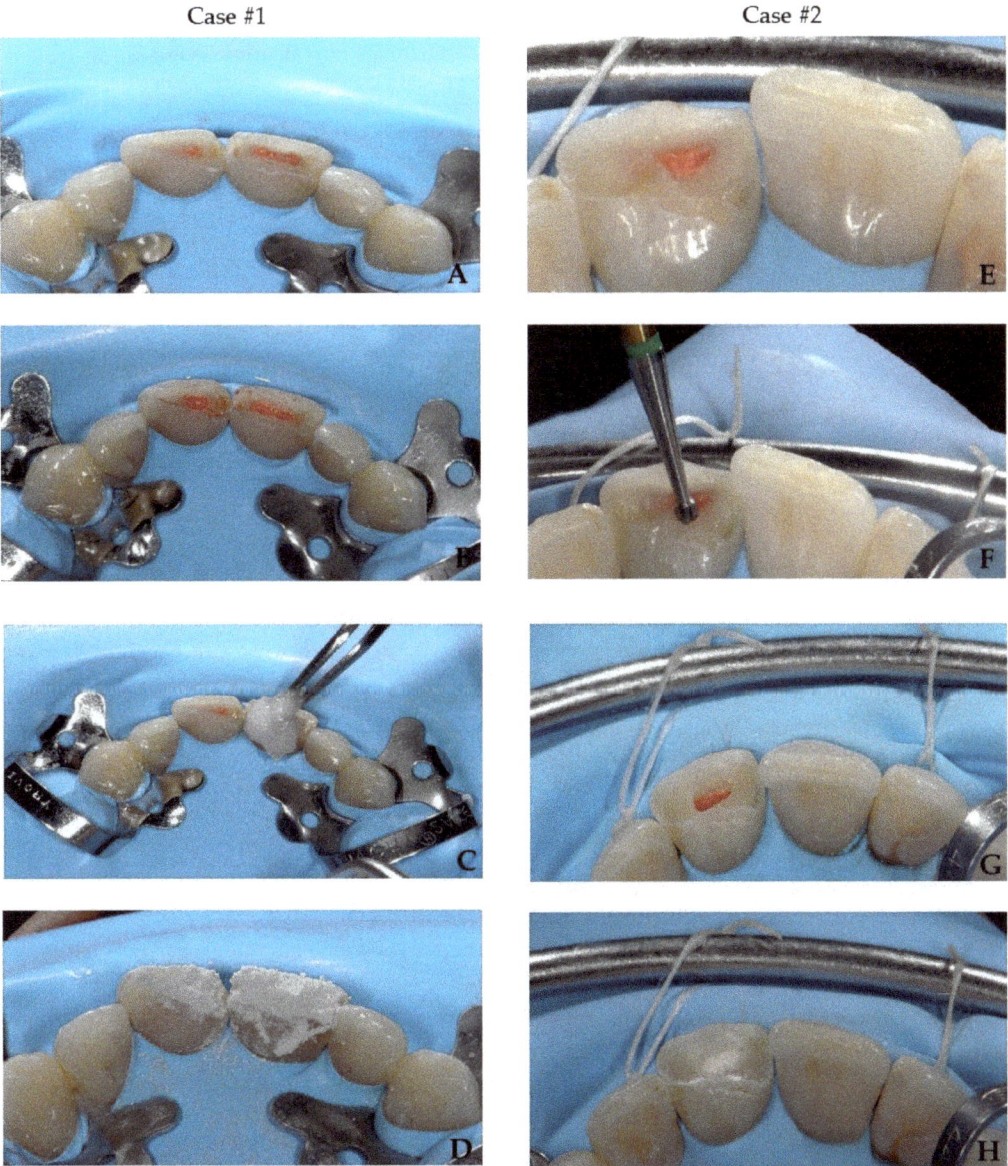

Figure 4. PP of teeth 11 and 21 (case #1) and PP of tooth 11 (case #2). (**A,E**)—clinical situation before pulpotomies; (**B,F**)—partial pulpotomies; (**C,G**)—hemostasis with cotton soaked with 1% sodium hypochlorite; (**D,H**)—capping with MTA.

The calcific metamorphosis is an adverse effect of the MTA and CH application [51,52]. It is associated with the induction of odontoblasts to form hard tissues and can only take place when the pulp is vital. The incidence of pulp obliteration after dental trauma amounts from 4 up to 24% [55]. The calcification is not considered a criterion of success or failure of treatment, and only the obliteration of the pulp chamber may increase the difficulty of endodontic treatment in the future, and may favor perforation when trying to locate the canal orifice.

2.5. Restorative Procedure

When a well-hydrated intact tooth fragment is available, which fits to the remaining crown without interfering with the patient's occlusion, the first-choice treatment should be adhesive reattachment of the fragment. It does not always have to be stored in a humid environment; a study shows that a dehydrated fragment was attached to the tooth with the use of additional retention elements, and after a 15 month follow-up, the tooth retained its vitality, functionality, and natural aesthetics [56]. However, the dehydration of the broken fragment may cause color disharmony with the tooth remnant, but such an issue disappears after about 12 months, due to the absorption of water by the fragment [57,58].

Compared to conventional restorative techniques, the reattachment of tooth fragments exhibits several advantages: the original shape, color, brightness, and texture of the enamel surface [59]. The incisal edges of reattached fragments tend to wear at a similar rate to adjacent natural teeth. This technique is less time-consuming, minimally invasive, and simple to perform [60]. The type of injury causing the crown fracture or the storage medium prior to reattachment can exert no effect on the survival, color, and bond strength of the treated teeth after reattaching the fragment [57]. It is very important to perform the reattachment procedure under a rubber dam to avoid contamination and deterioration of the adhesive layer [9].

Many different types of adhesive systems (total-etch, self-etch) and different intermediate materials e.g., paste and flowable composite materials, adhesives, or glass ionomer cements, can be applied [61–65]. There is no consensus in the literature regarding the ideal technique and material for reattachment of a tooth fragment [64].

Some authors recommend pre-reattachment/initial modification of remaining fragments, e.g., dentine grooves, over-contouring, chamfering, or beveling, to expand the enamel surface, increasing adhesion and ensuring higher fracture resistance of such restorations [66,67]. These additional retention elements should be considered if the broken fragment involves more than 50% of the clinical crown [68]. However, the most recent systemic review recommends simple reattachment without any modification to reduce the technical sensitivity of the procedure and the length of the clinical phase [64]. In addition, achieving imperceptible anterior restoration depends on operator clinical experience and knowledge of dental anatomy, rather than any previous preparation [69].

The bond strength between adhesive systems and calcium-silicate-based materials is also an important aspect. The in vitro results indicate that the bond strength of the resin-based materials to the MTA is favorable for the total-etch technique [70–72]. On the other hand, in the case of Biodentine, the bond strength when using self-etch or total-etch systems achieves similar results [73–76]. Due to the lack of evidence regarding the chemical interaction of self-etching materials with bioceramics, pre-treatment with phosphoric acid prior to the bonding procedure may be recommended [75].

In the present cases, no modification was carried out before the reattachment procedure. In both cases, the selective enamel etching both on the tooth and the fragment was performed using a 36% phosphoric acid gel (DeTrey Conditioner 36, Dentsply Sirona GmbH, Bensheim, Germany) under rubber dam isolation. Then, a self-etching two-component adhesive system (Clearfil™ Se Bond, Kuraray Noritake Dental Inc., Tokyo, Japan, CSE) was applied as per manufacturer's instruction, and air-dried with a strong stream of air for 5 s to completely remove the excess adhesive. This was finally light-cured for 20 s (Radii Xpert, Voco GmbH, Cuxhaven, Germany). Subsequently, a thin layer of enamel (Shade A2) mass composite (Asteria Tokuyama NE, Tokuyama Dental Corporation, Taitouku Tokyo, Japan) was applied directly on the tooth as an intermediate material to reattach the fragment to the tooth. The composite was heated up to 54 °C in a warming device (AdDent Calset™ Composite Warmer, AdDent Inc., Danbury, CT, USA) to increase the degree of polymerization, a better adaptation of the fragment on the tooth and to provide easier management of the excess removal [77]. Next, photopolymerization was carried out for 10 s. To avoid undesirable inhibition layer due to photopolymerization, the area was protected by covering the tooth with an oxygen inhibitor gel (Oxyguard II, Kuraray Europe GmbH, Frankfurt, Germany) and polymerized for 40 s. (Figure 5A–G).

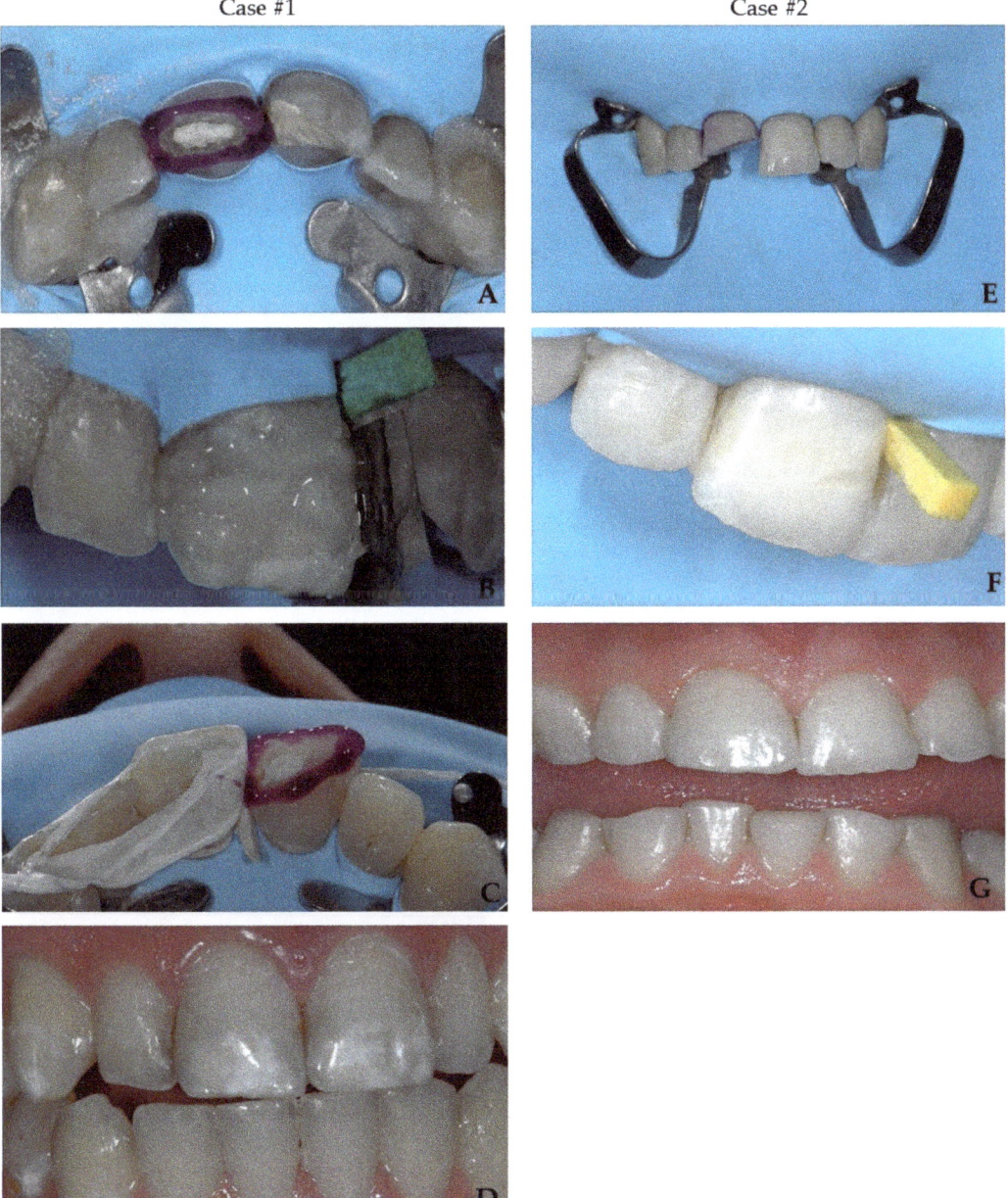

Figure 5. The reattachment of tooth 11 and 21 (case #1- up). (**A**)—selective etching of tooth 11; (**B**)—reattachment of coronal fragment of tooth 11; (**C**)—selective etching of tooth 21; (**D**)—buccal view after adhesive reattachment of teeth 11 and 21. The reattachment of tooth 11 (case #2- down). (**E**)—selective etching of tooth 11; (**F**)—reattachment of coronal fragment of tooth 11; (**G**)—buccal view after adhesive reattachment of tooth 11.

2.6. Occlusion Adjustment

Occlusal adjustment involves the development of an acceptable central relation contact position for the patient, ensuring acceptable lateral and protrusion guidance. This is necessary to eliminate premature contacts and bad guidance, which could contribute to excessive forces concentrating within the reattached fragment, thus, causing it to detach. Therefore, the presented cases were performed using a diamond bur (#3118F—KG Sorensen, Cotia, SP, Brazil). Due to the perfect fit of tooth fragments and prior excess removal, minimal occlusion adjustment was needed.

2.7. Finishing and Polishing

Polishing provides a smooth surface of the teeth, thus, reducing the accumulation of dental plaque. While it is important, polishing removes the fluorine-rich enamel layer and should, therefore, be carried out selectively [78].

The restored teeth were first finished using fine and extra-fine diamond burs (2135F and 2135FF, respectively (KG, Sorensen, Cotia, SP, Brazil)), and finally polished using either a Soflex discs coarse, medium, fine, and super-fine grit Sof-Lex disk (3M ESPE, St. Paul, MN, USA) in a slow-speed hand piece for 30 s each.

2.8. Follow-Up Visits and Prognosis

The follow-up visits after trauma injury are of paramount importance and, therefore, mandatory. The control should consist of an interview, radiological examination, and pulp sensitivity tests. It enables the early detection and implementation of appropriate treatment to avoid long-term complications. The most common post-traumatic problems include pulp infection and necrosis, pulp canal obliteration (PCO) or root resorptions.

In the case of the complicated crown fractures, the recommended follow-up visits are as follows: after 14 days, 6–8 weeks, 3 and 6 months, and one year after the injury. In the case of the presented cases, the check-ups were carried out in accordance with the recommended scheme, and the positive results obtained after one year by interview, radiological examination, and pulp sensitivity cold/hot test indicate the success of the treatment.

3. Prognosis and Future Perspectives

If the pulp is exposed, biological treatment procedures should be performed. It is of paramount importance in the case of patients with open apices, as the preservation of the vital pulp ensures further physiological root formation. The prognosis of direct pulp capping with use of CH shows a success rate of 54–90% [25,79]. In addition, partial pulpotomy with that material may present a greater success rate (86–100%) [14,79,80]. The use of hydraulic calcium-silicate-based cements might contribute to the better prognosis of VPT than application of CH [81]. Moreover, total pulpotomy using CSMs has a success rate of 74–100% after 1 to 5 years follow-up [25,82,83]. Currently, there are reports presenting the possibility of including irreversibly damaged pulp in the indications for VPT [84,85].

The reported success rate of partial pulpotomy in permanent dentition with complicated crown fractures ranges from 87.5% to 100% [12,53]. The initial condition of the pulp, the absence of its damage, or the presence of any other trauma, which may affect blood supply, play a key role in the long-term treatment success [53].

The employment of adhesive techniques increases the success rate of the reattachment procedure by up to 84–93% [57,59]. Cases of successful treatment after 5 or even 9 year follow-ups are reported [86,87]. The pulp treatment is not a factor that impaired the stability of the reattached fragments. When using the conventional etch and rinse technique, the bonding performance of the restoration mainly depends on the micromechanical retention between the composite resin and the etched enamel, as well as the hybrid layer. Therefore, the success rate is not affected by the pulp treatment [68]. Thus, the reattachment technique can be used both in uncomplicated and complicated crown fractures. Adhesive reattachment combined with vital pulp therapy procedures is a good first-choice treatment option in cases of complicated crown fractures.

Moreover, the use of toothpaste containing biomimetic hydroxyapatite for home management after reconstruction can reduce discoloration and hypersensitivity more effectively than conventional fluoride toothpaste [88,89].

Author Contributions: Conceptualization, S.S., C.C. and M.L.-S.; methodology, S.S., C.C. and M.L.-S.; software, M.R.; validation, S.S. and M.L.-S.; formal analysis, M.L.-S.; investigation, S.S. and C.C.; resources, M.L.-S. and M.R.; data curation, M.L.-S.; writing—original draft preparation, M.L.-S. and M.R.; writing—review and editing, S.S., A.L., M.L.-S. and M.R.; visualization, M.R.; supervision, S.S. and M.L.-S.; project administration, M.L.-S.; funding acquisition, C.C. and M.L.-S. All authors have read and agreed to the published version of the manuscript.

Funding: This research received no external funding.

Institutional Review Board Statement: Not applicable.

Informed Consent Statement: Informed consent was obtained from all subjects involved in the study.

Data Availability Statement: Not applicable.

Conflicts of Interest: The authors declare no conflict of interest.

References

1. Bourguignon, C.; Cohenca, N.; Lauridsen, E.; Flores, M.T.; O'Connell, A.C.; Day, P.F.; Tsilingaridis, G.; Abbott, P.V.; Fouad, A.F.; Hicks, L.; et al. International Association of Dental Traumatology Guidelines for the Management of Traumatic Dental Injuries: 1. Fractures and Luxations. *Dent. Traumatol.* **2020**, *36*, 314–330. [CrossRef] [PubMed]
2. Diangelis, A.J.; Andreasen, J.O.; Ebeleseder, K.A.; Kenny, D.J.; Trope, M.; Sigurdsson, A.; Andersson, L.; Bourguignon, C.; Flores, M.T.; Hicks, M.L.; et al. Guidelines for the Management of Traumatic Dental Injuries: 1. Fractures and Luxations of Permanent Teeth. *Pediatr. Dent.* **2017**, *39*, 401–411. [CrossRef] [PubMed]
3. Aggarwal, V.; Logani, A.; Shah, N. Complicated Crown Fractures—Management and Treatment Options. *Int. Endod. J.* **2009**, *42*, 740–753. [CrossRef] [PubMed]
4. Ojeda-Gutierrez, F.; Martinez-Marquez, B.; Arteaga-Larios, S.; Ruiz-Rodriguez, M.S.; Pozos-Guillen, A. Management and Followup of Complicated Crown Fractures in Young Patients Treated with Partial Pulpotomy. *Case Rep. Dent.* **2013**, *2013*, 597563. [CrossRef]
5. Dharmani, C.K.; Pathak, A.; Sidhu, H.S. Prevalence of Traumatic Dental Injuries to Anterior Teeth in 8-12-Year-Old Schoolchildren of Patiala City, Punjab, India: An Epidemiological Study. *Int. J. Clin. Pediatr. Dent.* **2019**, *12*, 25–29. [CrossRef]
6. Juneja, P.; Kulkarni, S.; Raje, S. Prevalence of Traumatic Dental Injuries and Their Relation with Predisposing Factors among 8-15 Years Old School Children of Indore City, India. *Clujul Med.* **2018**, *91*, 328–335. [CrossRef]
7. Levin, L.; Day, P.F.; Hicks, L.; O'Connell, A.; Fouad, A.F.; Bourguignon, C.; Abbott, P.V. International Association of Dental Traumatology Guidelines for the Management of Traumatic Dental Injuries: General Introduction. *Dent. Traumatol.* **2020**, *36*, 309–313. [CrossRef]
8. Gopikrishna, V.; Tinagupta, K.; Kandaswamy, D. Comparison of Electrical, Thermal, and Pulse Oximetry Methods for Assessing Pulp Vitality in Recently Traumatized Teeth. *J. Endod.* **2007**, *33*, 531–535. [CrossRef]
9. Marinčák, D.; Doležel, V.; Přibyl, M.; Voborná, I.; Marek, I.; Šedý, J.; Žižka, R. Conservative Treatment of Complicated Crown Fracture and Crown-Root Fracture of Young Permanent Incisor—A Case Report with 24-Month Follow-Up. *Children* **2021**, *8*, 725. [CrossRef]
10. Cohenca, N.; Silberman, A. Contemporary Imaging for the Diagnosis and Treatment of Traumatic Dental Injuries: A Review. *Dent. Traumatol. Off. Publ. Int. Assoc. Dent. Traumatol.* **2017**, *33*, 321–328. [CrossRef]
11. Matoug-Elwerfelli, M.; ElSheshtawy, A.S.; Duggal, M.; Tong, H.J.; Nazzal, H. Vital Pulp Treatment for Traumatized Permanent Teeth: A Systematic Review. *Int. Endod. J.* **2022**, 1–17. [CrossRef] [PubMed]
12. Yang, Y.T.; Xia, B.; Xu, Z.; Dou, G.; Lei, Y.; Yong, W. The Effect of Partial Pulpotomy with IRoot BP Plus in Traumatized Immature Permanent Teeth: A Randomized Prospective Controlled Trial. *Dent. Traumatol.* **2020**, *36*, 518–525. [CrossRef] [PubMed]
13. Krastl, G.; Weiger, R.; Filippi, A.; Van Waes, H.; Ebeleseder, K.; Ree, M.; Connert, T.; Widbiller, M.; Tjäderhane, L.; Dummer, P.M.H.; et al. Endodontic Management of Traumatized Permanent Teeth: A Comprehensive Review. *Int. Endod. J.* **2021**, *54*, 1221–1245. [CrossRef] [PubMed]
14. Cvek, M. Partial Pulpotomy in Crown—Fractured Incisors—Results 3 to 15 Years After Treatment. *Acta Stomatol. Croat.* **1993**, *27*, 167–173.
15. Aguilar, P.; Linsuwanont, P. Vital Pulp Therapy in Vital Permanent Teeth with Cariously Exposed Pulp: A Systematic Review. *J. Endod.* **2011**, *37*, 581–587. [CrossRef]
16. Haikal, L.; Ferraz Dos Santos, B.; Vu, D.-D.; Braniste, M.; Dabbagh, B. Biodentine Pulpotomies on Permanent Traumatized Teeth with Complicated Crown Fractures. *J. Endod.* **2020**, *46*, 1204–1209. [CrossRef]

17. da Rosa, W.L.O.; Piva, E.; da Silva, A.F. Disclosing the Physiology of Pulp Tissue for Vital Pulp Therapy. *Int. Endod. J.* **2018**, *51*, 829–846. [CrossRef]
18. Santos, J.M.; Pereira, J.F.; Marques, A.; Sequeira, D.B.; Friedman, S. Vital Pulp Therapy in Permanent Mature Posterior Teeth with Symptomatic Irreversible Pulpitis: A Systematic Review of Treatment Outcomes. *Medicina* **2021**, *57*, 573. [CrossRef]
19. Mutluay, M.; Arikan, V.; Sari, S.; Kisa, Ü. Does Achievement of Hemostasis after Pulp Exposure Provide an Accurate Assessment of Pulp Inflammation? *Pediatr. Dent.* **2018**, *40*, 37–42.
20. Asgary, S.; Parhizkar, A. Importance of 'Time' on 'Haemostasis' in Vital Pulp Therapy—Letter to the Editor. *Eur. Endod. J.* **2021**, *6*, 128–129. [CrossRef]
21. Zanini, M.; Hennequin, M.; Cousson, P.Y. Which Procedures and Materials Could Be Applied for Full Pulpotomy in Permanent Mature Teeth? A Systematic Review. *Acta Odontol. Scand.* **2019**, *77*, 541–551. [CrossRef] [PubMed]
22. Garcia-Godoy, F.; Murray, P. Systemic Evaluation of Various Haemostatic Agents Following Local Application Prior to Direct Pulp Capping. *Braz. J. Oral Sci.* **2005**, *4*, 791–797. [CrossRef]
23. AAE Position Statement on Vital Pulp Therapy. *J. Endod.* **2021**, *47*, 1340–1344. [CrossRef] [PubMed]
24. Chen, Y.; Chen, X.; Zhang, Y.; Zhou, F.; Deng, J.; Zou, J.; Wang, Y. Materials for Pulpotomy in Immature Permanent Teeth: A Systematic Review and Meta-Analysis. *BMC Oral Health* **2019**, *19*, 227. [CrossRef] [PubMed]
25. Till, D.; Galler, K. Current Recommendations for Vital Pulp Treatment. *Dtsch. Zahnärztliche Zeitschrift Int.* **2019**, *1*, 43–52.
26. Graham, L.; Cooper, P.R.; Cassidy, N.; Nor, J.E.; Sloan, A.J.; Smith, A.J. The Effect of Calcium Hydroxide on Solubilisation of Bio-Active Dentine Matrix Components. *Biomaterials* **2006**, *27*, 2865–2873. [CrossRef] [PubMed]
27. Hebling, J.; Lessa, F.C.R.; Nogueira, I.; Carvalho, R.M.; Costa, C.A.S. Cytotoxicity of Resin-Based Light-Cured Liners. *Am. J. Dent.* **2009**, *22*, 137–142.
28. Jalan, A.L.; Warhadpande, M.M.; Dakshindas, D.M. A Comparison of Human Dental Pulp Response to Calcium Hydroxide and Biodentine as Direct Pulp-Capping Agents. *J. Conserv. Dent.* **2017**, *20*, 129–133. [CrossRef]
29. Ravi, G.; Subramanyam, R. Possible Mechanisms of Lack of Dentin Bridge Formation in Response to Calcium Hydroxide in Primary Teeth. *Dent. Hypotheses* **2015**, *6*, 6–9. [CrossRef]
30. Kolasa, M.; Szczepańska, J. Direct Pulp Capping in Permanent Teeth in Children—Tertiary Dentin Formation, Materials Used. Part II. *Nowa Stomatol.* **2018**, *23*, 78–83. [CrossRef]
31. Malhotra, N.; Agarwal, A.; Mala, K. Mineral Trioxide Aggregate: A Review of Physical Properties. *Compend. Contin. Educ. Dent.* **2013**, *34*, e25–e32. [PubMed]
32. Abedi-Amin, A.; Luzi, A.; Giovarruscio, M.; Paolone, G.; Darvizeh, A.; Agulló, V.V.; Sauro, S. Innovative Root-End Filling Materials Based on Calcium-Silicates and Calcium-Phosphates. *J. Mater. Sci. Mater. Med.* **2017**, *28*, 31. [CrossRef] [PubMed]
33. Islam, I.; Chng, H.K.; Yap, A.U.J. Comparison of the Physical and Mechanical Properties of MTA and Portland Cement. *J. Endod.* **2006**, *32*, 193–197. [CrossRef] [PubMed]
34. Kunert, M.; Lukomska-Szymanska, M. Bio-Inductive Materials in Direct and Indirect Pulp Capping—A Review Article. *Materials* **2020**, *13*, 1204. [CrossRef] [PubMed]
35. Parirokh, M.; Torabinejad, M. Mineral Trioxide Aggregate: A Comprehensive Literature Review—Part III: Clinical Applications, Drawbacks, and Mechanism of Action. *J. Endod.* **2010**, *36*, 400–413. [CrossRef] [PubMed]
36. Pelepenko, L.E.; Saavedra, F.; Bombarda, G.F.; Gomes, B.P.F.D.A.; De-Jesus-Soares, A.; Zaia, A.A.; Duarte, M.A.H.; Tanomaru-Filho, M.; Marciano, M.A. Dental Discoloration Caused by Grey-Mtaflow Cement: Analysis of Its Physicochemical, Biological and Antimicrobial Properties. *J. Appl. Oral Sci.* **2020**, *28*, 1–15. [CrossRef] [PubMed]
37. Salem-Milani, A.; Ghasemi, S.; Rahimi, S.; Ardalan-Abdollahi, A.; Asghari-Jafarabadi, M. The Discoloration Effect of White Mineral Trioxide Aggregate (WMTA), Calcium Enriched Mixture (CEM), and Portland Cement (PC) on Human Teeth. *J. Clin. Exp. Dent.* **2017**, *9*, e1397–e1401. [CrossRef]
38. Możyńska, J.; Metlerski, M.; Lipski, M.; Nowicka, A. Tooth Discoloration Induced by Different Calcium Silicate-Based Cements: A Systematic Review of In Vitro Studies. *J. Endod.* **2017**, *43*, 1593–1601. [CrossRef]
39. Camilleri, J. Color Stability of White Mineral Trioxide Aggregate in Contact with Hypochlorite Solution. *J. Endod.* **2014**, *40*, 436–440. [CrossRef]
40. Jang, J.-H.; Kang, M.; Ahn, S.; Kim, S.; Kim, W.; Kim, Y.; Kim, E. Tooth Discoloration after the Use of New Pozzolan Cement (Endocem) and Mineral Trioxide Aggregate and the Effects of Internal Bleaching. *J. Endod.* **2013**, *39*, 1598–1602. [CrossRef]
41. Marciano, M.A.; Camilleri, J.; Lucateli, R.L.; Costa, R.M.; Matsumoto, M.A.; Duarte, M.A.H. Physical, Chemical, and Biological Properties of White MTA with Additions of AlF(3). *Clin. Oral Investig.* **2019**, *23*, 33–41. [CrossRef] [PubMed]
42. Marciano, M.A.; Camilleri, J.; Costa, R.M.; Matsumoto, M.A.; Guimarães, B.M.; Duarte, M.A.H. Zinc Oxide Inhibits Dental Discoloration Caused by White Mineral Trioxide Aggregate Angelus. *J. Endod.* **2017**, *43*, 1001–1007. [CrossRef] [PubMed]
43. Meraji, N.; Bolhari, B.; Sefideh, M.; Niavarzi, S. Prevention of Tooth Discoloration Due to Calcium-Silicate Cements: A Review. *Dent. Hypotheses* **2019**, *10*, 4–8. [CrossRef]
44. Choi, Y.L.; Jang, Y.E.; Kim, B.S.; Kim, J.W.; Kim, Y. Pre-Application of Dentin Bonding Agent Prevents Discoloration Caused by Mineral Trioxide Aggregate. *BMC Oral Health* **2020**, *20*, 163. [CrossRef]
45. Kadali, N.; Alla, R.K.; Guduri, V.; AV, R.; MC, S.S.; Raju, R.V. Mineral Trioxide Aggregate: An Overview of Composition, Properties and Clinical Applications. *Int. J. Dent. Mater.* **2020**, *02*, 11–18. [CrossRef]

46. Arruda, R.A.A.; Cunha, R.S.; Miguita, K.B.; Silveira, C.F.M.; De Martin, A.S.; Pinheiro, S.L.; Rocha, D.G.P.; Bueno, C.E.S. Sealing Ability of Mineral Trioxide Aggregate (MTA) Combined with Distilled Water, Chlorhexidine, and Doxycycline. *J. Oral Sci.* **2012**, *54*, 233–239. [CrossRef]
47. Jacinto, R.C.; Linhares-Farina, G.; da Sposito, O.S.; Zanchi, C.H.; Cenci, M.S. Influence of 2% Chlorhexidine on PH, Calcium Release and Setting Time of a Resinous MTA-Based Root-End Filling Material. *Braz. Oral Res.* **2015**, *29*, 1–6. [CrossRef]
48. Nekoofar, M.H.; Adusei, G.; Sheykhrezae, M.S.; Hayes, S.J.; Bryant, S.T.; Dummer, P.M.H. The Effect of Condensation Pressure on Selected Physical Properties of Mineral Trioxide Aggregate. *Int. Endod. J.* **2007**, *40*, 453–461. [CrossRef]
49. Musale, P.K.; Kothare, S.S.; Soni, A.S. Mineral Trioxide Aggregate Pulpotomy: Patient Selection and Perspectives. *Clin. Cosmet. Investig. Dent.* **2018**, *10*, 37–43. [CrossRef]
50. Alqaderi, H.; Lee, C.-T.; Borzangy, S.; Pagonis, T.C. Coronal Pulpotomy for Cariously Exposed Permanent Posterior Teeth with Closed Apices: A Systematic Review and Meta-Analysis. *J. Dent.* **2016**, *44*, 1–7. [CrossRef]
51. El-Meligy, O.A.S.; Avery, D.R. Comparison of Mineral Trioxide Aggregate and Calcium Hydroxide as Pulpotomy Agents in Young Permanent Teeth (Apexogenesis). *Pediatr. Dent.* **2006**, *28*, 399–404. [PubMed]
52. Özgür, B.; Uysal, S.; Güngör, H.C. Partial Pulpotomy in Immature Permanent Molars After Carious Exposures Using Different Hemorrhage Control and Capping Materials. *Pediatr. Dent.* **2017**, *39*, 364–370. [PubMed]
53. Witherspoon, D.E. Vital Pulp Therapy with New Materials: New Directions and Treatment Perspectives—Permanent Teeth. *J. Endod.* **2008**, *34*, S25–S28. [CrossRef] [PubMed]
54. Qudeimat, M.A.; Barrieshi-Nusair, K.M.; Owais, A.I. Calcium Hydroxide vs Mineral Trioxide Aggregates for Partial Pulpotomy of Permanent Molars with Deep Caries. *Eur. Arch. Paediatr. Dent. Off. J. Eur. Acad. Paediatr. Dent.* **2007**, *8*, 99–104. [CrossRef]
55. Siddiqui, S.H.; Mohamed, A.N. Calcific Metamorphosis: A Review. *Int. J. Health Sci.* **2016**, *10*, 437–442. [CrossRef]
56. AlQhtani, F.A. Reattachment of a Dehydrated Tooth Fragment Using Retentive Holes. *Cureus* **2020**, *12*, e6640. [CrossRef] [PubMed]
57. Yilmaz, Y.; Guler, C.; Sahin, H.; Eyuboglu, O. Evaluation of Tooth-Fragment Reattachment: A Clinical and Laboratory Study. *Dent. Traumatol.* **2010**, *26*, 308–314. [CrossRef] [PubMed]
58. Toshihiro, K.; Rintaro, T. Rehydration of Crown Fragment 1 Year after Reattachment: A Case Report. *Dent. Traumatol. Off. Publ. Int. Assoc. Dent. Traumatol.* **2005**, *21*, 297–300. [CrossRef] [PubMed]
59. Bissinger, R.; Müller, D.D.; Hickel, R.; Kühnisch, J. Survival Analysis of Adhesive Reattachments in Permanent Teeth with Crown Fractures after Dental Trauma. *Dent. Traumatol.* **2021**, *37*, 208–214. [CrossRef]
60. Madhubala, A.; Tewari, N.; Mathur, V.P.; Bansal, K. Comparative Evaluation of Fracture Resistance Using Two Rehydration Protocols for Fragment Reattachment in Uncomplicated Crown Fractures. *Dent. Traumatol.* **2019**, *35*, 199–203. [CrossRef]
61. Reis, A.; Kraul, A.; Francci, C.; de Assis, T.G.R.; Crivelli, D.D.; Oda, M.; Loguercio, A.D. Re-Attachment of Anterior Fractured Teeth: Fracture Strength Using Different Materials. *Oper. Dent.* **2002**, *27*, 621–627. [PubMed]
62. Demarco, F.F.; Fay, R.-M.; Pinzon, L.M.; Powers, J.M. Fracture Resistance of Re-Attached Coronal Fragments—Influence of Different Adhesive Materials and Bevel Preparation. *Dent. Traumatol.* **2004**, *20*, 157–163. [CrossRef]
63. Poubel, D.L.N.; Almeida, J.C.F.; Dias Ribeiro, A.P.; Maia, G.B.; Martinez, J.M.G.; Garcia, F.C.P. Effect of Dehydration and Rehydration Intervals on Fracture Resistance of Reattached Tooth Fragments Using a Multimode Adhesive. *Dent. Traumatol.* **2017**, *33*, 451–457. [CrossRef] [PubMed]
64. Garcia, F.C.P.; Poubel, D.L.N.; Almeida, J.C.F.; Toledo, I.P.; Poi, W.R.; Guerra, E.N.S.; Rezende, L.V.M.L. Tooth Fragment Reattachment Techniques—A Systematic Review. *Dent. Traumatol.* **2018**, *34*, 135–143. [CrossRef] [PubMed]
65. Bruschi-Alonso, R.C.; Alonso, R.C.B.; Correr, G.M.; Alves, M.C.; Lewgoy, H.R.; Sinhoreti, M.A.C.; Puppin-Rontani, R.M.; Correr-Sobrinho, L. Reattachment of Anterior Fractured Teeth: Effect of Materials and Techniques on Impact Strength. *Dent. Traumatol.* **2010**, *26*, 315–322. [CrossRef]
66. Chazine, M.; Sedda, M.; Ounsi, H.F.; Paragliola, R.; Ferrari, M.; Grandini, S. Evaluation of the Fracture Resistance of Reattached Incisal Fragments Using Different Materials and Techniques. *Dent. Traumatol.* **2011**, *27*, 15–18. [CrossRef] [PubMed]
67. Reis, A.; Francci, C.; Loguercio, A.D.; Carrilho, M.R.; Rodriques Filho, L.E. Re-Attachment of Anterior Fractured Teeth: Fracture Strength Using Different Techniques. *Oper. Dent.* **2001**, *26*, 287–294.
68. Kang, H.; Chae, Y.; Lee, K.; Lee, H.; Choi, S.; Nam, O. Long-Term Outcome of Reattached Tooth Fragment in Permanent Anterior Teeth of Children and Adolescents. *J. Korean Acad Pediatr. Dent.* **2021**, *48*, 42–49. [CrossRef]
69. Patni, P.; Jain, D.; Goel, G. A Holistic Approach to Management of Fractured Teeth Fragments: A Case Report. *Oral Surg. Oral Med. Oral Pathol. Oral Radiol. Endod.* **2010**, *109*, e70–e74. [CrossRef]
70. Sulwińska, M.; Szczesio, A.; Bołtacz-Rzepkowska, E. Bond Strength of a Resin Composite to MTA at Various Time Intervals and with Different Adhesive Strategies. *Dent. Med. Probl.* **2017**, *54*, 155–160. [CrossRef]
71. Tunç, E.Ş.; Bayrak, Ş.; Eğilmez, T. The Evaluation of Bond Strength of a Composite and a Compomer to White Mineral Trioxide Aggregate with Two Different Bonding Systems. *J. Endod.* **2008**, *34*, 603–605. [CrossRef] [PubMed]
72. Bayrak, S.; Tunç, E.S.; Saroglu, I.; Egilmez, T. Shear Bond Strengths of Different Adhesive Systems to White Mineral Trioxide Aggregate. *Dent. Mater. J.* **2009**, *28*, 62–67. [CrossRef] [PubMed]
73. Krawczyk-Stuss, M.; Nowak, J.; Bołtacz-Rzepkowska, E. Bond Strength of Biodentine to a Resin-Based Composite at Various Acid Etching Times and with Different Adhesive Strategies. *Dent. Med. Probl.* **2019**, *56*, 39–44. [CrossRef] [PubMed]

74. Odabaş, M.E.; Bani, M.; Tirali, R.E. Shear Bond Strengths of Different Adhesive Systems to Biodentine. *Sci. World J.* **2013**, *2013*, 626103. [CrossRef]
75. Hardan, L.; Mancino, D.; Bourgi, R.; Alvarado-Orozco, A.; Rodríguez-Vilchis, L.E.; Flores-Ledesma, A.; Cuevas-Suárez, C.E.; Lukomska-Szymanska, M.; Eid, A.; Danhache, M.-L.; et al. Bond Strength of Adhesive Systems to Calcium Silicate-Based Materials: A Systematic Review and Meta-Analysis of In Vitro Studies. *Gels* **2022**, *8*, 311. [CrossRef]
76. Carretero, V.; Giner-Tarrida, L.; Peñate, L.; Arregui, M. Shear Bond Strength of Nanohybrid Composite to Biodentine with Three Different Adhesives. *Coatings* **2019**, *9*, 783. [CrossRef]
77. Lopes, L.C.P.; Terada, R.S.S.; Tsuzuki, F.M.; Giannini, M.; Hirata, R. Heating and Preheating of Dental Restorative Materials-a Systematic Review. *Clin. Oral Investig.* **2020**, *24*, 4225–4235. [CrossRef]
78. Sawai, M.A.; Bhardwaj, A.; Jafri, Z.; Sultan, N.; Daing, A. Tooth Polishing: The Current Status. *J. Indian Soc. Periodontol.* **2015**, *19*, 375–380. [CrossRef]
79. Hecova, H.; Tzigkounakis, V.; Merglova, V.; Netolicky, J. A Retrospective Study of 889 Injured Permanent Teeth. *Dent. Traumatol. Off. Publ. Int. Assoc. Dent. Traumatol.* **2010**, *26*, 466–475. [CrossRef]
80. Wang, G.; Wang, C.; Qin, M. Pulp Prognosis Following Conservative Pulp Treatment in Teeth with Complicated Crown Fractures-A Retrospective Study. *Dent. Traumatol. Off. Publ. Int. Assoc. Dent. Traumatol.* **2017**, *33*, 255–260. [CrossRef]
81. Krastl, G.; Weiger, R. Vital Pulp Therapy after Trauma. *Endod. Pract. Today* **2014**, *8*, 293–300.
82. Linsuwanont, P.; Wimonsutthikul, K.; Pothimoke, U.; Santiwong, B. Treatment Outcomes of Mineral Trioxide Aggregate Pulpotomy in Vital Permanent Teeth with Carious Pulp Exposure: The Retrospective Study. *J. Endod.* **2017**, *43*, 225–230. [CrossRef] [PubMed]
83. Taha, N.A.; Ahmad, M.B.; Ghanim, A. Assessment of Mineral Trioxide Aggregate Pulpotomy in Mature Permanent Teeth with Carious Exposures. *Int. Endod. J.* **2017**, *50*, 117–125. [CrossRef] [PubMed]
84. Qudeimat, M.A.; Alyahya, A.; Hasan, A.A. Mineral Trioxide Aggregate Pulpotomy for Permanent Molars with Clinical Signs Indicative of Irreversible Pulpitis: A Preliminary Study. *Int. Endod. J.* **2017**, *50*, 126–134. [CrossRef] [PubMed]
85. Taha, N.A.; Khazali, M.A. Partial Pulpotomy in Mature Permanent Teeth with Clinical Signs Indicative of Irreversible Pulpitis: A Randomized Clinical Trial. *J. Endod.* **2017**, *43*, 1417–1421. [CrossRef]
86. Martos, J.; Koller, C.D.; Silveira, L.F.M.; Cesar-Neto, J.B. Crown Fragment Reattachment in Anterior-Fractured Tooth: A Five-Year Follow-Up. *Eur. J. Gen. Dent.* **2012**, *1*, 112–115. [CrossRef]
87. de Lima, M.D.; Martins, J.F.; de Moura, M.S.; de Area Leao, V.L.; de Deus, L.D.F.A.; Moura, D.D.S. Reattachment of Fractured Fragment of an Anterior Tooth: Case Report and Nine-Year Follow-Up. *Gen. Dent.* **2011**, *59*, e192–e195.
88. Scribante, A.; Dermenaki Farahani, M.R.; Marino, G.; Matera, C.; Rodriguez y Baena, R.; Lanteri, V.; Butera, A. Biomimetic Effect of Nano-Hydroxyapatite in Demineralized Enamel before Orthodontic Bonding of Brackets and Attachments: Visual, Adhesion Strength, and Hardness in In Vitro Tests. *Biomed Res. Int.* **2020**, *2020*, 6747498. [CrossRef]
89. Butera, A.; Gallo, S.; Pascadopoli, M.; Montasser, M.A.; Abd El Latief, M.H.; Modica, G.G.; Scribante, A. Home Oral Care with Biomimetic Hydroxyapatite vs. Conventional Fluoridated Toothpaste for the Remineralization and Desensitizing of White Spot Lesions: Randomized Clinical Trial. *Int. J. Environ. Res. Public Health* **2022**, *19*, 8676. [CrossRef]

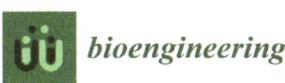 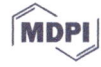

Article

The Assessment of Quality of the Root Canal Filling and the Number of Visits Needed for Completing Primary Root Canal Treatment by Operators with Different Experience

Krystyna Pietrzycka [1], Mateusz Radwanski [1], Louis Hardan [2], Rim Bourgi [2], Davide Mancino [3,4,5], Youssef Haikel [3,4,5] and Monika Lukomska-Szymanska [6,*]

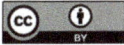

Citation: Pietrzycka, K.; Radwanski, M.; Hardan, L.; Bourgi, R.; Mancino, D.; Haikel, Y.; Lukomska-Szymanska, M. The Assessment of Quality of the Root Canal Filling and the Number of Visits Needed for Completing Primary Root Canal Treatment by Operators with Different Experience. *Bioengineering* 2022, 9, 468. https://doi.org/10.3390/bioengineering9090468

Academic Editors: Chengfei Zhang and Liang Luo

Received: 10 July 2022
Accepted: 10 September 2022
Published: 13 September 2022

Publisher's Note: MDPI stays neutral with regard to jurisdictional claims in published maps and institutional affiliations.

Copyright: © 2022 by the authors. Licensee MDPI, Basel, Switzerland. This article is an open access article distributed under the terms and conditions of the Creative Commons Attribution (CC BY) license (https://creativecommons.org/licenses/by/4.0/).

[1] Department of Endodontics, Medical University of Lodz, 251 Pomorska Str., 92-213 Lodz, Poland
[2] Department of Restorative Dentistry, School of Dentistry, Saint-Joseph University, Beirut 1107 2180, Lebanon
[3] Department of Biomaterials and Bioengineering, INSERM UMR_S 1121, Biomaterials and Bioengineering, 67000 Strasbourg, France
[4] Department of Endodontics, Faculty of Dental Medicine, Strasbourg University, 67000 Strasbourg, France
[5] Pôle de Médecine et Chirurgie Bucco-Dentaire, Hôpital Civil, Hôpitaux Universitaire de Strasbourg, 67000 Strasbourg, France
[6] Department of General Dentistry, Medical University of Lodz, 251 Pomorska Str., 92-213 Lodz, Poland
* Correspondence: monika.lukomska-szymanska@umed.lodz.pl; Tel.: +48-426-757-429

Abstract: The main goal of root canal treatment (RCT) is to eradicate or essentially diminish the microbial population within the root canal system and to prevent reinfection by a proper chemo-mechanical preparation and hermetic final obturation of the root canal space. The aim of this study was to assess the quality of the root canal filling and the number of visits needed for completing RCT by operators with different experience, including dentistry students (4th and 5th year), general dental practitioners (GDPs), and endodontists. Data from medical records of 798 patients were analyzed, obtaining 900 teeth and 1773 obturated canals according to the inclusion and exclusion criteria. A similar number of teeth was assessed in each group in terms of density and length of root canal filling and number of visits. The larger number of visits and the lower quality of treatment was observed for 4th year students than for other groups ($p < 0.05$); in contrast, the endodontists needed the lowest number of visits to complete RCT and more often overfilled teeth than other operator groups ($p < 0.05$). Interestingly, no statistical difference in quality of root canal filling was noted between 5th year students, GPDs and endodontists. The treatment of lower teeth demanded statistically more visits than that of upper teeth ($p < 0.05$). The results of the study emphasize that most of the root canal filling performed by operators was considered adequate, regardless of tooth type, files used and number of visits.

Keywords: endodontists; general practicing dentists; root canal treatment; quality; undergraduate students

1. Introduction

The purpose of root canal treatment (RCT) is to maintain the function of a tooth, cure disorders of the pulp, prevent and treat the diseases of periapical tissue. Apical periodontitis is mainly caused by the colonization of microorganisms due to dental caries, dental trauma, or iatrogenic exposure of the pulp tissue to various oral microbiota [1]. Therefore, the main goal of RCT is to eradicate or essentially diminish the microbial population within the root canal system and to prevent reinfection by a proper chemo-mechanical preparation and hermetic final obturation of the root canal space [2,3].

The results of endodontic treatment are evaluated with the use of clinical and radiological examination [4]. The clinical findings should define whether signs and symptoms of infection are present. The radiological examination allows assessing the quality of filling of the canal system and periapical tissue.

The success of RCT amounts up to 68–95% [5–8]. According to Schilder [2], it depends not only on the cleaning of the canal and its cone-shaped preparation but also on the proper filling of the entire canal system. The standards of RCT were described in the recommendations for endodontic treatment: consensus report of the European Society of Endodontology (ESE) [9]. On the other hand, the scope of knowledge and skills that an European dentist should demonstrate upon graduation was published by De Moor in the Undergraduate Curriculum Guidelines [10]. According to both documents, the correct filling of the canal should be homogeneous, without any voids within the canal filling (internal voids), but also between the filling and the walls of the root canal (external voids). Moreover, the root canal filling should end at the length of 0.5 to 2.0 mm from the apex of the tooth root [9]. On the postoperative radiograph, the light of the root canal between the end of the filling and the radiological apex should not be visible [9].

There are different models of teaching across the globe. Endodontics at the Medical University of Lodz is taught in the third (6th semester—15 h of theory and 30 h of practical training), fourth (7th and 8th semester—34 h of theory and 96h of practical training) and fifth year (9th semester—24 h of theory and 49 h of practical training) of the five-year course of dentistry. In clinical classes (4th and 5th year), the assistant—student ratio amounts up to 1:6. In German-speaking countries, endodontic education at dental schools is differentiated. Theory classes range from 1 to 70 h (15 h mean), and practical classes range from 3 to 78 h (39 h mean) [11]. The staff–student ratio varies between 1:4 and 1:38 (mean—1:15). In the UK and Spain, students spend 20 h on preclinical training and 50 h on clinical training [12,13]. In Spanish dental schools, the staff–student ratio during preclinical endodontic training ranges from 1:6 to 1:20 and from 1:6 to 1:10 during clinical practice [12]. In UK dental schools, the staff–student ratio in preclinical training ranges from 1:5 to 1:20, and supervising staff mainly consists of general dental practitioners (GDPs) with/without a special interest and training in endodontics. During clinical training, the ratio is from 1:4 to 1:6, and students are supervised by GDPs with a special interest and training in endodontics and endodontists [13].

According to the ESE, postgraduate specialty training programs in endodontology within Europe should last 3 years [14]. In Poland, endodontics along with conservative dentistry is recognized as a specialty after 3 years of training. In Spain, endodontics is not recognized as a dental specialty, and the postgraduate program in endodontics lasts 2 or 3 years [12]. The duration of the full-time course in endodontics takes usually 2 (University of Glasgow, University of Birmingham) or 3 years (University of London, University of Plymouth, The University of Manchester, King's College London, Queen Mary University of London) in the UK. The average duration of the Advanced Dental Education Program in Endodontics in USA lasts two (University of Illinois, University of Pennsylvania) or three years (Indiana University School of Dentistry, New York University). The three-year program of endodontics takes place in The University of Hong Kong, British Columbia (Canada), Queensland in Australia and Amrita University Coimbatore in India.

The quality of primary RCT may differ among dentistry students, GDPs, and endodontists. These discrepancies are associated with different levels of knowledge, experiences, and dexterity. To our best knowledge, there is no study comparing the quality of primary RCT performed by operators with differentiated experience in Poland.

The aim of this study was to compare the quality of the final filling and number of visits needed for completing primary root treatment performed by operators with different experience. The null hypothesis is that there are no differences in the quality of the filling and number of visits after treatment in evaluated groups.

2. Materials and Methods

2.1. Study Group

The study was approved by the Bioethics Committee of the Medical University of Lodz (RNN/04/18/KE). All patient's data remain confidential and have been used for research purposes only. Information on the performed treatment was introduced to a clinical patient card entered an electronic database with a restricted access code. Before the analysis, the data were anonymized. Patients were admitted from October 2017 to February 2019. RCT was carried out with the patients' informed consent to participate in the study.

Sample size estimation revealed 377 patients needed for the survey. Calculations were completed with a margin of error of 5% and confidence level of 95%. The inclusion criteria consisted of single- or multi-rooted teeth demanding primary root treatment. Teeth with complex anatomy, roots with severe apical resorption, external or internal resorption, open apex and calcifications were excluded from the study. X-rays of low quality or with additional artifacts were not included in the study. According to inclusion and exclusion criteria, the final sample group included data from medical records of 798 patients, including 900 teeth and 1773 obturated canals.

All treated patients were admitted by dentistry students (Medical University of Lodz), GPDs at the Endodontics Department, and by endodontists at the Endodontics Clinic of Clinical Hospital in Lodz. Both institutions have the same location and equipment in terms of the dental materials used during endodontic treatment.

2.2. Root Canal Treatment Protocol

Only primary RCT was included in the study. All treatment procedures were carried out following the standards of the ESE [9]. After the examination, and preoperative X-ray in two angulations was made to confirm diagnosis. Next, RCT protocol was initiated. All procedures were performed under local anesthesia and isolation with the use of a rubber dam (Rubber-Dam, size medium, Cerkamed, Stalowa Wola, Polska). The choice of anesthetic depended on the patient's health condition; articaine with a vasoconstrictor (Ubistesin 4%, Molteni, 3M, St. Paul, MN, USA) was used for healthy individuals, and when this anesthetic was contraindicated, mepivacaine was applied (Mepivastesin 3% Molteni, 3M, St. Paul, MN, USA). When trepanation of pulp cavity was accomplished, the chamber was prepared, and the canals were found. Loupes ($2.5\times$) and microscope ($8\times$) were applied when orifices could not be localized. The canal orifices were prepared to assure a straight line access to the canals; then, the working length (WL) was determined with sodium hypochlorite (NaOCl) in root canal and a C-PILOT file (VDW, Munich, Germany) using a Raypex 5 apex locator (VDW, Munich, Germany).

All root canals were shaped by the students with the step-back technique using RT files (Mani, Tochigi, Japan), and the Master Apical File (MAF) was #30–35 for all canals (determined after evaluation of the initial size of the physiological foramen). GDPs and endodontists used nickel–titanium (NiTi) rotary files. Depending on the anatomical characteristics of the teeth and clinicians' preferences rotary NiTi files: ProTaper Next (Dentsply Maillefer, Ballaigues, Switzerland), Mtwo (VDW, Munich, Germany), E3 Azure (Poldent, Warszawa, Poland) and DC-taper 2H (SS White, Lakewood, NJ, USA) according to the manufacturer's instructions were used. The canals were shaped with the X-smart Endodontic Motor (Dentsply Sirona Endodontics, Ballaigues, Switzerland) using continuous clockwise rotation at 300 rpm and 2.5 Ncm. In all rotary systems, the final instruments used for canal preparation correspond to a tip size of 30.

All groups followed the same rising protocol using 5 mL disposable plastic syringes with 27-gauge needles that were close-ended and had rounded tips with side holes (Endo—Top, Cerkamed, Stalowa Wola, Poland). For each canal, after each instrument, 1 mL of 5.25% NaOCl (CHLORAXiD 5.25%, NaOCl, Cerkamed, Stalowa Wola, Poland) was applied, and as final irrigation, canals were flushed with 5 mL 17% ethylenediaminetetraacetic acid (EDTA), 2.5 mL physiological saline, 5 mL 5.25% NaOCl followed by a final rinse with 2.5 mL of physiological saline. The solutions were manually activated with the use of a gutta-percha (GP) cone reaching 1 mm shorter than the established WL.

In the case of multi-visit treatment, if necessary, calcium hydroxide (Calcipast, Cerkamed, Stalowa Wola, Poland) was used as an intracanal dressing. In the absence of symptoms of infection and pain, canals were rinsed with protocol described for a single visit appointment.

After drying canals with paper points, the final root canal obturation was performed with GP and AH plus (Dentsply Maillefer, Ballaigues, Switzerland) as a sealant using the cold lateral compaction technique. Next, the GP was cut off with a heated plugger, and the cavity was cleaned with isopropyl alcohol. The cavity was temporarily restored with a Fuji IX glass ionomer (GC, Tokyo, Japan) between the visits.

2.3. Assessment of the Root Canal Filling

A retrospective randomized double-blind comparison study was conducted to assess the quality of the RCT. An X-ray with an X-ray positioning holder was performed before the final restoration of the tooth. X-ray images were taken with GENDEX Expert DC (KaVo, Biberach/Riss, Germany). The images were evaluated using the VixWin Platinum software (KaVo, Biberach/Riss, Germany). The distance between the end of the canal filling and the radiographic apex of the tooth root was measured. All data were coded and blindly assessed by two endodontists (K.P., M.R.). The two examining operators were calibrated before the examination. The calibration was performed on 30 cases. The quality of the filling on the X-ray was assessed according to ESE standards [9]. The assessment method of radiographs was a modified version of the technique introduced by Balto et al. [15]. The quality of root filling was evaluated according to two parameters: length and density (Table 1, Figure 1). A root canal filling was identified as acceptable when both parameters were satisfactory.

Table 1. Evaluation of parameters of root canal filling.

Parameter of Root Canal Filling	Criteria	Definition
Length	Adequate	Root filling ≤2 mm from radiographic apex
	Overfilling	Root filling beyond the radiographic apex (gutta percha cones or/and sealer)
	Short-filling	Root filling >2 mm from radiographic apex
Density	Adequate	Voids absent, homogeneous root filling
	Inadequate	Voids present, heterogeneous root filling

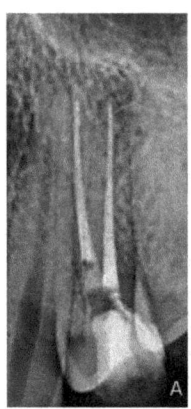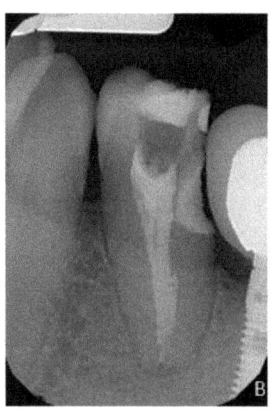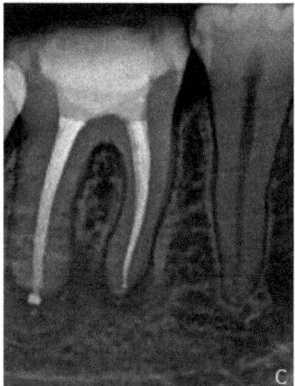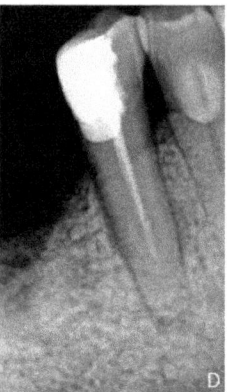

Figure 1. RVG images showing evaluation parameters. (**A**) Adequate length and density, (**B**) Inadequate density, (**C**) Overfilling, (**D**) Short-filling.

2.4. Statistical Analysis

All statistical analyses were performed with the statistical software package Statistica v. 13.1 (StatSoft, Inc., Tulsa, OK, USA). The normality test was performed using a Shapiro–Wilk test. The analysis of distribution of teeth and diagnoses between groups and differences in number of visits were conducted with use of a Kruskal–Wallis test. The statistical analysis of length and homogeneity of root canal filling was performed using the chi-squared test. The comparison between two groups (maxilla/mandible) without normal distribution and the gender and age of patients included in the study was analyzed with the Mann–Whitney U test. In all cases, statistical significance was considered at $p < 0.05$.

3. Results

3.1. Quality of Root Canal Filling

3.1.1. Length

A total of 1733 obturated canals of 900 treated teeth were evaluated. The overfilling was observed most frequently in the palatal canal of first maxillary molars, while short-filling was observed in the mesio-buccal canal of first mandibular molars. Moreover, the material was extended beyond the apex more often in the case of diagnosis of periapical tissue inflammation. The number of adequate obturated canals was statistically significantly higher than the short- and overfilled ($p < 0.05$) (Table 2). The analysis of the discrepancy between the observed and expected numbers showed that in the case of endodontists, the material was overfilled more often than in the case of other groups. In the group of 4th year students, short-filling of the canals was observed significantly more often than in other groups ($p < 0.05$).

Table 2. The distribution of root canal filling length in each group.

Group/Diagnoses	Number of Root Canals			
	Adequate	Overfilling	Short-Filling	Total
4th year students	286 (81.71%)	40 (11.4%)	24 (6.86%)	350
5th year students	325 (86.67%)	41 (10.9%)	9 (2.40%)	375
GPDs	367 (85.75%)	43 (10.0%)	18 (4.21%)	428
Endodontists	432 (74.48%)	129 (22.2%)	19 (3.28%)	580
Total	1410 (81.36%)	253 (14.60%)	70 (4.04%)	1733

3.1.2. Homogeneity

The analysis showed a statistically significant relationship between the inadequate filling of the canal in the studied groups ($p < 0.0001$). In the group of 4th year students, non-homogeneous filling of the treated canals was observed significantly more often than in other groups. The distribution of density in individual groups is shown in Figure 2.

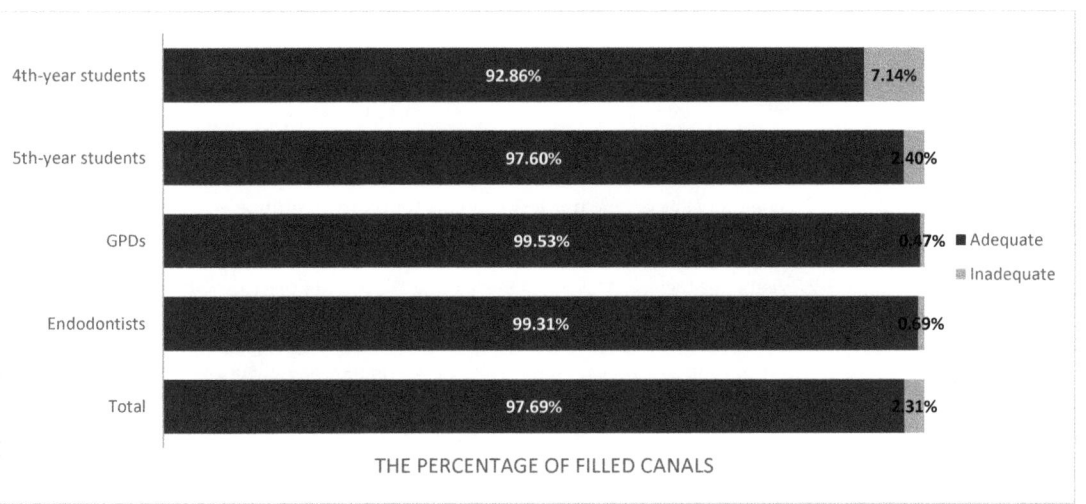

Figure 2. The distribution of density of canal filling in evaluated groups.

Moreover, no statistical relationship was determined between the homogeneity and the length of the root canal filling in all evaluated groups.

3.2. Number of Visits

The mean value of visit is presented in Figure 3. The Mann–Whitney U test revealed that endodontists needed statistically significant fewer visits than other groups ($p < 0.001$). Moreover, GPDs needed statistically significant fewer visits than 4th year students ($p < 0.001$). The mean number of visits was significantly higher in the mandible (2.12 visits per tooth) than in the maxilla (2.01 visits per tooth) ($p < 0.05$). One-visit treatment was carried out in 12.04% of cases treated by 4th year students, in 26.15%—by 5th year students, in 32.06%—by GPDs, and in 51.36%—by endodontists.

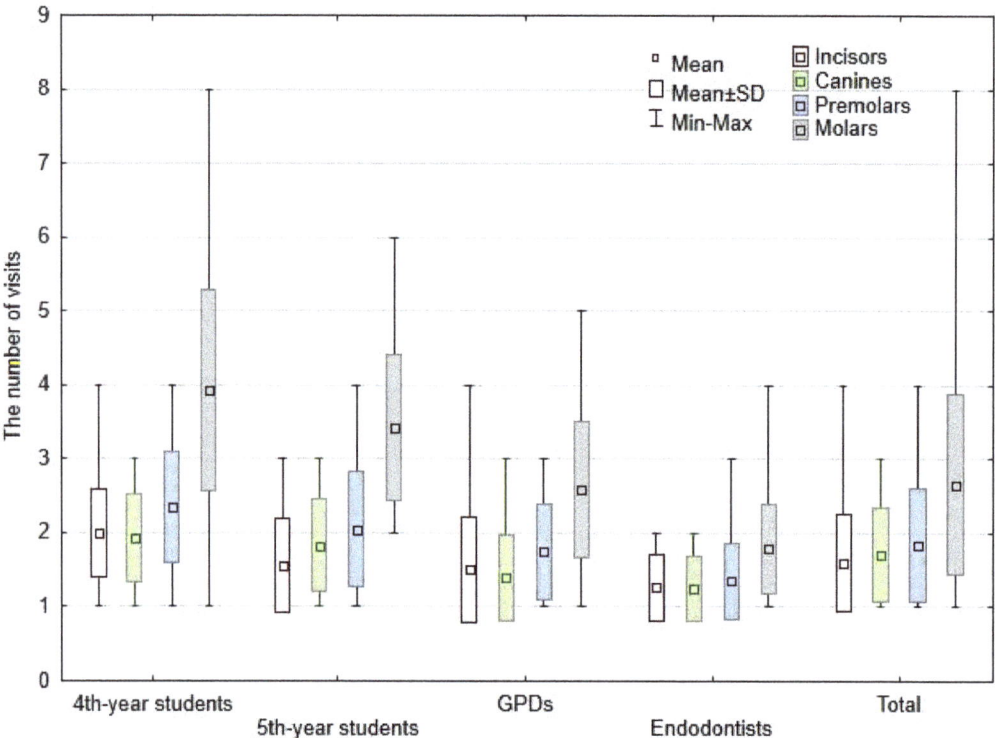

Figure 3. The mean value of number of visits in evaluated groups.

The highest average number of visits for all teeth groups was recorded for 4th year students: 2.00 visits per incisor, 1.93 visits per canine, 2.34 visits per premolar, and 3.93 visits per molar. On the other hand, the lowest number of visits was noted for endodontists: 1.27 visits per incisor, 1.25 visits per canine, 1.35 visits per premolar, and 1.79 visits per molar. The treatment of incisors performed by 4th year students demanded statistically significantly the most visits when compared with other groups ($p < 0.001$). Next, the mean number of visits to treat canines by 4th year students was statistically greater in comparison to GPDs and endodontists ($p < 0.05$). In addition, the number of visits to treat canines was statistically larger for 5th year students when compared to endodontists ($p < 0.05$). However, the number of visits to treat premolars was significantly lower for endodontists than for the other study groups ($p < 0.001$). Moreover, the treatment of premolars by 4th year students demanded statistically larger numbers of visits than by GPDs ($p < 0.01$). Next, the mean number of visits to treat molars by students (4th and 5th year) was statistically greater in comparison to GPDs and endodontists ($p < 0.001$). The treatment of molars by GPDs demanded a statistically larger number of visits than by endodontists ($p < 0.001$). Moreover, no statistical relationship was determined between the number of visits and the homogeneity/the length of the root canal filling in all evaluated groups.

3.3. Type of Instruments

In total, 434 of the 900 teeth were prepared with hand files, and 466 were prepared using rotary instruments. The rotary systems were used only in the group of GPDs and endodontists. The distribution of rotary systems used is presented in Table 3. The ProTaper Next files were statistically more often used than other rotary instruments ($p < 0.05$).

Table 3. The rotary systems used during RCT.

Group/Rotary System	ProTaper Next (Dentsply Maillefer)	Mtwo (VDW)	E3 Azure (Poldent)	DC-Taper 2H (SS White)
		Number of Teeth		
GPDs	184	6	1	18
Endodontists	208	48	1	0

3.4. Distribution of Teeth and Diagnoses

The age of the patients ranged from 6 to 86 years (mean amounted up to 47.61), with a gender distribution of 42.36% male and 57.64% female. Gender and age were not statistically significant ($p > 0.05$).

During the assessed period (2017–2019), a total of 900 primary RCTs were performed. The distribution of tooth groups and diagnoses in each group are presented in Tables 4 and 5, respectively. No significant statistical differences were found between study groups regarding the distribution of teeth and diagnoses ($p > 0.05$).

Table 4. The distribution of teeth in each group.

Group/Teeth	Incisors	Canines	Premolars	Molars	Total
4th year students	64 (29.63%)	43 (19.91%)	63 (29.17%)	46 (21.30%)	216
5th year students	67 (30.73%)	41 (18.81%)	44 (20.18%)	66 (30.28%)	218
GPDs	41 (19.62%)	25 (11.96%)	53 (25.36%)	90 (43.06%)	209
Endodontists	52 (20.23%)	16 (6.23%)	73 (28.40%)	116 (45.14%)	257
Total	224 (24.89%)	125 (13.89%)	233 (25.89%)	318 (35.33%)	900

Table 5. The distribution of diagnoses in each group.

Group/Diagnoses	Pulp	Periapical	Endo-Perio	Total
		Number of teeth		
4th year students	133 (61.57%)	83 (38.43%)	0	216
5th year students	113 (51.83%)	105 (48.17%)	0	218
GPDs	107 (51.20%)	97 (46.41%)	5 (2.39%)	209
Endodontists	149 (57.98%)	108 (42.02%)	0	257
Total	502 (55.78%)	393 (43.67%)	5 (0.56%)	900

4. Discussion

The present study compared the quality of the final root canal filling after primary root treatment performed by 4th and 5th year dentistry students, GPDs and endodontists. The quality of the final obturation on the X-ray was estimated according to the guidelines of the ESE [12]. The study evaluated length and density. Additionally, the number of visits, type of instruments used, and demographic data (distribution of teeth and diagnoses) were assessed.

4.1. Quality of Root Canal Filling

The quality assessment of the endodontic treatment carried out by dentistry students as well as GPDs and endodontists was evaluated in the literature [12,16–41].

Electronic and radiographic methods are recommended to determine the WL. According to the ESE, the WL should normally be confirmed with radiographs [9]. In the present study, the WL was confirmed both radiographically and with apex locators. The accuracy of modern apex locators measurement is undisputable [42,43]. Additionally, WL measurements with an apex locator showed higher accuracy than conventional periapical radiographs [43,44]. However, periapical lesions seemed to influence the measurements with apex locators [45]. According to another study, the precision of electronic measurement depends on the generation of apex locator and the type of irrigation used during RCT and is not affected by the status of the pulp tissue [46]. In the present study, the working length was confirmed using an apex locator with 5.25% NaOCl in root canal, similarly as in other studies [13,16].

The main criteria used in assessing the quality of RCT are the length and density of final obturation [9,10]. In the current study, the overall quality of RCT amounted up to 81.36%—for length and 97.69%—for density. In total, 14.60% and 4.04% of cases were overfilled and short-filled, respectively. In this investigation, not only the extrusion of gutta-percha cones but also any amount of sealer beyond apex was considered as overfilling. Various studies have investigated the radiographic quality of root canal fillings performed by clinical dental students [17,37–41]. In this research, the adequate length and density of RCT performed by 4th-year students were found in 81.71% and 92.86%, respectively. These results are in contrast with others showing higher [18,19] or lower percentages [20,39]. In the mentioned studies, the RCT of maxillary and mandibular teeth was performed [18–20,39], root canal shaping was carried out with the step-back technique [19,20] and root canal obturation was accomplished with the lateral condensation technique of gutta-percha [18–20,39] or with a single-cone technique [18]. In the current study, for 5th year students, the adequate dentistry and homogeneity were observed in 86.67% and 97.60%, respectively. Unlike in other research, the percentage of acceptable length and density performed by senior dental students was lower (59.48% vs. 50.76%) [21]. However, for incisors and molars, the proper length (81.71–86.67%) and density (92.86–97.60%) in the present and other studies were similar [22–24]. The observed discrepancies in outcomes may be only explained by the different types of endodontically treated teeth and the assistant–student ratio because endodontic procedures (canal preparation, MAF, WL measurement, rinsing solutions) were the same as in the present survey. Another study contradicts these results, where the lower percentage of adequate length (69%) and homogeneity (42.7%) was reported [34]. The lower results of that study [34] could be influenced by the type of treated teeth (mainly premolars and molars) and the combination of endodontic procedures with restorative treatment carried out in a multidisciplinary clinic (including prosthodontics). Therefore, all procedures performed during RCTs might not have been directly supervised by trained endodontists.

In the current study, the adequate length and density were noted in 85.75% and 99.53% for GPDs, respectively. The lower percentage (70.1%) of the adequate length of root canal filling was found for students of the postgraduate program in endodontics [16]. This difference could be associated with the different instrumentation and obturation techniques used in RCT in both studies. The inferior results of the mentioned survey could result from the lower number of treated molars in the present study (43.06% vs. 56.2%). In another research study where molars were treated in a group of GPDs, the adequate length and density were noted in 31.3% and 62.7%, respectively [27]. Interestingly, another study reported 90.3% cases with adequate obturation in the GDPs group [25]. However, in the present study, the results were similar to those reported by others (length—84.3% and dentistry—98%), where RCT was performed by postgraduate students [23,39]. These data are in contrast with the results reported in a retrospective study assessing the obturation quality of primary RCTs of molar teeth performed by GPD, where an acceptable quality of root filling was only found in 31.3% [27]. In contrast, in Saudi Arabia, GPDs performed RCT with adequate length and density in 46.4% and 75.8%, respectively.

In this investigation, the adequate length for endodontists was noted in 74.48%, which is in agreement with other research [26], but it is in contrast with others showing higher (86–93.55%) [28,29] or lower percentages (41.2–62.5%) [27,47]. Similarly to these results, the adequate quality of root fillings (length and density) performed by Australian endodontists was found in 77.4–91.0% [30]. These discrepancies can be related to different NiTi rotary systems, obturation methods (lateral condensation of cold gutta-percha vs. single cone technique) and number of operators who performed RCT (one vs. more). In the present study, the short-filling of root canals among endodontists was reported in 3.28% of cases, similarly to others [26,28]. However, it is in contrast with the studies where mainly posterior teeth were treated (short-filling in 17.7–18.8%) [27,47]. The short-filling may occur due to the anatomical complexity of mandibular molars, underestimation of working length, inconsistent reading of the apex locator in a canal with lateral canals and deltas, instrumentation mishaps (ledges, blocking, failure to maintain apical patency), inadequate chemo-mechanical preparation and an incorrectly matched master apical cone [27]. In this study, overfilled canals were found in 22.2%, similarly to other research [26,47]. More favorable results (overfilled canals in 6.45%) were found in the study where only one specialist performed the RCT (2000 RCTs) [29]. However, the lower percentage of overfilled canals was reported by others (4.4%) [27]. Further analysis of teeth groups in the above-mentioned study [27] indicated that overfilling was observed more often in maxillary molar teeth, whereas short-filling was observed in mandibular molar teeth, which is supported by the current study. The overfilling can be observed due to the overestimation of working length, the apex locator may give false results in roots with apical resorption, overpreparing of the canal, incorrectly matched master apical cones, and excessive pressure on the spreader during the lateral condensation technique, especially after rotary instrumentation [27]. Additionally, the final obturation of the root canals beyond the apex may occur more often in the case of periapical tissue inflammation [48]. It should be emphasized that the small extrusion of a sealer is generally well-tolerated by the periapical tissues [49–51]. However, some authors found a higher risk of non-healing lesions in cases with sealer extrusion [52,53].

According to the literature, inadequate root canal filling with voids was the most affected by bacterial leakage [1]. Residual microorganisms inducing the root canal infection were associated with apical periodontitis [54]. In the present study, the adequate density for endodontists was found in 99.31%. However, poorer results were reported in previous studies (49.6–81.3%) [27,28,47]. Interestingly, 97% of cases with adequate obturation (no voids and proper length) were treated by endodontists [25], while in this study, a lower percentage was (76.26%) observed. This might be related to the different generation of NiTi rotary systems used, where all operators (six endodontists) used rotary NiTi instruments [30] and had different experience (4–26 years). However, the retrospective study assessing the obturation quality of primary RCTs of molar teeth performed by endodontists reported an acceptable quality of root filling in 50.4% [27]. These unfavorable results might be attributed to the filling method (single cone technique) and subsequent misfit between cone and master file size and taper causing voids [27].

4.2. Number of Visits

In the current study, the 4th and 5th year students conducted multi-visit treatments in 87.96% and 73.85%, respectively. Comparable results of multi-visit treatments (86.3%) carried out by the undergraduate students were reported [55]. However, another study noted a 1:1 ratio between single-visit and multi-visit treatment performed by undergraduate students [20]. In the present study, the treatment of lower teeth demanded more visits than that of upper teeth. This might be attributable to the anatomical difficulties and difficulties related with an ineffective inferior alveolar nerve block of mandibular molars with pulpitis.

The multi-visit treatment was also mainly performed by GDPs (67.94%), which was in contrast with other studies (92.2–96.2%) [32,56]. In the present study, the one-visit treatment was carried out by endodontists in 51.36%. However, a significantly lower percentage was reported in the literature (4.7–37.15%) [29,30,32,56]. In the present study, most of the one-visit treatment was performed by endodontists, while other operators preferred the multi-visit treatment. The rotary systems used in the group of GDPs and endodontists might have shortened the number of visits in this study.

The issue of one- and multi-visit endodontic treatment has been under dispute for a long time. There is still no consensus regarding this matter [57–59]. However, with the introduction of new heat-treated files and techniques, it seemed that the single-visit procedure has become a good treatment option [58,60,61]. According to the literature, both procedures had similar success rates of RCT regardless of the diagnosis (pulp vs. periapical tissue) [61–63]. During multiple-visit RCT, usually, an antiseptic medication (calcium hydroxide) is placed in the root canal system for further disinfection of the canals between treatment appointments [64,65]. In contrast, in single-visit RCT, the root canal system is obturated directly after shaping and cleaning without any antibacterial medication. The higher concentration (5.25%) of NaOCl presents faster and greater capacity in dissolving the organic matter, lubrication, and bactericidal effect. In addition, the number of visits might also depend on the dexterity and skills of the operator [32,66]. It is a well-known the fact that experience and specialty training strongly influenced the decision making during RCT provided by GDPs and endodontists [67,68]; the data also showed that root morphology was significant [69]. Other common reasons why GDPs and endodontists choose multiple-visit treatment were the healing effect of inter-appointment medications, lessening the symptoms of apical periodontitis and the shorter duration of the appointment [32].

4.3. Type of Instruments

According to ESE general guidelines [9], the root canal after preparation should be tapered, microorganisms should be eliminated, and debris should be removed [2]. The crucial goal of RCT is the reduction in intracanal infection. It could be accomplished by means of a proper chemo-mechanical preparation with irrigation, hand files or rotary systems [2,70]. The rotary canal instrumentation exhibited a similar clinical and radiographic success rate, diminished procedural errors, more predictable canal shape and an increased pace of work when compared to the manual instrumentation technique [71–73].

It was suggested that the RCT performed by undergraduate students as unexperienced operators should be performed only in cases with minimal complexity at the beginning of clinical practice [13,27,74–76]. Similarly, in the present study, students performed manual instrumentation with the step back technique [40,74,77,78]. In contrast, according to other studies, undergraduate students utilized NiTi rotary instruments and the crown-down technique [12,13,33,35].

In the present study, 48.22% of endodontically treated teeth were prepared with hand files, while 51.78% were prepared with rotary instruments. The rotary systems were used only by GDPs and endodontists. However, in a previous study [16], postgraduate students of program in endodontics performed RCT with manual and rotary instrumentation in 20.2% and 79.8%, respectively. The technique used by the endodontists and the GDPs for chemo-mechanical preparation in the current study was the crown-down or single length technique, which is in accordance with other research [27,28,79]. However, another study reported that all canals were prepared with stainless steel files and the step-back technique [29]. However, the current literature indicates that endodontists conducted only difficult cases of RCT using rotary instruments [28,30,80].

4.4. Distribution of Teeth

In the present study, the 4th year students treated more often incisors (29.63%) and premolars (29.17%), while the 5th year students treated more often incisors (30.73%) and molars (30.28%). A very similar distribution was presented by other scientists [24,36,81]. According to other studies, two-thirds of treated teeth by 4th and 5th year students were premolars and molars [23,37], while one study presented a uniform distribution of teeth treated by students [38]. According to the ESE undergraduate curriculum guidelines for endodontology [10], students should gain adequate experience in the treatment of anterior, premolar, and uncomplicated molar teeth. The quality of RCT performed by students depended on the number of endodontic procedures performed during pre- and clinical training, the treatment protocol used, and the assistant–student ratio [10,12,13]. Moreover, the teaching staff should be specialists or have a special interest in endodontology [10]. It was claimed that dentistry students should perform only RCT with minimal complexity [13,27,74–76]. However, upon graduation, dentists should demonstrate both in-depth theoretical knowledge and appropriate clinical skills acquired during preclinical and clinical classes in the field of endodontics.

In this study, premolars and molars were the most frequently treated teeth by GDPs and endodontists; similar data were presented by previous authors [30,36,47,80,82]. However, other researchers indicated that GDP more often conducted RCT of anterior teeth [77], and endodontists treated only posterior teeth [25]. Moreover, simple cases of RCT were more often performed by GDP than by endodontists [31,82–84]. Interestingly, another study claimed that anterior teeth were treated endodontically by a specialist in 52.1% [30]. According the ESE report, a dental practitioner is expected to treat effectively pulpal and periapical diseases and have a basic knowledge of endodontology [10]. In contrast, a specialist should possess highly developed technical and clinical skills to perform complex primary root canal treatment, re-treatment or endodontic surgery [14].

4.5. Distribution of Diagnoses

The most common diagnosis prior to primary RCT in the current study was pulpitis (55.78%), less often was periapical tissue disease (43.67%) and the least frequent was endo-perio lesion (0.56%). These data coincided with the available literature [29,38,39]. Various studies reported that primary RCT was performed by postgraduate students of the program in endodontics, and additionally, pulpitis was diagnosed more often than non-vital pulp [16,80]. However, other studies did not support these findings [38,78]. Interestingly, it was claimed that one-third of endodontically treated teeth were diagnosed as irreversible pulpitis, while half were diagnosed as pulp necrosis associated with periapical radiolucency [38,40], and endodontic–periodontic lesions were diagnosed rarely (2%) [38]. According to the undergraduate curriculum guidelines for endodontology [10], GDPs should be familiar with the management of pulp and periradicular disease and be able to perform RCT of uncomplicated anterior and posterior teeth. An endodontist is a clinically competent practitioner who performs primary and secondary RCT of teeth with complicated anatomy, infected root canal systems, and periapical infection, with the use of magnification (dental operating microscope) [35] and modern endodontic tools and devices.

Moreover, the limitations of the present study should be acknowledged. The distribution of teeth in the study groups should be more consistent. Premolars and molars were the most frequently treated teeth by GDP and endodontists; meanwhile, anterior teeth were the most frequently treated teeth by the undergraduate students. Another limitation is the skill of the operator and the analysis of the RCT quality in two-dimensional images. Conventional radiographs compress three-dimensional anatomical structures into a two-dimensional image, greatly limiting diagnostic performance. Additionally, root canals are visualized in the mesio-distal plane only, and the bucco-lingual plane may not be completely appreciated [85]. Furthermore, anatomical noise, geometrical malformation, and two-dimensional imaging may cause impaired diagnosis [86]. Another limitation of the present study is the differentiated instrumentation technique. RCT performed by undergraduate students was conducted with manual instrumentation, while by GPDs and endodontists, it was conducted with rotary instrumentation techniques. Moreover, further studies comparing other evaluation methods, instruments, canal shaping and obturation techniques should be carried out. Next, corresponding research, investigating the quality of endodontic retreatment, and respective comparisons should be performed.

5. Conclusions

Within limitations of the study, the following can be stated:

1. The larger number of visits and the lower quality of treatment was observed for 4th-year students than for other groups; in contrast, endodontists needed the lowest number of visits to complete RCT and more often overfilled teeth than the other operator groups.
2. Interestingly, no difference in quality (homogeneity and length) of root canal filling between 5th-year students, GPDs, and endodontics was noted.
3. Endodontists and GDPs more often performed RCT of teeth with more complicated anatomy (premolars and molars).
4. The overfilling was observed most frequently in the palatal canal of first maxillary molars and in the case of periapical tissue inflammation, while short-filling was observed most frequently in the mesio-buccal canal of first mandibular molars.
5. The treatment of lower teeth demanded more visits than that of upper teeth.

Author Contributions: Conceptualization, K.P.; methodology, K.P. and M.L.-S.; investigation, K.P. and M.L.-S.; resources, K.P.; data curation, K.P. and M.R.; writing—original draft preparation, K.P. and M.R.; writing—review and editing, K.P., M.R., L.H., R.B., Y.H., D.M. and M.L.-S.; visualization, M.R., L.H., Y.H., R.B. and D.M.; supervision, M.L.-S.; funding acquisition, K.P. All authors have read and agreed to the published version of the manuscript.

Funding: This work was funded by grant No. 503/2-044-02/503-21-001-19-00 from the Medical University of Lodz.

Institutional Review Board Statement: The study was conducted according to the guidelines of the Declaration of Helsinki and approved by the Bioethics Committee of the Medical University of Lodz (RNN/04/18/KE).

Informed Consent Statement: Informed consent was obtained from all subjects involved in the study.

Data Availability Statement: Not applicable.

Conflicts of Interest: The authors declare no conflict of interest.

References

1. Siqueira, J.F., Jr.; Rôças, I.N. Clinical Implications and Microbiology of Bacterial Persistence after Treatment Procedures. *J. Endod.* **2008**, *34*, 1291–1301.e3. [CrossRef]
2. Schilder, H. Cleaning and Shaping the Root Canal. *Dent. Clin. N. Am.* **1974**, *18*, 269–296. [CrossRef]
3. Kharouf, N.; Arntz, Y.; Eid, A.; Zghal, J.; Sauro, S.; Haikel, Y.; Mancino, D. Physicochemical and Antibacterial Properties of Novel, Premixed Calcium Silicate-Based Sealer Compared to Powder–Liquid Bioceramic Sealer. *J. Clin. Med.* **2020**, *9*, 3096. [CrossRef] [PubMed]
4. Fernández, R.; Cadavid, D.; Zapata, S.M.; Alvarez, L.G.; Restrepo, F.A. Impact of Three Radiographic Methods in the Outcome of Nonsurgical Endodontic Treatment: A Five-Year Follow-Up. *J. Endod.* **2013**, *39*, 1097–1103. [CrossRef] [PubMed]
5. Ng, Y.-L.; Mann, V.; Rahbaran, S.; Lewsey, J.; Gulabivala, K. Outcome of Primary Root Canal Treatment: Systematic Review of the Literature—Part 1. Effects of Study Characteristics on Probability of Success. *Int. Endod. J.* **2007**, *40*, 921–939. [CrossRef] [PubMed]
6. Ng, Y.-L.; Mann, V.; Gulabivala, K. Outcome of Secondary Root Canal Treatment: A Systematic Review of the Literature. *Int. Endod. J.* **2008**, *41*, 1026–1046. [CrossRef]
7. Ng, Y.-L.; Mann, V.; Gulabivala, K. A Prospective Study of the Factors Affecting Outcomes of Nonsurgical Root Canal Treatment: Part 1: Periapical Health. *Int. Endod. J.* **2011**, *44*, 583–609. [CrossRef]
8. Olcay, K.; Eyüboglu, T.F.; Özcan, M. Clinical Outcomes of Non-Surgical Multiple-Visit Root Canal Retreatment: A Retrospective Cohort Study. *Odontology* **2019**, *107*, 536–545. [CrossRef]

9. European Society of Endodontology. Quality Guidelines for Endodontic Treatment: Consensus Report of the European Society of Endodontology. *Int. Endod. J.* **2006**, *39*, 921–930. [CrossRef]
10. De Moor, R.; Hülsmann, M.; Kirkevang, L.L.; Tanalp, J.; Whitworth, J. Undergraduate Curriculum Guidelines for Endodontology. *Int. Endod. J.* **2013**, *46*, 1105–1114. [CrossRef]
11. Sacha, S.R.; Sonntag, D.; Burmeister, U.; Rüttermann, S.; Gerhardt-Szép, S. A Multicentric Survey to Evaluate Preclinical Education in Endodontology in German-speaking Countries. *Int. Endod. J.* **2021**, *54*, 1957–1964. [CrossRef] [PubMed]
12. Segura-Egea, J.J.; Zarza-Rebollo, A.; Jiménez-Sánchez, M.C.; Cabanillas-Balsera, D.; Areal-Quecuty, V.; Martín-González, J. Evaluation of Undergraduate Endodontic Teaching in Dental Schools within Spain. *Int. Endod. J.* **2021**, *54*, 454–463. [CrossRef] [PubMed]
13. Al Raisi, H.; Dummer, P.M.H.; Vianna, M.E. How Is Endodontics Taught? A Survey to Evaluate Undergraduate Endodontic Teaching in Dental Schools within the United Kingdom. *Int. Endod. J.* **2019**, *52*, 1077–1085. [CrossRef] [PubMed]
14. European Society of Endodontology. Accreditation of Postgraduate Speciality Training Programmes in Endodontology. Minimum Criteria for Training Specialists in Endodontology within Europe. *Int. Endod. J.* **2010**, *43*, 725–737. [CrossRef] [PubMed]
15. Balto, H.; Al Khalifah, S.; Al Mugairin, S.; Al Deeb, M.; Al-Madi, E. Technical Quality of Root Fillings Performed by Undergraduate Students in Saudi Arabia. *Int. Endod. J.* **2010**, *43*, 292–300. [CrossRef] [PubMed]
16. Llena, C.; Nicolescu, T.; Perez, S.; de Pereda, S.; Gonzalez, A.; Alarcon, I.; Monzo, A.; Sanz, J.L.; Melo, M.; Forner, L. Outcome of Root Canal Treatments Provided by Endodontic Postgraduate Students. A Retrospective Study. *J. Clin. Med.* **2020**, *9*, 1994. [CrossRef]
17. Awooda, E.M.; Siddig, R.I.; Alturki, R.S.; Sanhouri, N.M. Radiographic Technical Quality of Root Canal Treatment Performed by Undergraduate. *J. Int. Soc. Prev. Community Dent.* **2016**, *6*, 554–558. [CrossRef]
18. Hayes, S.J.; Gibson, M.; Hammond, M.; Bryant, S.T.; Dummer, P.M. An Audit of Root Canal Treatment Performed by Undergraduate Students. *Int. Endod. J.* **2001**, *34*, 501–505. [CrossRef]
19. AlRahabi, M.K. Evaluation of Complications of Root Canal Treatment Performed by Undergraduate Dental Students. *Libyan J. Med.* **2017**, *12*, 1345582. [CrossRef]
20. Al-Manei, K.K. Radiographic Quality of Single vs. Multiple-Visit Root Canal Treatment Performed by Dental Students: A Case Control Study. *Iran. Endod. J.* **2018**, *13*, 149–154. [CrossRef]
21. Habib, A.A.; Doumani, M.D.; Nassani, M.Z.; Shamsy, E.; Jto, B.S.; Arwadİ, H.A.; Mohamed, S.A. Radiographic Assessment of the Quality of Root Canal Fillings Performed by Senior Dental Students. *Eur. Endod. J.* **2018**, *3*, 101–106. [CrossRef] [PubMed]
22. Donnelly, A.; Coffey, D.; Duncan, H.F. A Re-Audit of the Technical Quality of Undergraduate Root Canal Treatment after the Introduction of New Technology and Teaching Practices. *Int. Endod. J.* **2017**, *50*, 941–950. [CrossRef] [PubMed]
23. Unal, G.C.; Kececi, A.D.; Kaya, B.U.; Tac, A.G. Quality of Root Canal Fillings Performed by Undergraduate Dental Students. *Eur. J. Dent.* **2011**, *5*, 324–330. [CrossRef] [PubMed]
24. Vukadinov, T.; Blažić, L.; Kantardžić, I.; Lainović, T. Technical Quality of Root Fillings Performed by Undergraduate Students: A Radiographic Study. *Sci. World J.* **2014**, *2014*, 751274. [CrossRef]
25. Ramey, K.; Yaccino, J.; Wealleans, J. A Retrospective, Radiographic Outcomes Assessment of 1960 Initial Posterior Root Canal Treatments Performed by Endodontists and Dentists. *J. Endod.* **2017**, *43*, 1250–1254. [CrossRef]
26. Ricucci, D.; Russo, J.; Rutberg, M.; Burleson, J.A.; Spångberg, L.S. A Prospective Cohort Study of Endodontic Treatments of 1369 Root Canals: Results after 5 Years. *Oral Surg. Oral Med. Oral Pathol. Oral Radiol. Endod.* **2011**, *112*, 825–842. [CrossRef]
27. Yusufoglu, S.İ.; Sarıçam, E. Comparison of Endodontic Treatment Qualities of Molar Teeth Performed by Endodontists and Practitioners: A Radiographic Analysis. *Selcuk Dent. J.* **2021**, *8*, 127–132. [CrossRef]
28. Berrezouga, L.; Bouguezzi, A.; Belkhir, M.S. Outcome of Initial Endodontic Treatment Performed, by One Specialist, in 122 Tunisian Patients: A Retrospective Study. *Int. J. Dent.* **2018**, *2018*, 3504245. [CrossRef]
29. Imura, N.; Pinheiro, E.T.; Gomes, B.P.; Zaia, A.A.; Ferraz, C.C.; Souza-Filho, F.J. The Outcome of Endodontic Treatment: A Retrospective Study of 2000 Cases Performed by a Specialist. *J. Endod.* **2007**, *33*, 1278–1282. [CrossRef]
30. Bierenkrant, D.E.; Parashos, P.; Messer, H.H. The Technical Quality of Nonsurgical Root Canal Treatment Performed by a Selected Cohort of Australian Endodontists. *Int. Endod. J.* **2008**, *41*, 561–570. [CrossRef]
31. Burry, J.C.; Stover, S.; Eichmiller, F.; Bhagavatula, P. Outcomes of Primary Endodontic Therapy Provided by Endodontic Specialists Compared with Other Providers. *J. Endod.* **2016**, *42*, 702–705. [CrossRef] [PubMed]
32. Wong, A.W.-Y.; Zhang, S.; Zhang, C.-F.; Chu, C.-H. Perceptions of Single-Visit and Multiple-Visit Endodontic Treatment: A Survey of Endodontic Specialists and General Dentists in Hong Kong. *J. Investig. Clin. Dent.* **2016**, *7*, 263–271. [CrossRef] [PubMed]
33. Baharin, S.A.; Omar, S.H. Undergraduate Endodontic Clinical Training in Malaysia: A National Survey. *Eur. J. Dent. Educ.* **2021**, *25*, 168–174. [CrossRef] [PubMed]
34. Moussa-Badran, S.; Roy, B.; du Parc, A.S.; Bruyant, M.; Lefevre, B.; Maurin, J.C. Technical Quality of Root Fillings Performed by Dental Students at the Dental Teaching Centre in Reims, France. *Int. Endod. J.* **2008**, *41*, 679–684. [CrossRef]
35. Kharouf, N.; Hemmerlé, J.; Haikel, Y.; Mancino, D. Technical Quality of Root Canal Filling in Preclinical Training at Strasbourg University Using Two Teaching Protocols. *Eur. J. Dent.* **2019**, *13*, 521–526. [CrossRef]
36. Ertas, E.T.; Ertas, H.; Sisman, Y.; Sagsen, B.; Er, O. Radiographic Assessment of the Technical Quality and Periapical Health of Root-Filled Teeth Performed by General Practitioners in a Turkish Subpopulation. *Sci. World J.* **2013**, *2013*, 514841. [CrossRef]

37. İlgüy, D.; İlgüy, M.; Fişekçioğlu, E.; Ersan, N.; Tanalp, J.; Dölekoğlu, S. Assessment of Root Canal Treatment Outcomes Performed by Turkish Dental Students: Results After Two Years. *J. Dent. Educ.* **2013**, *77*, 502–509. [CrossRef]
38. Fong, W.; Heidarifar, O.; Killough, S.; Lappin, M.J.; El Karim, I.A. An Audit on Technical Quality of Root Fillings Performed by Undergraduate Students. *Int. Endod. J.* **2018**, *51* (Suppl. S3), e197–e203. [CrossRef]
39. Ribeiro, D.M.; Henckel, M.D.; Mello, F.W.; Felippe, M.C.S.; Felippe, W.T. Radiographic Analysis the Obturation's Quality in Root Canal Treatment Performed by a South Brazilian Sample of Undergraduate Students. *Rev. Gaúcha Odontol.* **2019**, *67*, e20190040. [CrossRef]
40. Ribeiro, D.M.; Réus, J.C.; Felippe, W.T.; Pacheco-Pereira, C.; Dutra, K.L.; Santos, J.N.; Porporatti, A.L.; De Luca Canto, G. Technical Quality of Root Canal Treatment Performed by Undergraduate Students Using Hand Instrumentation: A Meta-Analysis. *Int. Endod. J.* **2018**, *51*, 269–283. [CrossRef]
41. Rafeek, R.N.; Smith, W.A.; Mankee, M.S.; Coldero, L.G. Radiographic Evaluation of the Technical Quality of Root Canal Fillings Performed by Dental Students. *Aust. Endod. J.* **2012**, *38*, 64–69. [CrossRef] [PubMed]
42. Pratten, D.H.; McDonald, N.J. Comparison of Radiographic and Electronic Working Lengths. *J. Endod.* **1996**, *22*, 173–176. [CrossRef]
43. Mahmoud, O.; Abdelmagied, M.H.A.; Dandashi, A.H.; Jasim, B.N.; Kayali, H.A.T.; Al Shehadat, S. Comparative Evaluation of Accuracy of Different Apex Locators: Propex IQ, Raypex 6, Root ZX, and Apex ID with CBCT and Periapical Radiograph—In Vitro Study. *Int. J. Dent.* **2021**, *2021*, 5563426. [CrossRef]
44. Adriano, L.Z.; Barasuol, J.C.; Cardoso, M.; Bolan, M. In Vitro Comparison between Apex Locators, Direct and Radiographic Techniques for Determining the Root Canal Length in Primary Teeth. *Eur. Arch. Paediatr. Dent.* **2019**, *20*, 403–408. [CrossRef] [PubMed]
45. Adorno, C.G.; Solaeche, S.M.; Ferreira, I.E.; Pedrozo, A.; Escobar, P.M.; Fretes, V.R. The Influence of Periapical Lesions on the Repeatability of Two Electronic Apex Locators in Vivo. *Clin. Oral Investig.* **2021**, *25*, 5239–5245. [CrossRef]
46. Tsesis, I.; Blazer, T.; Ben-Izhack, G.; Taschieri, S.; Del Fabbro, M.; Corbella, S.; Rosen, E. The Precision of Electronic Apex Locators in Working Length Determination: A Systematic Review and Meta-Analysis of the Literature. *J. Endod.* **2015**, *41*, 1818–1823. [CrossRef] [PubMed]
47. Bajawi, A.; AL-Sagoor, S.; Alhadi, A.; Alhadi, M.; Almasrahi, M.; AL-Ghazali, N.; Al Moaleem, M. Radiographic Assessment of the Quality of Root Canal Treatments Performed by Practitioners with Different Levels of Experience. *Biomed. Pharmacol. J.* **2018**, *11*, 1609–1616. [CrossRef]
48. Malagnino, V.A.; Pappalardo, A.; Plotino, G.; Carlesi, T. The Fate of Overfilling in Root Canal Treatments with Long-Term Follow-up: A Case Series. *Restor. Dent. Endod.* **2021**, *46*, e27. [CrossRef]
49. Ghanaati, S.; Willershausen, I.; Barbeck, M.; Unger, R.; Joergens, M.; Sader, R.; Kirkpatrick, C.; Willershausen, B. Tissue Reaction to Sealing Materials: Different View at Biocompatibility. *Eur. J. Med. Res.* **2010**, *15*, 483. [CrossRef]
50. Szczurko, G.; Pawińska, M.; Łuczaj-Cepowicz, E.; Kierklo, A.; Marczuk-Kolada, G.; Hołownia, A. Effect of Root Canal Sealers on Human Periodontal Ligament Fibroblast Viability: Ex Vivo Study. *Odontology* **2018**, *106*, 245–256. [CrossRef]
51. Goldberg, F.; Cantarini, C.; Alfie, D.; Macchi, R.L.; Arias, A. Relationship between Unintentional Canal Overfilling and the Long-term Outcome of Primary Root Canal Treatments and Nonsurgical Retreatments: A Retrospective Radiographic Assessment. *Int. Endod. J.* **2020**, *53*, 19–26. [CrossRef] [PubMed]
52. Gutiérrez, J.H.; Brizuela, C.; Villota, E. Human Teeth with Periapical Pathosis after Overinstrumentation and Overfilling of the Root Canals: A Scanning Electron Microscopic Study. *Int. Endod. J.* **1999**, *32*, 40–48. [CrossRef] [PubMed]
53. Aminoshariae, A.; Kulild, J.C. The Impact of Sealer Extrusion on Endodontic Outcome: A Systematic Review with Meta-analysis. *Aust. Endod. J.* **2020**, *46*, 123–129. [CrossRef]
54. Chugal, N.M.; Clive, J.M.; Spångberg, L.S. Endodontic Infection: Some Biologic and Treatment Factors Associated with Outcome. *Oral Surg. Oral Med. Oral Pathol. Oral Radiol. Endodontol.* **2003**, *96*, 81–90. [CrossRef]
55. ElMubarak, A.H.H.; Abu-bakr, N.H.; Ibrahim, Y.E. Postoperative Pain in Multiple-Visit and Single-Visit Root Canal Treatment. *J. Endod.* **2010**, *36*, 36–39. [CrossRef] [PubMed]
56. Madarati, A.A. Preferences of Dentists and Endodontists, in Saudi Arabia, on Management of Necrotic Pulp with Acute Apical Abscess. *BMC Oral Health* **2018**, *18*, 110. [CrossRef]
57. Vera, J.; Siqueira, J.F., Jr.; Ricucci, D.; Loghin, S.; Fernández, N.; Flores, B.; Cruz, A.G. One- versus Two-Visit Endodontic Treatment of Teeth with Apical Periodontitis: A Histobacteriologic Study. *J. Endod.* **2012**, *38*, 1040–1052. [CrossRef]
58. Schwendicke, F.; Göstemeyer, G. Single-Visit or Multiple-Visit Root Canal Treatment: Systematic Review, Meta-Analysis and Trial Sequential Analysis. *BMJ Open* **2017**, *7*, e013115. [CrossRef]
59. Tirupathi, S.P.; Krishna, N.; Rajasekhar, S.; Nuvvula, S. Clinical Efficacy of Single-Visit Pulpectomy over Multiple-Visit Pulpectomy in Primary Teeth: A Systematic Review. *Int. J. Clin. Pediatr. Dent.* **2019**, *12*, 453–459. [CrossRef]
60. Pietrzycka, K.; Pawlicka, H. Effectiveness of One-Visit Treatment of Teeth with Infected Root Canals with and without Ozonotherapy. *J. Stomatol.* **2011**, *64*, 37–49.
61. Pietrzycka, K.; Pawlicka, H. Effectiveness of One-Visit and Two-Visit Treatment of Teeth with Infected Root Canals. *J. Stomatol.* **2013**, *66*, 351–365. [CrossRef]
62. Moreira, M.S.; Anuar, A.S.N.-S.; Tedesco, T.K.; dos Santos, M.; Morimoto, S. Endodontic Treatment in Single and Multiple Visits: An Overview of Systematic Reviews. *J. Endod.* **2017**, *43*, 864–870. [CrossRef] [PubMed]

63. Paredes-Vieyra, J.; Enriquez, F.J.J. Success Rate of Single- versus Two-Visit Root Canal Treatment of Teeth with Apical Periodontitis: A Randomized Controlled Trial. *J. Endod.* **2012**, *38*, 1164–1169. [CrossRef] [PubMed]
64. Kim, D.; Kim, E. Antimicrobial Effect of Calcium Hydroxide as an Intracanal Medicament in Root Canal Treatment: A Literature Review—Part I. In Vitro Studies. *Restor. Dent. Endod.* **2014**, *39*, 241–252. [CrossRef]
65. Zancan, R.F.; Vivan, R.R.; Lopes, M.R.M.; Weckwerth, P.H.; de Andrade, F.B.; Ponce, J.B.; Duarte, M.A.H. Antimicrobial Activity and Physicochemical Properties of Calcium Hydroxide Pastes Used as Intracanal Medication. *J. Endod.* **2016**, *42*, 1822–1828. [CrossRef]
66. Dechouniotis, G.; Petridis, X.M.; Georgopoulou, M.K. Influence of Specialty Training and Experience on Endodontic Decision Making. *J. Endod.* **2010**, *36*, 1130–1134. [CrossRef]
67. Lee, J.; Kang, S.; Jung, H.-I.; Kim, S.; Karabucak, B.; Kim, E. Dentists' Clinical Decision-Making about Teeth with Apical Periodontitis Using a Variable-Controlled Survey Model in South Korea. *BMC Oral Health* **2020**, *20*, 23. [CrossRef]
68. McCaul, L.K.; McHugh, S.; Saunders, W.P. The Influence of Specialty Training and Experience on Decision Making in Endodontic Diagnosis and Treatment Planning. *Int. Endod. J.* **2001**, *34*, 594–606. [CrossRef]
69. Sul, H.; Liao, H.-F.; Fiorellini, J.; Kim, S.; Korostoff, J. Factors Affecting Treatment Planning Decisions for Compromised Anterior Teeth. *Int. J. Periodontics Restor. Dent.* **2014**, *34*, 389–398. [CrossRef]
70. Hulsmann, M.; Peters, O.A.; Dummer, P.M.H. Mechanical Preparation of Root Canals: Shaping Goals, Techniques and Means. *Endod. Top.* **2005**, *10*, 30–76. [CrossRef]
71. Peralta-Mamani, M.; Rios, D.; Duarte, M.A.H.; Santiago, J.F., Jr.; Honório, H.M. Manual vs. Rotary Instrumentation in Endodontic Treatment of Permanent Teeth: A Systematic Review and Meta-Analysis. *Am. J. Dent.* **2019**, *32*, 311–324. [PubMed]
72. Chu, D.; Lockwood, C. The Effectiveness of Nickel-Titanium versus Stainless Steel Instrumentation for Non-Surgical Endodontic Therapy: A Systematic Review Protocol. *JBI Database Syst. Rev. Implement. Rep.* **2015**, *13*, 127–138. [CrossRef]
73. Radwański, M.; Łęski, M.; Puszkarz, A.K.; Krucińska, I. Shaping Ability of ProTaper Next, Hyflex CM, and V-Taper 2H Nickel-Titanium Files in Mandibular Molars: A Micro-Computed Tomographic Study. *Iran. Endod. J.* **2021**, *16*, 103–108. [CrossRef]
74. Alsulaimani, R.; Al-Manei, K.; Alsubait, S.; AlAqeely, R.; Al-Shehri, S.; Al-Madi, E.M. Effects of Clinical Training and Case Difficulty on the Radiographic Quality of Root Canal Fillings Performed by Dental Students in Saudi Arabia. *Iran. Endod. J.* **2015**, *10*, 268–273. [CrossRef]
75. Farooq, M.; Kyani, S.G.; Hassan, F.; Toosy, W.J.; Malik, S.; Jabeen, W. Evaluation of Complications of Root Canal Treatment Performed by BDS Fresh Graduates. *Med. Forum Mon.* **2019**, *30*, 20–32.
76. Grock, C.H.; Luz, L.B.; Oliveira, V.F.; Ardenghi, T.M.; Bizarro, L.; Ferreira, M.B.C.; Montagner, F. Experiences during the Execution of Emergency Endodontic Treatment and Levels of Anxiety in Dental Students. *Eur. J. Dent. Educ.* **2018**, *22*, e715–e723. [CrossRef]
77. Adebayo, E.T.; Ahaji, L.E.; Nnachetta, R.N.; Nwankwo, O.; Akabogu-Okpeseyi, N.; Yaya, M.O.; Hussain, N.A. Technical Quality of Root Canal Fillings Done in a Nigerian General Dental Clinic. *BMC Oral Health* **2012**, *12*, 42. [CrossRef]
78. Polyzos, N.K.; Sarris, K.G.; Pita, A.I.; Mikrogeorgis, G.V.; Lyroudia, K.M. Factors Affecting the Outcome of Non-Surgical Endodontic Treatments Performed by Undergraduate Students in a Greek Dental School. *Eur. Endod. J.* **2018**, *3*, 93–100. [CrossRef]
79. Hamasha, A.A.; Hatiwsh, A. Quality of Life and Satisfaction of Patients after Nonsurgical Primary Root Canal Treatment Provided by Undergraduate Students, Graduate Students and Endodontic Specialists. *Int. Endod. J.* **2013**, *46*, 1131–1139. [CrossRef]
80. Touboul, V.; Germa, A.; Lasfargues, J.J.; Bonte, E. Outcome of Endodontic Treatments Made by Postgraduate Students in the Dental Clinic of Bretonneau Hospital. *Int. J. Dent.* **2014**, *2014*, 684979. [CrossRef]
81. Khabbaz, M.G.; Protogerou, E.; Douka, E. Radiographic Quality of Root Fillings Performed by Undergraduate Students. *Int. Endod. J.* **2010**, *43*, 499–508. [CrossRef] [PubMed]
82. Borén, D.L.; Jonasson, P.; Kvist, T. Long-Term Survival of Endodontically Treated Teeth at a Public Dental Specialist Clinic. *J. Endod.* **2015**, *41*, 176–181. [CrossRef] [PubMed]
83. Alley, B.S.; Kitchens, G.G.; Alley, L.W.; Eleazer, P.D. A Comparison of Survival of Teeth Following Endodontic Treatment Performed by General Dentists or by Specialists. *Oral Surg. Oral Med. Oral Pathol. Oral Radiol. Endodontol.* **2004**, *98*, 115–118. [CrossRef] [PubMed]
84. Pietrzycka, K.; Wujec, P.; Olczyk, I.; Pawlicka, H. Endodontic Procedures Used by Dental Practitioners in Daily Dental Practice—Questionnaire Study. *J. Stomatol.* **2016**, *69*, 183–200. [CrossRef]
85. Patel, S.; Dawood, A.; Whaites, E.; Ford, T.P. New Dimensions in Endodontic Imaging: Part 1. Conventional and Alternative Radiographic Systems. *Int. Endod. J.* **2009**, *42*, 447–462. [CrossRef]
86. Davies, A.; Patel, S.; Foschi, F.; Andiappan, M.; Mitchell, P.J.; Mannocci, F. The Detection of Periapical Pathoses Using Digital Periapical Radiography and Cone Beam Computed Tomography in Endodontically Retreated Teeth—Part 2: A 1 Year Post-Treatment Follow-Up. *Int. Endod. J.* **2016**, *49*, 623–635. [CrossRef]

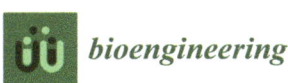

Article

Comparison of Wear of Interim Crowns in Accordance with the Build Angle of Digital Light Processing 3D Printing: A Preliminary In Vivo Study

Hakjun Lee [1,†], Keunbada Son [2,†], Du-Hyeong Lee [1], So-Yeun Kim [1] and Kyu-Bok Lee [1,*]

1. Department of Prosthodontics, School of Dentistry, Kyungpook National University, Daegu 41940, Korea
2. Advanced Dental Device Development Institute (A3DI), Kyungpook National University, Daegu 41940, Korea
* Correspondence: kblee@knu.ac.kr; Tel.: +82-32-660-6925
† These authors (H.L. and K.S.) have contributed equally to this work.

Abstract: The aim of this study is to evaluate the wear volume of interim crowns fabricated using digital light processing 3D printing according to the printing angle. A total of five patients undergoing the placement of a single crown on the mandibular molar were included. Interim crowns were fabricated directly in the oral cavity using the conventional method. A digital light processing 3D printer was then used to fabricate crowns with build angles of 0, 45, and 90 degrees. Therefore, four fabricated interim crowns were randomly delivered to the patients, and each was used for one week. Before and after use, the intaglio surfaces of the interim crowns were scanned using a 3D scanner. The volume changes before and after use were measured, and changes in the height of the occlusal surface were evaluated using the root mean square value. Data normality was verified by statistical analysis, and the wear volume in each group was evaluated using a one-way analysis of variance and Tukey's honestly significant difference test ($\alpha = 0.05$). Compared with the RMS values of the conventional method (11.88 ± 2.69 µm) and the 3D-printing method at 0 degrees (12.14 ± 2.38 µm), the RMS values were significantly high at 90 degrees (16.46 ± 2.39 µm) ($p < 0.05$). Likewise, there was a significant difference in the change in volume between the groups ($p = 0.002$), with a significantly higher volume change value at 90 degrees (1.74 ± 0.41 mm^3) than in the conventional method (0.70 ± 0.15 mm^3) ($p < 0.05$). A printing angle of 90 degrees is not recommended when interim crowns are fabricated using digital light processing 3D printing.

Keywords: 3D printing; digital light processing; interim crown; in vivo study; wear

1. Introduction

Interim crowns are important for successful prosthetic restoration. Interim crowns provide essential functional support, including proper maintenance of the occlusal relationship, prevention of tooth movement, and protection of the dental pulp and periodontal tissue [1,2]. The appropriate wear resistance of interim crowns is required to maintain these functions. If wear is excessive, there may be a change in the functionality of the masticatory movement as the occlusal vertical dimension decreases. In addition, masticatory efficiency may decrease, and premature contact may occur in the anterior teeth [3].

The conventional direct technique for an interim crown is a method of manufacturing using a material in which resin polymerization occurs only by chemical catalysis without heat or light, and 3D printing with photopolymerization technology is a method of activating a photo initiator through a light source [4]. In the conventional method, interim crowns are directly manufactured in the oral cavity [5]. However, such interim crowns may be affected by high rates of contraction and heat production and lack mechanical characteristics, unlike crowns fabricated using the indirect method with computer-aided design and computer-aided manufacturing (CAD/CAM) technologies, known as the milling

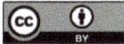

production method [6–8]. Crowns fabricated using the milling production method have superior wear and flexure strength [9], short chair time placement, and superior marginal and internal fit compared with those of crowns fabricated using the conventional method [8]. Recently, studies on the production of interim crowns using 3D printing have been conducted. Among these methods, a stereolithography apparatus (SLA) and digital light processing (DLP) are representative methods [10]. The main difference between an SLA and DLP is the light source. An SLA applies a laser beam from point to point, while DLP uses a digital micromirror to cure a complete resin layer-by-layer [11]. Unkovskiy et al. [12] reported for accuracy that an SLA may produce an intaglio denture surface with a better trueness than DLP. Li et al. [11] reported that the surface roughness was significantly influenced by the build angle rather than by the AM method. However, DLP has a faster printing speed because the entire layer of liquid resin is polymerized at once, and the DLP method is more actively utilized in the dental field [13].

Various in vitro studies have been conducted on the wear of DLP-printed interim crowns. Kessler et al. [14] investigated the three-body wear of different additively manufactured temporary materials and concluded they had comparative wear resistance to already-established materials. Myagmar et al. [15] measured the wear of DLP-printed and CAD/CAM-milled interim resin materials using a mastication simulator and found these 3D-printing digital technologies exhibited less wear volume loss than the conventional interim resin. These studies on the wear resistance of interim crowns have been conducted in vitro using a mastication simulator because controlling various variables can be difficult [16]. Prause et al. [17] reviewed the wear resistance of 3D-printed materials and could not find any in vivo studies.

A mastication simulator can reflect a variety of elements, such as force, sliding distance, testing medium, pH cycling, and temperature cycling, to imitate the masticatory system of the oral cavity. However, wear is not a simple material property but a system property arising from complex interactions between various factors. The capacity of an in vitro study to take all these factors into account is limited [18]. Indeed, Sari et al. [19] compared in vitro and in vivo wear data of temporary crowns fabricated by a CAD/CAM milling system and a cartridge system. Although the maximum wear differences between in vitro and in vivo were not significant, the mean wear differences between in vitro and in vivo were significant for CAD material. Thus, the clinical wear resistances of 3D-printed interim crowns should be verified in the oral cavity in addition to a mastication simulator.

With the DLP method, the mechanical properties of restoration are affected by the build angle [20]. The difference in physical properties according to the build angle is called anisotropy. Various physical properties of anisotropy have been reported, such as marginal and internal fit [8,21], surface roughness [22], and flexural strength [23]; thus, an optimum printing angle according to each characteristic is recommended. However, few studies on wear according to build angle have been conducted. Hanon et al. [24] studied the effect of build angle on the wear resistance of 3D-printed polymers using a DLP method and concluded no relationship between wear behavior and build angle in a cylinder-shaped specimen. However, in an X-axis experiment, the output direction of the layer and the actual sliding direction did not match. Therefore, to date, studies on the relationship between wear and the build angle of interim crowns are still rare.

In summary, there is no in vivo study on the wear resistance of DLP-printed interim crowns. In addition, there are few studies on wear resistance according to the build angle of DLP-printed interim crowns. Therefore, the purpose of this study is to evaluate the wear volume of DLP-printed interim crowns in vivo and to find the build angle with the highest wear resistance among 0, 45, and 90 degrees. In addition, compared with the existing traditional method, the clinical feasibility of DLP-printed interim crowns was demonstrated. The null hypothesis is that the wear volume of DLP-printed interim crowns does not differ according to the build angle.

2. Materials and Methods

This clinical study was approved by the Kyungpook National University Dental Hospital Institutional Review Board (Approval number: KNUDH-2021-11-02-01) (Figure 1). Informed consent was obtained from all participants. Patients who visited the Department of Prosthodontics at Kyungpook National University Dental Hospital for single-crown treatment and consented to participate in the present study were recruited. The selection criteria were as follows: patients who needed single-crown restoration treatment in the mandibular molar teeth, who had no decay or periodontal abnormalities in the abutment tooth, and who had no occlusal problems. Owing to a possible impact on wear or other potential side effects, the following patients were excluded: (1) those requiring restoration of the antagonist teeth, (2) those with a possible cracked tooth, and (3) those with bruxism or clenching habits. Based on the results of a previous study [15], the sample size was calculated to be a minimum of three participants per group (G*Power version 3.1.9.2; Heinrich-Heine-Universität, Düsseldorf, Germany) (actual power = 99.98%; power = 99%; $\alpha = 0.05$). For the present study, the sample size was determined to be five participants. Anticipating a 20% dropout rate, a total of six patients were recruited. The profiles of the participants are listed in Table 1. To control the variables, each person was asked to use all four types of interim crown so that the same person's masticatory force was applied to the interim crown for each angle. In addition, patients who need treatment on same area were recruited, and the order of use of interim crown was randomly allocated for each angle. One participant dropped out of the study owing to frequent fractures of the temporary tooth.

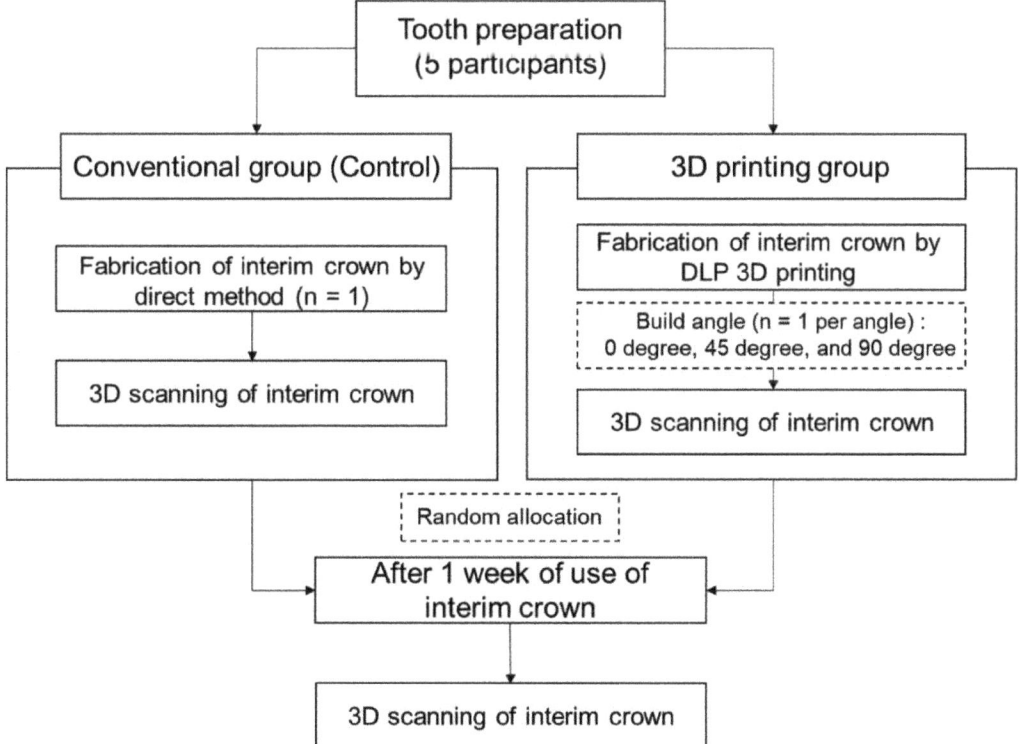

Figure 1. Study design.

Table 1. The profiles of the participants.

No.	Sex	Age	Abutment	Antagonist	Endo.	Etc.
1	F	23	#46	#15, 16	O	-
2	M	31	#36	#25, 26	O	-
3	F	57	#37	#26, 27	O	-
4	F	20	#47	#16, 17	O	-
5	F	41	#36	#25, 26	O	-
6	M	24	#37	#26, 27	O	Dropped out owing to frequent crown fracture.

At the first visit, mandibular molar teeth were prepared by a skilled technician using a diamond bur (102R bur, Shofu, Kyoto, Japan). During tooth preparation, a supragingival chamfer margin was formed, and 1.5 mm of the occlusal surface was reduced. A skilled operator then obtained a virtual working cast of the abutment tooth, proximal teeth, and antagonist teeth and performed an occlusal scan using an intraoral scanner (CS3600; Carestream Dental, Rochester, NY, USA).

Immediately after tooth preparation, interim crowns were fabricated at the chairside using self-cured resin (Unifast III; GC Corporation, Tokyo, Japan) by the direct conventional method (Table 2). Occlusal adjustment and final polishing were performed by a skilled clinician using the same process for all groups. The interim crowns were polished with silicon carbide papers of 600- and 1200-grit grain on a rotary machine with water cooling. A 21 μm thick check bit (Check-Film II—Red/Black; Caicedo Group Inc., Brooklyn, NY, USA) and an 8 μm thick shimstock (ARI SHIMSTOCK; TAEKWANG, Seoul, Korea) were used to determine whether the occlusal point and height were appropriate. After the final polishing process and immediately before cementation, the interim crown surface was scanned extraorally using an intraoral scanner (CS3600, Carestream Dental). The crowns were temporarily cemented (Temp-bond NE, Kerr, Orange, CA, USA) for one week to avoid sticky or hard foods that might cause falls or fractures of the interim crowns.

Table 2. Interim crown material.

Group	Product Name	Method	Manufacturer	LOT Number
Conventional group	UNIFAST III	Self-cured	GC Corporation, Tokyo, Japan	2004171
3D-printing group	RAYDENT C&B	DLP 3D printing	Ray Co., Ltd., Hwaseong-si, Korea	RCB209082B

The acquired virtual working cast was exported in the standard tesselation language (STL) format using an intraoral scanner. In addition, using CAD software (3Shape Dental Designer; 3Shape A/S, Copenhagen, Denmark), interim crowns were designed in a 60 μm cement space condition. After the CAD process, the virtual interim crowns were exported in the STL format, and the build angles for printing were set to 0, 45, and 90 degrees using 3D printer software (Megagen, Daegu, Korea) (Figure 2). The 3D-printing support was set to the software-recommended value. The crowns were printed using a 3D printer with DLP technology (MEG-PRINTER 3D II; Megagen, Daegu, Korea) under the following conditions: 50 μm XY resolution and 50 μm layer thickness (Table 2). Resin (Raydent C&B; Ray Co., Ltd., Hwaseong-si, Korea) was selected as the 3D-printing material. The printed interim crowns were washed using 83% ethanol, and all residual resin was removed for 60 s using an ultrasonic cleaner (SAEHAN, Seoul, Republic of Korea). All moisture and ethanol on the surface of the interim crown was dried. Finally, after the posttreatment process, a photocuring process was performed for 300 s using a curing unit (CUREDEN; Kwang Myung DAICOM, Seoul, Republic of Korea), and they were stored in distilled water at 37 °C until cementation.

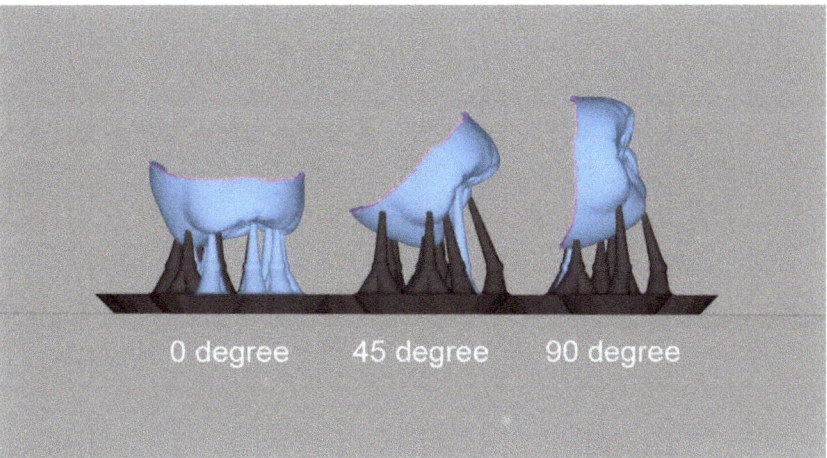

Figure 2. Digital light processing 3D-printing build angles.

The patients revisited the hospital one week after the first interim crown was placed. The existing interim crown was removed, and the surface was scanned extraorally using an intraoral scanner (CS3600, Carestream Dental, Atlanta, GA, USA).

The patients were provided with a new interim crown, which was randomly selected from the following printing angles: 0, 45, and 90 degrees. The patients underwent relining, occlusal adjustment, and polishing of the oral cavity. For relining, self-cured resin (Unifast III; GC Korea, Seoul, Korea) was used. The interim crown surface was scanned before use. The patients had the new interim crown in place for one week. At the next hospital visit, the existing interim crown surface was scanned, and one of the remaining interim crowns was chosen at random and placed. This step was repeated for the placement of the final crown.

The patients, thus, used four crowns in total (conventional method, n = 1; 3D-printing method, n = 3) for one week each. The surfaces of the interim crowns were scanned before and after use. Finally, the technician made a final impression and set the final prosthesis.

Using 3D inspection software (Geomagic Control X; 3D Systems, Cary, NC, USA), STL file changes of the interim crowns before and after wear were imported (Figure 3). The volume and height of the interim crowns were measured. The interim crowns before wear were designated as the reference, and the best-fit alignment of those after wear was determined based on the outer surface area of the interim crown, excluding the occlusal surface area before wear (Figure 3). To verify the coincidence of the outer surface area in which the interim crowns overlapped before and after wear, 3D inspection software was used (Geomagic Control X; 3D Systems). The overlapping areas of the two models were found to have a very high coincidence (3.60 ± 0.80 µm). The volume loss was calculated by comparing the volume before and after wear. The root mean square (RMS) was used to calculate the interval between the data points before and after wear (Figure 3) using the following formula:

$$RMS = \frac{1}{\sqrt{n}} \cdot \sqrt{\sum_{i=1}^{n}(X_{1,i} - X_{2,i})^2} \qquad (1)$$

where $X_{1,i}$ is the interim crown's point cloud before wear, $X_{2,i}$ is the point cloud after wear (which indicates the 3D position of the ith measurement point), and n is the number of all point clouds evaluated.

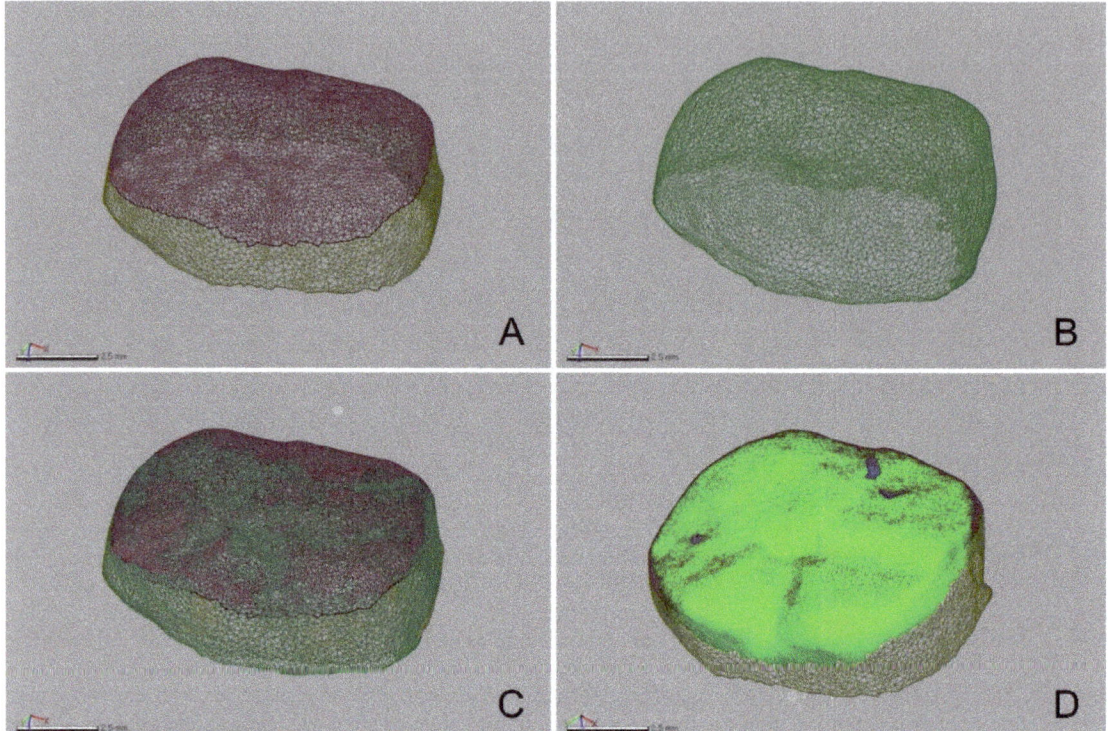

Figure 3. 3D analysis procedure. (**A**) Segmented virtual model of the interim crown before wear. (**B**) Virtual model of the interim crown after wear. (**C**) Superimposition. (**D**) Evaluation of wear on the segmented occlusal surface of (**A**).

The RMS value showed the difference in the deviation from zero between the two datasets. Thus, a low RMS value indicated a high degree of 3D agreement with the overlapped data. A 3D comparison is shown using a color difference map, and a range of −100 μm and a tolerance range of −10 μm were designated (green).

The statistical analyses in this study were conducted using SPSS Statistics (IBM Co., Armonk, NY, USA). The normal data distribution was first investigated using the Shapiro–Wilk test, and the data were found to be normally distributed. Each group's wear volume was compared using a one-way analysis of variance test, and an ex-post analysis was conducted using Tukey's honestly significant difference (HSD) test ($\alpha = 0.05$).

3. Results

Significant differences in the RMS values between the groups were found ($p = 0.002$; Table 3, Figure 4). Compared with the RMS values of the conventional method (11.88 ± 2.69 μm) and the 3D-printing method at 0 degrees (12.14 ± 2.38 μm), the RMS values were significantly higher at 90 degrees (16.46 ± 2.39 μm) ($p < 0.05$; Table 3, Figure 4). Likewise, there was a significant difference in the change in volume between the groups ($p = 0.002$; Table 3, Figure 4), with a significantly higher volume change value at 90 degrees (1.74 ± 0.41 mm^3) than in the conventional method (0.70 ± 0.15 mm^3) ($p < 0.05$; Table 3, Figure 4). In addition, the interim crowns fabricated using the conventional method showed significantly lower RMS and volume change values than those fabricated using 3D printing ($p < 0.05$; Tables 3 and 4, Figure 4).

Table 3. Comparison of the wear of interim crowns fabricated according to build angle (RMS (μm)).

Build angle	Mean	SD	95% Confidence Interval		Minimum	Maximum	Comparison **
			Lower	Upper			
Conventional method	11.88	2.69	8.53	15.22	7.70	14.80	A
0 degree	12.14	2.38	9.17	15.10	9.7	15.50	A
45 degrees	13.78	1.29	12.17	15.38	11.80	15.10	AB
90 degrees	16.46	2.39	13.49	19.42	13.20	18.90	B
F				4.363			
p				0.02 *			

RMS, root mean square; SD, standard deviation. * Significance was determined using one-way ANOVA; $p < 0.05$.
** The letters (A and B) were determined using Tukey's HSD test; $p < 0.05$.

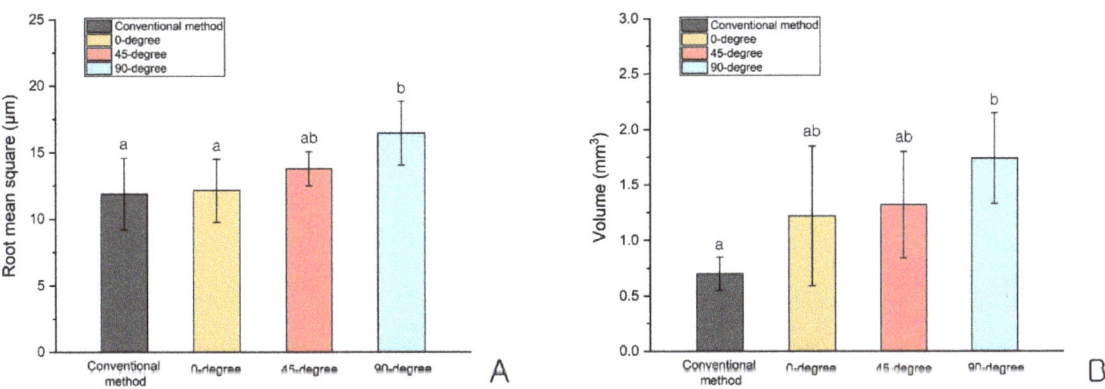

Figure 4. Comparison of the root mean square and wear volume according to build angle: (**A**) root mean square and (**B**) wear volume. The letters (a and b) were determined using Tukey's HSD test; $p < 0.05$.

Table 4. Comparison of the wear of interim crowns fabricated according to build angle (volume (mm^3)).

Build Angle	Mean	SD	95% Confidence Interval		Minimum	Maximum	Comparison **
			Lower	Upper			
Conventional method	0.70	0.15	0.50	0.89	0.50	0.90	A
0 degree	1.22	0.63	0.43	2.00	0.20	1.70	AB
45 degrees	1.32	0.48	0.71	1.92	0.60	1.90	AB
90 degrees	1.74	0.41	1.22	2.25	1.30	2.4	B
F				4.367			
p				0.020 *			

RMS, root mean square; SD, standard deviation. * Significance was determined using one-way ANOVA; $p < 0.05$.
** The letters (A and B) were determined using Tukey's HSD test; $p < 0.05$.

The color difference map according to the build angle showed relatively smaller areas of wear with the conventional method, whereas, with the 3D-printing method, the areas of wear tended to broaden from 0 to 90 degrees (Figure 5). The areas of wear in the color difference map corresponded with the occlusal points found in the oral cavity.

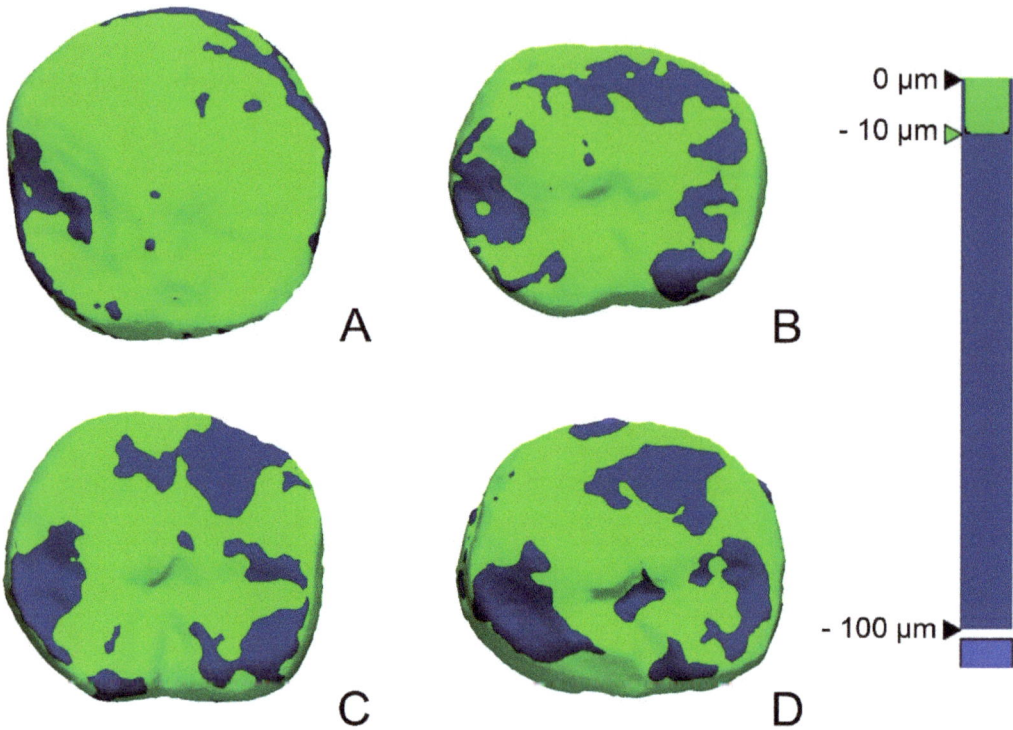

Figure 5. Comparison of 3D wear according to build angle. (**A**) Conventional method. (**B**) 3D-printing build angle of 0 degree. (**C**) 3D-printing build angle of 45 degrees. (**D**) 3D-printing build angle of 90 degrees.

4. Discussion

The purpose of this study was to examine wear volume differences according to the printing angle of interim crowns using a DLP 3D-printing method in vivo. We found a significant difference in the RMS values but no significant differences in wear volumes for the 3D-printed interim crowns according to the angle. Additionally, compared with those of the conventional method, there were significantly higher RMS values and wear volumes at 90 degrees ($p < 0.05$). Thus, the null hypothesis that the wear volume of the interim crowns would not be significantly different according to the build angle was rejected.

In this study, a difference in the wear of the interim crowns between the conventional and 3D-printing methods was found ($p = 0.020$). Loss in vertical height can be estimated using the RMS value, while the absolute wear volume can be measured using the volume loss value. The height and wear volume of the interim crowns printed at 0 degrees for the two criteria were the smallest, while the height and wear volume of the interim crowns printed at 90 degrees were the largest. In other words, the greater the printing angle, the greater the wear.

If the volumetric variation is large due to wear, it may cause a loss in vertical dimension and movement of the antagonist in cases of poor periodontal condition. In addition, in cases of anterior restoration, changes in occlusal scheme, including frontal and lateral guidance, may occur, and unnecessary interference may occur. Therefore, the properties of an interim crown require adequate wear resistance.

Differing physical properties according to angle are called anisotropy. A previous study found anisotropy in 3D-printed restorations using a DLP method [20]. However, conflicting results have been reported. One study showed a potentially weak area of polymerization owing to a shadow area between pixels [25]. Additionally, Monzon et al. [25] reported that a resin bar printed at 90 degrees showed superior mechanical properties in terms of flexural modulus and flexural stress compared to those printed at 0 degrees. However, others have suggested that anisotropy is caused by the difference in bonding strength between the inter- and intra-layers [13,26]. Park et al. [13] noted that a three-unit interim bridge printed at 90 degrees had the lowest flexural strength. In addition, in a study of bar-shaped interim material conducted by Kessler et al. [26], the interlayer was found to be the weakest link, and a specimen printed at 90 degrees was more vulnerable to fracture. Thus, our results are similar to those of both Park et al. [13] and Kessler et al. [26], which together suggest that wear decreases as the printing angle decreases and the mechanical properties become stronger. However, additional studies are needed to examine the tendency of wear according to physical properties for more robust conclusions to be drawn.

In the previous study, Kessler et al. [14] reported that the mean wear depth of a DLP-printed interim crown against a metal wheel was between 13 and 66 μm after 50,000 cycles of chewing simulation. Ahn et al. [16] reported that steatite, similar to the surface hardness of enamel, was used as an antagonist, and the wear volume loss of a DLP-printed interim crown was 1.507 mm^3 after 30,000 cycles of chewing simulation. Hanon et al. [24] reported that the wear depth of non-colored, post-processed DLP cylinder against a steel counterpart was measured between 9 μm and 12 μm among samples of each build angle. Sari. et al. [19] studied an in vivo wear test of interim crowns by milling type and cartridge type on the mandibular first molar for 14 days, and the mean wear data were 296.9 μm (milling type) and 244.4 μm (Cartridge type). However, considering that the thickness of the check film was 21 μm, it could be said that the number of Sari et al.'s experiments was large compared to other articles. As such, the wear data so far have varied depending on the type of opposing tooth, whether they are in vivo or in vitro, the shape of the specimen, and the test period. The results of this experiment were also within the general variation range, and it was possible to show the tendency of the difference in wear in accordance with the build angle.

There are two types of wear: (1) two-body wear caused by direct friction between the cusps and (2) three-body wear caused indirectly by food between the two cusps. In this study, both types of wear were observed. Two-body wear can be observed through the interim crown's occlusal points, and the size and number were found to decrease after use in the present study. This can be explained by a decrease in the area where the cusps contacted each other as wear progressed, while the overall occlusal vertical dimension was maintained. However, three-body wear may decrease or increase according to the debris, and the wear volume may be either very small or may not always occur [27]. In fact, after excluding the two-body wear points around the occlusal points, almost no wear could be seen on the color map in the remaining areas (Figure 5), suggesting that the impact of three-body wear was insignificant in this study. In addition, on the color map (Figure 5), the wear areas tended to broaden from 0 to 90 degrees. This again indicated that the greater the printing angle, the greater the wear.

In a study conducted by Beleidy et al. [28], no difference in the wear analysis between 3D scanning and optical digital profilometry (the conventional method) was reported. In the present study, the coincidence of the overlapping outer surface areas of the interim crowns before and after wear was 3.60 ± 0.80 μm, and the two models' overlapping areas showed very high coincidence.

If the experiment condition in the oral cavity is limited, wear can be evaluated virtually using a finite element method. As a preclinical study, it can reduce the cost and the discomfort of the patient from the clinical trial. For example, Jamari et al. [29] simulated the contact pressure between the metal femoral head and the acetabular cup of an artificial hip joint using a finite element method and proposed a design to reduce cumulative contact pressure and wear in consideration of the physical characteristics of each metal material. Tribst et al. [30] simulated the effect of filling materials and pulp chamber extension on the biomechanical response of an endocrown through a finite element method and proposed an optimal divergence angle with preferred materials to seal the orifice.

To apply this method to interim crown design, it should be preceded by figuring out the physical characteristics of the interim crown, in addition to the build angle and mastication pattern of the jaws. Tian et al. [31] reviewed the factors affecting 3D-printed products as build angle, layer thickness, post-curing, and material composition. Alshamrani et al. [32] reported that a 100 μm layer thickness with a dry storage postprocessing group has the highest flexural strength. Kessler et al. [14] reported that the filler content influenced the wear behavior. As a result, it would be possible to make an optimal crown design for each angle by reflecting the properties of the materials and printing process in a computational simulation.

In the present study, there was no statistical difference in wear volume between the interim crowns fabricated using the conventional method and those printed at 0 degrees ($p > 0.05$). In general, interim crowns fabricated using a DLP method are printed at 0 degrees. Previous studies have shown weaker wear resistance with the DLP method than with conventional fabrication, milling, and SLA methods [33,34]. Nevertheless, other studies have shown wear resistance to be the same [6,14] or better [15,16] with the DLP method than with conventional fabrication, milling, and SLA methods. Even if the interim crowns are fabricated using the same method, wear might differ according to the composition of the resin material used. Kessler et al. [14] reported significant differences in wear among various 3D-printed materials, and therefore, products with a high filler content were recommended. Kessler et al. [26] also studied an evaluation of the flexural strength of three products and noted that, among the various factors assessed, the product characteristics were the most important. Thus, the results of the present study were limited by the products used. Additional studies are needed to evaluate the wear associated with various products.

This study has several major limitations as an in vivo pilot study. First, the scan data used to evaluate wear were acquired using an intraoral scanner. However, since the volumes of crowns were measured outside the oral cavity rather than intraorally, it was generally more accurate than the degree of suspension presented by an intraoral scanner. In fact, Huang et al. [35] reported 8.66 ± 0.40 μm trueness and 5.44 ± 0.52 μm precision when using the same scanner (CS3600) extraorally. Additionally, Ahn et al. [16] also measured the wear volume of specimens using an intraoral scanner outside the oral cavity. Nevertheless, if a lab scanner was used, it would have been possible to measure the amount of wear more accurately. Second, the wear test was conducted for one week on each interim crown. Previous in vitro studies have been variously tested at levels such as 10,000, 30,000, and 50,000 cycles, as well as up to 200,000 cycles for long term use. In general, 20,000 cycles of a chewing simulator is equivalent to 1 month of use [14,15,36]. Thus, although the wear volume loss for one week would be small, in actual clinical practice, the period of use of an interim crown for a single crown is generally from one to two weeks. In addition, as each participant had to test for each of the four groups in this experiment, the period of use was limited to the shortest period as one week. Third, this experiment was for single-crown restoration. As the overall occlusal vertical dimension was always maintained, it was difficult for the two-body wear to occur continuously by the antagonist, even if the period were further extended. Therefore, the actual measurable change in wear volume was limited. Fourth, anatomical interim crowns were used in this study. While the actual printing angle may have been 45 degrees, for instance, the actual contact angle between the tooth and the temporary restoration could have been greater than or less than 45 degrees considering the cusp shape and direction of jaw movement. In other words, the actual angle may have been altered from the intended angle. Lastly, the masticatory force, dietary habits, and oral habits were individually different. Koc et al. [37] reported that the maximum bite force is higher in males than in females. In addition, although the correlation between age and bite force seems to be significant, it might be assumed that the effect of age on bite force is relatively small. It is practically impossible to avoid individual differences, but to control the variables, each participant in this study was asked to use all four types of interim crown so that the same person's masticatory force was applied to the interim crown for each angle. In addition, patients who need a treatment on same area were recruited, and the order of use of interim crown was randomly allocated for each angle.

It is recommended that further studies reflect the following. First, patients who need a long-term restoration or a full-arch restoration with changeable vertical dimensions should be recruited. Second, by increasing the number of samples, participants should be divided into four groups, and interim crowns of one type of angle should be assigned. Thereafter, the wear amount for each group could be compared. Alternatively, patients could be recruited based on the same age and gender. Third, it is necessary to verify the wear resistance by each restoration area. Compared to the posterior teeth, the anterior teeth have a different contact angle on the lingual surface because more complex occlusal contacts, such as lateral guidance, occur. Lastly, since the product content is different for each commercial product, verification is required.

This study was the first in vivo study on the wear resistance of DLP-printed interim crowns that investigated wear resistance in accordance with the build angle of the DLP-printed interim crowns. The clinical feasibility of DLP-printed interim crowns was verified, and a build angle for wear resistance was suggested. In the future, it could be used to manufacture more complex prostheses, such as anterior restorations and full-arch restorations.

5. Conclusions

The interim crowns fabricated using the conventional method showed wear resistance similar (at 0 degree) or superior to those fabricated using the DLP 3D-printing method. The clinical feasibility of DLP-printed interim crowns was verified. To ensure high wear resistance, a printing angle of 90 degrees is not recommended when an interim crown is fabricated using DLP 3D printing; rather, a printing angle of 0 degrees is recommended. Further experiments with longer periods of use, larger numbers of participants, more complex and multi-positioned restorations, the use of precise scanners, and more diverse product groups are needed.

Author Contributions: H.L. and K.S. contributed to the conception and design, data acquisition, analysis, and writing of the original draft; D.-H.L. contributed to the data acquisition and interpretation; S.-Y.K. contributed to the data acquisition and interpretation; and K.-B.L. contributed to the supervision and project administration. All authors have read and agreed to the published version of the manuscript.

Funding: This work was supported by a National Research Foundation of Korea (NRF) grant funded by the Korean government (MSIT) (No. 2022R1C1C2007040).

Institutional Review Board Statement: The study protocol was approved by the Kyungpook National University Dental Hospital Institutional Review Board (approval number: KNUDH-2021-11-02-01). All methods were carried out in accordance with relevant guidelines and regulations. Informed consent was obtained from all the participants.

Informed Consent Statement: Informed consent was obtained from all the participants involved in the study. Written informed consent was obtained from the patients to publish this paper.

Data Availability Statement: The datasets used and analyzed during the current study are available from the corresponding author on reasonable request.

Acknowledgments: The authors thank the researchers at the Advanced Dental Device Development Institute (A3DI) of Kyungpook National University, for their time and contributions to the study. This work was supported by a National Research Foundation of Korea (NRF) grant funded by the Korean government (MSIT) (No. 2022R1C1C2007040).

Conflicts of Interest: The authors declare no conflict of interest.

References

1. Gough, M. A Review of Temporary Crowns and Bridges. *Dent. Update* **1994**, *21*, 203–207. [PubMed]
2. Fisher, D.W.; Shillingburg, H.T., Jr.; Dewhirst, R.B. Indirect Temporary Restorations. *J. Am. Dent. Assoc.* **1971**, *82*, 160–163. [CrossRef] [PubMed]
3. Stober, T.; Henninger, M.; Schmitter, M.; Pritsch, M.; Rammelsberg, P. Three-Body Wear of Resin Denture Teeth with and without Nanofillers. *J. Prosthet. Dent.* **2010**, *103*, 108–117. [CrossRef]
4. Giudice, R.L.; Famà, F. Health Care and Health Service Digital Revolution. *Int. J. Environ. Res. Public Health* **2020**, *17*, 4913. [CrossRef]
5. Tom, T.N.; Uthappa, M.A.; Sunny, K.; Begum, F.; Nautiyal, M.; Tamore, S. Provisional Restorations: An Overview of Materials Used. *J. Adv. Clin. Res. Insights* **2016**, *3*, 212–214. [CrossRef]
6. Park, J.M.; Ahn, J.S.; Cha, H.S.; Lee, J.H. Wear Resistance of 3D Printing Resin Material Opposing Zirconia and Metal Antagonists. *Materials* **2018**, *11*, 1043. [CrossRef]
7. Singh, J.P.; Gupta, A.K.; Dhiman, R.K.; Roy Chowdhury, S.K. Comparative Study of Immediate Functional Loading and Immediate Non-functional Loading of Monocortical Implants. *Med. J. Armed. Forces India* **2015**, *71*, 333–339. [CrossRef]
8. Ryu, J.E.; Kim, Y.L.; Kong, H.J.; Chang, H.S.; Jung, J.H. Marginal and Internal Fit of 3D Printed Provisional Crowns According to Build Directions. *J. Adv. Prosthodont.* **2020**, *12*, 225–232. [CrossRef]
9. Rayyan, M.M.; Aboushelib, M.; Sayed, N.M.; Ibrahim, A.; Jimbo, R. Comparison of Interim Restorations Fabricated by CAD/CAM with Those Fabricated Manually. *J. Prosthet. Dent.* **2015**, *114*, 414–419. [CrossRef]
10. Lee, S. Prospect for 3D Printing Technology in Medical, Dental, and Pediatric Dental Field. *J. Korean Acad. Pediatr. Dent.* **2016**, *43*, 93–108. [CrossRef]
11. Li, P.; Fernandez, P.K.; Spintzyk, S.; Schmidt, F.; Beuer, F.; Unkovskiy, A. Effect of Additive Manufacturing Method and Build Angle on Surface Characteristics and Candida Albicans Adhesion to 3D printed Denture Base Polymers. *J. Dent.* **2022**, *116*, 103889. [CrossRef]
12. Unkovskiy, A.; Schmidt, F.; Beuer, F.; Li, P.; Spintzyk, S.; Fernandez, P.K. Stereolithography vs. Direct Light Processing for Rapid Manufacturing of Complete Denture Bases: An In Vitro Accuracy Analysis. *J. Clin. Med.* **2021**, *10*, 1070. [CrossRef]
13. Park, S.M.; Park, J.M.; Kim, S.K.; Heo, S.J.; Koak, J.Y. Comparison of Flexural Strength of Three-Dimensional Printed Three-Unit Provisional Fixed Dental Prostheses according to Build Directions. *J. Korean. Dent. Sci.* **2019**, *12*, 13–19. [CrossRef]
14. Keßler, A.; Reymus, M.; Hickel, R.; Kunzelmann, K.H. Three-Body Wear of 3D Printed Temporary Materials. *Dent. Mater.* **2019**, *35*, 1805–1812. [CrossRef]
15. Myagmar, G.; Lee, J.H.; Ahn, J.S.; Yeo, I.L.; Yoon, H.I.; Han, J.S. Wear of 3D Printed and CAD/CAM Milled Interim Resin Materials after Chewing Simulation. *J. Adv. Prosthodont.* **2021**, *13*, 144–151. [CrossRef]
16. Ahn, J.J.; Huh, J.B.; Choi, J.W. In Vitro Evaluation of Wear Resistance of Provisional Resin Materials Fabricated by Different Methods. *J. Korean Acad. Prosthodont.* **2019**, *57*, 110–117. [CrossRef]
17. Prause, E.; Hey, J.; Beuer, F.; Schmidt, F. Wear Resistance of 3D-printed Materials: A Systematic Review. *Dent. Rev.* **2022**, *2*, 100051. [CrossRef]
18. Lawson, N.C.; Janyavula, S.; Cakir, D.; Burgess, J.O. An Analysis of the Physiologic Parameters of Intraoral Wear: A Review. *J. Phys. D Appl. Phys.* **2013**, *46*, 404007. [CrossRef]
19. Sari, T.; Usumez, A.; Strasser, T.; Şahinbas, A.; Rosentritt, M. Temporary Materials: Comparison of In Vivo and In Vitro Performance. *Clin. Oral Investig.* **2020**, *24*, 4061–4068. [CrossRef]
20. Dizon, J.R.C.; Espera, A.H., Jr.; Chen, Q.; Advincula, R.C. Mechanical Characterization of 3D-Printed Polymers. *Addit. Manuf.* **2018**, *20*, 44–67. [CrossRef]
21. Yu, B.Y.; Son, K.B.D.; Lee, K.B. Evaluation of Intaglio Surface Trueness and Margin Quality of Interim Crowns in Accordance with the Build Angle of Stereolithography Apparatus 3-Dimensional Printing. *J. Prosthet. Dent.* **2021**, *126*, 231–237. [CrossRef] [PubMed]
22. Alharbi, N.; Osman, R.B. Does Build Angle Have an Influence on Surface Roughness of Anterior 3D-Printed Restorations? An In-Vitro Study. *Int. J. Prosthodont.* **2021**, *34*, 505–510. [CrossRef] [PubMed]
23. Shim, J.S.; Kim, J.E.; Jeong, S.H.; Choi, Y.J.; Ryu, J.J. Printing Accuracy, Mechanical Properties, Surface Characteristics, and Microbial Adhesion of 3D-Printed Resins with Various Printing Orientations. *J. Prosthet. Dent.* **2020**, *124*, 468–475. [CrossRef] [PubMed]
24. Hanon, M.M.; Zsidai, L. Tribological and Mechanical Properties Investigation of 3D Printed Polymers Using DLP Technique. *AIP Conf. Proc.* **2020**, *2213*, 020205. [CrossRef]
25. Monzon, M.; Ortega, Z.; Hernández, A.; Paz, R.; Ortega, F. Anisotropy of Photopolymer Parts Made by Digital Light Processing. *Materials* **2017**, *10*, 64. [CrossRef] [PubMed]
26. Keßler, A.; Hickel, R.; Ilie, N. In Vitro Investigation of the Influence of Printing Direction on the Flexural Strength, Flexural Modulus and Fractographic Analysis of 3D-Printed Temporary Materials. *Dent. Mater. J.* **2021**, *40*, 641–649. [CrossRef] [PubMed]
27. Abdelbary, A. Sliding Mechanics of Polymers. In *Wear of Polymers and Composites*; Woodhead Publishing: Oxford, UK, 2014; pp. 37–66, ISBN 978-1-78242-177-1.
28. Beleidy, M.; Ziada, A. 3D Surface Deviation Wear Analysis of Veneered Peek Crowns and Its Correlation with Optical Digital Profilometry. *J. Prosthodont.* **2022**. [CrossRef]
29. Jamari, J.; Ammarullah, M.I.; Santoso, G.; Sugiharto, S.; Supriyono, T.; Prakoso, A.T.; Basri, H.; van der Heide, E. Computational Contact Pressure Prediction of CoCrMo, SS 316L and Ti6Al4V Femoral Head against UHMWPE Acetabular Cup under Gait Cycle. *J. Funct. Biomater.* **2022**, *13*, 64. [CrossRef]

30. Tribst, J.P.M.; Lo Giudice, R.; dos Santos, A.F.C.; Borges, A.L.S.; Silva-Concílio, L.R.; Amaral, M.; Lo Giudice, G. Lithium Disilicate Ceramic Endocrown Biomechanical Response According to Different Pulp Chamber Extension Angles and Filling Materials. *Materials* **2021**, *14*, 1307. [CrossRef]
31. Tian, Y.; Chen, C.; Xu, X.; Wang, J.; Hou, X.; Li, K.; Lu, X.; Shi, H.; Lee, E.; Jiang, H.B. A Review of 3D Printing in Dentistry: Technologies, Affecting Factors, and Applications. *Scanning* **2021**, *2021*, 9950131. [CrossRef]
32. Alshamrani, A.A.; Raju, R.; Ellakwa, A. Effect of Printing Layer Thickness and Postprinting Conditions on the Flexural Strength and Hardness of a 3D-Printed Resin. *Biomed. Res. Int.* **2022**, *2022*, 8353137. [CrossRef]
33. Lutz, A.M.; Hampe, R.; Roos, M.; Lumkemann, N.; Eichberger, M.; Stawarczyk, B. Fracture Resistance and 2-Body Wear of 3-Dimensional-Printed Occlusal Devices. *J. Prosthet. Dent.* **2019**, *121*, 166–172. [CrossRef]
34. Wesemann, C.; Spies, B.C.; Sterzenbach, G.; Beuer, F.; Kohal, R.; Wemken, G.; Krügel, M.; Pieralli, S. Polymers for Conventional, Subtractive, and Additive Manufacturing of Occlusal Devices Differ in Hardness and Flexural Properties but not in Wear Resistance. *Dent. Mater.* **2021**, *37*, 432–442. [CrossRef]
35. Huang, M.Y.; Son, K.; Lee, W.S.; Lee, K.B. Comparison of the Accuracy of Intraoral Scanner by Three-Dimensional Analysis in Single and 3-Unit Bridge Abutment Model: In Vitro Study. *J. Korean. Acad. Prosthodont.* **2019**, *57*, 102–109. [CrossRef]
36. Dayan, C.; Kiseri, B.; Gencel, B.; Kurt, H.; Tuncer, N. Wear Resistance and Microhardness of Various Interim Fixed Prosthesis Materials. *J. Oral. Sci.* **2019**, *61*, 447–453. [CrossRef]
37. Koc, D.; Dogan, A.; Bek, B. Bite Force and Influential Factors on Bite Force Measurements: A Literature Review. *Eur. J. Dent.* **2010**, *4*, 223–232. [CrossRef]

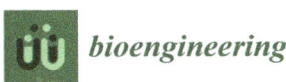

Article

Effect of Different Desensitizers on Shear Bond Strength of Self-Adhesive Resin Cements to Dentin

Alejandro Elizalde-Hernández [1,†], Louis Hardan [2,†], Rim Bourgi [2], Cristina Pereira Isolan [3], Andressa Goicochea Moreira [1], J. Eliezer Zamarripa-Calderón [4], Evandro Piva [1], Carlos Enrique Cuevas-Suárez [5,*], Walter Devoto [6], Ahmed Saad [7], Patrycja Proc [8] and Monika Lukomska-Szymanska [9,*]

1. Graduate Program in Dentistry, Federal University of Pelotas, Pelotas 96015-560, RS, Brazil
2. Department of Restorative Dentistry, School of Dentistry, Saint-Joseph University, Beirut 1107 2180, Lebanon
3. School of Dentistry, Federal University of Jequitinhonha and Mucuri Valleys (UFVJM), Diamantina 39803-371, MG, Brazil
4. Academic Area of Dentistry, Autonomous University of Hidalgo Sate, Pachuca 42083, Mexico
5. Dental Materials Laboratory, Academic Area of Dentistry, Autonomous University of Hidalgo State, Circuito ex Hacienda la Concepción S/N, San Agustín Tlaxiaca 42160, Mexico
6. Independent Researcher, 16030 Sestri Levante, Italy
7. Department of Restorative Dentistry, College of Dentistry, Al-Bayan University, Baghdad 100013, Iraq
8. Department of Pediatric Dentistry, Medical University of Lodz, 92213 Lodz, Poland
9. Department of General Dentistry, Medical University of Lodz, 92213 Lodz, Poland
* Correspondence: cecuevas@uaeh.edu.mx (C.E.C.-S.); monika.lukomska-szymanska@umed.lodz.pl (M.L.-S.); Tel.: +52-177172000 (C.E.C.-S.); +48-42-675-74-64 (M.L.-S.)
† These authors contributed equally to this work.

Abstract: The sealing and bonding characteristics of luting cements may be affected by the application of desensitizers containing ingredients that induce chemical interaction with dentin organic matrix. This study evaluated the effect of different desensitizers on the immediate and long-term shear bond strength (SBS) of a self-adhesive resin cement (SARC) to dentin. Healthy bovine dentin specimens were used for the study. Gluma® Desensitizer, Desensibilize Nano P®, and Soothe® desensitizer were used in study groups, while the control group did not receive any treatment. Next, SARC (RelyXTM U200) in cylindrical mold was applied to the sample surface. All specimens were stored at 37 °C for 24 h or six months and tested for SBS. Additionally, water contact angle was measured using an optical tensiometer. Results were analyzed by analysis of variance and Student-*t* tests ($p < 0.05$). Application of the different types of desensitizers had no significant influence on immediate or long-term SBS of SARC to dentin ($p > 0.05$). Differences for water contact angle were not statistically significant among the tested groups ($p = 0.450$). Within the limitations of the present study, it can be concluded that the application of the different types of desensitizers had no significant influence on the SBS of a SARC to dentin.

Keywords: bond strength; contact angle; dentin; desensitizers; resin cements

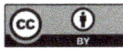

1. Introduction

Dentin hypersensitivity following tooth preparation for crown reduction is a common problem in dentistry, however very rarely documented [1]. Previous in vitro study revealed that reducing the amount of water cooling or increasing the air pressure and load during cavity preparation increases the temperature of the pulp chamber, which could result in hypersensitivity or even pulp necrosis [2]. Other factors, such as aggressive tooth grinding or preparation, preparation time, preparation thickness, method of manufacture and adjustment of provisional, bacterial contamination, and dehydration of dentin, are also implicated [3].

Brannström's hydrodynamic theory posits that dentinal hypersensitivity is promoted by external stimuli, such as thermal, tactile, chemical, or osmotic pressure, that cause movement of intratubular dentinal fluids in exposed dentin [4]. Such fluid movement is capable of exciting the nerve fibers that induce hypersensitivity or pain [5].

The treatment of dentin sensitivity after tooth preparation is intended to offer immediate and permanent pain relief. However, many of these treatments may be unsatisfactory, since most of the conventionally used desensitizers are related to the occlusion of the dentinal tubules without considering the causal factors that have triggered the problem [6]. Therefore, the initial therapeutic strategies should aim to eliminate predisposing factors, such as abrasion, erosive components, and abfraction, thus avoiding recurrence of symptoms [7]. The therapeutic procedures options for reducing dental hypersensitivity are based on substances that depress transmission, such as potassium salts or potassium nitrate, substances that occlude the dentin tubules by stimulating mineral deposits, such as fluorides, oxalates, varnishes, adhesive resins, Bioglass®, and Portland cement, while low power (Helium-Neonium; He-Ne, Aluminum Gallium Arsenide; AsGaAl) and high power laser treatments (Neodymium Yttrium Aluminum Granate; Nd:YAG, carbon dioxide;CO_2) are considered therapeutic treatments [8].

Clinical studies have evaluated the use of fluorides for the treatment of tooth sensitivity. Kielbassa et al. [9] evaluated two types of a commercial fluoride lacquers, one that contained 6% sodium fluoride (NaF) and calcium fluoride (CaF_2), and another one used as a control that only consisted of 6% NaF. In their subsequent evaluations at six and 12 months, the hypersensitivity scores decreased after treatment. There was a pain relief, however none of the treatments completely eliminated the problem. Easily soluble NaF provides a rapid release of fluoride ions, which are converted to CaF_2 on the tooth surface to effectively assist in remineralization. The CaF_2 was slowly soluble in saliva, which would justify the transient action of a chemical barrier that provides a lasting retention on the surface of the tooth. This guarantees a long-lasting fluoridation. It was concluded that a lacquer containing CaF_2/NaF in treating dentin hypersensitivity is effective in the initial reduction of dentin hypersensitivity. The combination of CaF_2/NaF can be recommended for clinical use. On the other hand, when comparing the desensitizing effects of a gallium–aluminum–arsenide (GaAlAs) laser and NaF, an immediate reduction in the visual analog scale (VAS) score was observed. However, the NaF group showed an increase in the VAS scale at three and six months in comparison to one week and one month. The authors concluded that GaAlAs laser irradiation was effective in treating tooth sensitivity and was considered a more comfortable and faster procedure when compared to traditional treatment [10]. Nowadays, these are the main mechanisms through which desensitizers adequately manage pain.

The clinical success of an indirect restorative procedure depends on several factors; however, cementation technique is a crucial step for long-term clinical success, which favors retention and prevents micro-leakage, secondary caries, and restoration loss [11]. Cementation could be performed using either conventional water-based cements or resin-based cements; among the latter, self-adhesive resin-based cements have been introduced into the market to facilitate the cementation of fixed restorations. These cements do not require any pretreatment of the tooth surface, thus reducing the application time and the technique sensitivity [12]. The self-adhesive resin cements (SARCs) are able to effectively diffuse and decalcify the underlying dentin due to increasing viscosity occurring after paste-to-paste mixing (owing to an acid-based reaction) [13]. Additionally, a greater contact with dental tissues to react with hydroxyapatite is observed, possibly resulting in an enhanced monomer dentinal interaction with the dental tissues [13]. Moreover, a high hydrophilicity enhances wetting of the tooth surface and a low pH—etching of the tooth substrates [14]. As a consequence, dentin and enamel demineralization takes place. Next, the carboxylic and phosphoric acid-groups of the modified methacrylate monomer present in the SARCs interact with the calcium from the hydroxyapatite (enamel and dentin) [12,15]. As the adhesion to the tooth structure has been established the acidity of the SARCs is being neutralized (from 2.8 to 7.0 after 24 h) [13]. These materials are structurally similar to compomers, the main difference being the concentration of acid monomer. Most of these SARCs may contain somewhat lower filler particles compared to compomers. Therefore, hydrated substrates more efficiently facilitate the ionization of acid monomers followed by acid-base neutralization reactions involving the tooth and the basic filling. For this reason, SARCs may demonstrate adhesion to dentin. In summary, due to the composition of SARCs that do not contain water, the dentin surface treatment must not dry out excessively before the application of this cement. However, over-wetting of the adherent dentin surface can hinder polymerization and reduce the integrity of the bonding interface. For this reason, the chemical interactions between the functional acid monomers of the SARCs and the dental substrate (dentin and enamel) are important mechanisms for adhesion. In addition, the ability of self-adhesive systems to release fluoride has been investigated, and they were found not to provide postoperative sensitivity [16].

The sealing and bonding characteristics of these luting cements may be affected by the application of desensitizers containing ingredients that induce chemical interaction with dentin organic matrix. Nevertheless, few studies have evaluated the effect of desensitizers on the shear bond strength (SBS) of the self-adhesive resin cement (SARC) to dentin. Therefore, this study aimed to evaluate the effect of three different desensitizers on the immediate and long-term SBS of SARC to dentin. The null hypothesis tested was that the application of desensitizers will not affect the immediate or long-term SBS of a SARC to dentin.

2. Materials and Methods

2.1. Experimental Design

In this work, the bond strength between a SARC (Rely X U200; 3M ESPE, St. Louis, MI, USA) and bovine dentin was evaluated according to the following factors: (1) previous application of a desensitizer agent at three levels (Gluma® Desensitizer, Nano P®, and Soothe®); and (2) storing time at two levels (24 h and 6 months). These aging times were chosen following the directions of the ISO/TS 11406 International Standard [17]. A group without the application of a desensitizer agent was used as control. The chemical composition and application protocols of the desensitizing agents used in this study are described in Table 1.

Table 1. Chemical composition and application protocols of the materials used in this study.

Study Group	Desensitizer Agent	Chemical Composition *	Application Protocol
Gluma	Gluma® Desensitizer (Kulzer, Hanau, Germany)	(2-hydroxyethyl) methacrylate glutardialdehyde, purified water	Apply to the dentin for 60 s with a microbrush and dry with dry air until it disappears (observe a non-shiny surface) and then wash with water
Nano P	Nano P® (FGM, Joinville, Brazil)	Potassium nitrate and sodium fluoride	Apply with microbrush on the dentin surface, rub the product with a rubber cup for 10 s, leave the product to rest for 5 min and finally remove the excess with a cotton pad
Soothe	Soothe® (SDI, Victoria, Australia)	6% potassium nitrate and 0.1% fluoride gel	Apply on the surface for 2 min
Cement used: Rely X U200		Base paste: Methacrylate monomers containing phosphoric acid groups, methacrylate monomers, silanated fillers, initiator components, stabilizers, rheological additives	Mix base paste and catalyst paste into a homogenous paste within 20 s. Spread cement within the restoration and apply moderate pressure
		Catalyst: Methacrylate monomers, Alkaline (basic) fillers, Silanated fillers, Initiator components, Stabilizers, Pigments, Rheological additives	

* Information according to the manufacturer's datasheet.

2.2. Specimen Preparation

Healthy bovine incisors were sectioned at the cemento-enamel junction using a low-speed motor (MotorTurbo & E-ASP1, Eighteeth, Changzhou, China) with cooling. Crowns were embedded in cylindrical plastic molds using cold-cure acrylic resin, which allowed the buccal enamel surface to be exposed. Next, the buccal enamel was abraded with an orthodontic grinder until a flat medium dentin surface was exposed. Then, samples were standardized by polishing with 600 grit silicon carbide sandpaper for 1 min. Afterward, each sample was examined under a light stereomicroscope at a magnification of $40\times$ to verify the exposed dentin.

The desensitizers were applied four times with one-week intervals on the surface of samples according to manufacturer's instructions. Between each surface treatment, specimens were stored (for 7 days) in artificial saliva at the temperature of 37 °C, thereby simulating clinical conditions. The control group did not receive any treatment was stored in artificial saliva at 37 °C for four weeks.

Next, specimens were washed with distilled water and excess dentin moisture was removed. Elastomer molds with two cylindrical opening (1.5 mm diameter, 0.5 mm thickness) were placed at the center of the sample. The SARC Rely X U200 was applied (according to manufacturer instructions) and polymerized for 40 s with Curing Pen (Eighteeth, Changzhou, China) at 1000 mW/cm^2.

The sample size (n = 10) was estimated based on the data of other study [18], considering a comparative study design of four independent groups, a minimum detectable difference in SBS of 3.1, a standard deviation (SD) of 1.9, a power of 0.8, and α = 0.05.

2.3. Shear Bond Strength Test

Samples in each study group were tested after aging in distilled water at 37 °C for 24 h and for 6 months. The plastic molds containing the specimens were fixed to a microshear test device (Odeme Dental Research, Luzerna-SC, Brazil). Next, a thin steel wire (0.2 mm diameter) was looped around the cylinder and aligned with the bonding interface. The steel wire was then pushed upwards applying a tensile force (Figure 1). SBS test was conducted at a crosshead speed of 0.5 mm/min until failure in a universal testing machine (EMIC®, DL 500; São José dos Pinhais, Brazil). SBS (in MPa) was calculated by dividing the maximum force achieved by the area (1.77 mm^2) of the bonded specimen.

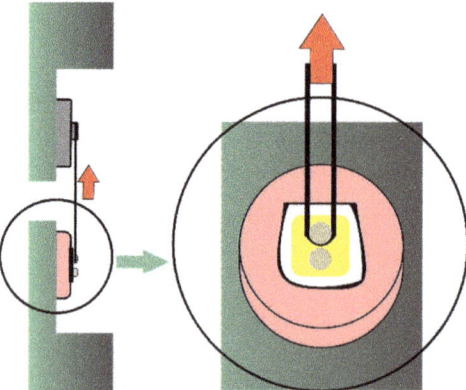

Figure 1. Diagram of the shear bond strength test. Red arrows indicate the direction of the force.

Additionally, the bonding surface was analyzed with a stereomicroscope ($50\times$) to determine the failure mode: adhesive, cohesive in dentin, cohesive in resin, and mixed [19].

2.4. Contact Angle

The water contact angle of the dentin after application of the desensitizing agents was measured with an optical tensiometer (Theta Lite TL101, Biolin Scientific Inc; Stockholms Lan, Finland) following a sessile drop method. For each study group, the dentin surface was prepared as previously described. Standardized drops of the distilled water (5 µL) were directly dispensed onto the dentin surface. Immediately after placing the drop onto the dentin surface, a dynamic reading of the right and left contact angle was measured in real time with One Attension software (Biolin Scientific Inc, Stockholms Lan, Sweden) using 20 frames per second for 20 s. The contact angle (°) was estimated as the mean between the right and left readings ($n = 3$).

2.5. Statistical Analysis

Data were analyzed using SigmaPlot 14.0 software at a statistical significance of $\alpha = 0.05$. Approximate normality of data distribution was determined by Kolmogorov–Smirnov and Shapiro–Wilk tests. For each storage period, one-way analysis of variance, followed by Tukey post-hoc test was used to detect significant differences between the desensitizer groups. The effect of aging condition was analyzed by two-sample Student's t-test.

3. Results

3.1. Shear Bond Strength and Failure Mode

Means and standard deviations of SBS values at 24 h and six months aging are shown in Figure 2. At 24 h, the only statistically significant difference detected was for the comparison between Gluma® Desensitizer and Soothe® SDI ($p = 0.049$). When compared to the control, none of the desensitizers showed statistically significant differences ($p > 0.05$). The highest value was observed for Gluma® Desensitizer (7.8 ± 0.99), while the lowest was for Soothe® SDI (5.95 ± 1.26). At six months, the lowest SBS value was obtained for the Nano P® desensitizer group (3.23 ± 0.73 MPa) and the highest value was observed for Gluma® Desensitizer (4.55 ± 0.62). However, the only statistically significant difference in SBS at six months was found between Gluma® and Nano P® ($p = 0.033$). The comparisons of the SBS values after 24 h and six months of aging by Student's t-test showed statistically significant differences in the SBS means between all the groups ($p < 0.05$) (Figure 3). The failure mode in all study groups was adhesive (Figure 4).

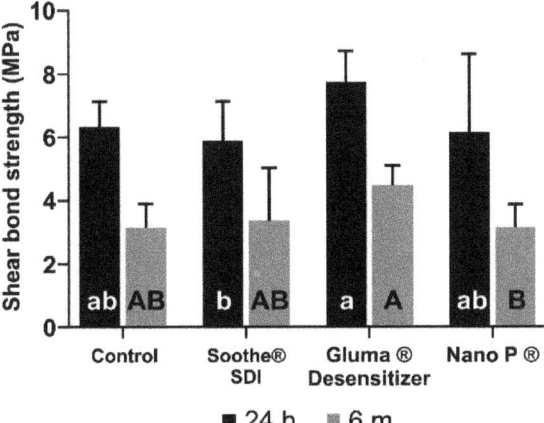

Figure 2. Shear bond strength for study groups (surface treatment and aging times). The same lowercase letters indicate no difference between desensitizers at 24 h. The same uppercase letters indicate no difference between desensitizers at 6 months.

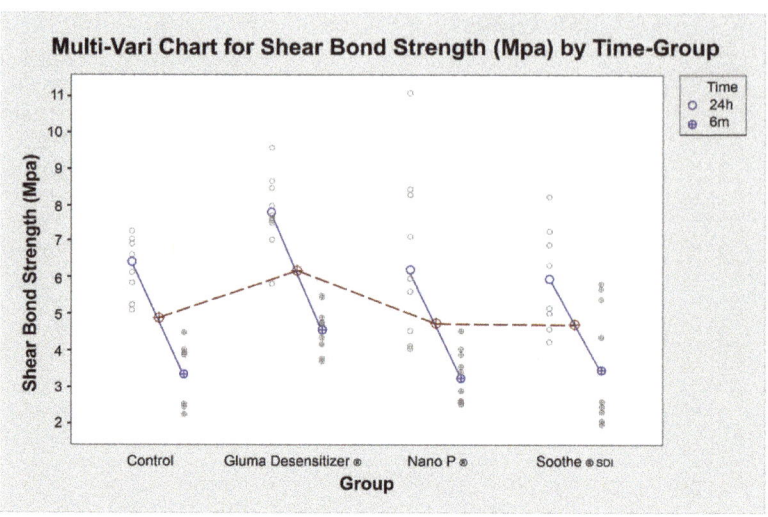

Figure 3. Shear bond strength (MPa) values at 24 h and 6 months. Red circles indicate mean for both aging times.

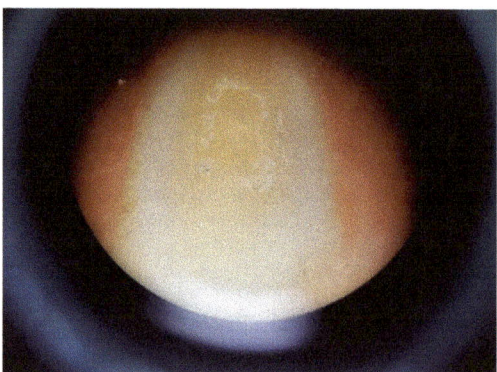

Figure 4. Representative image of the adhesive failure mode of the specimens.

3.2. Contact Angle

Contact angle measurements are shown in Figure 5. Differences in water contact angle were not statistically significant among the study groups ($p = 0.450$).

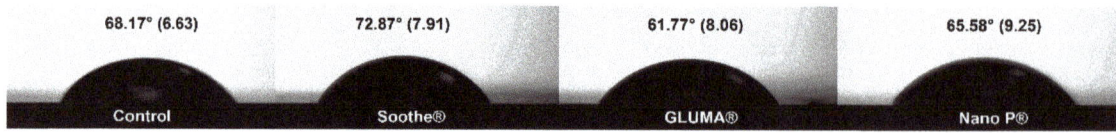

Figure 5. Water contact angle [Mean ± (SD)] for dentin surfaces treated with the desensitizer agents.

4. Discussion

In this study, the immediate and long-term SBS of a SARC to bovine dentin after application of different desensitizers was evaluated. The results suggest that the use of the desensitizers had no influence on the SBS. Therefore, the hypothesis that the application of desensitizers will not affect the immediate or long-term SBS of a SARC was not rejected.

It has been previously reported that the SBS of resin cements depends on several factors, such as the type of dentin (coronal, apical, caries-affected, and sclerotic), preparation depth (superficial or close to the pulp), and tooth surface management [20–23]. For SARCs, no conditioning of dentin with a bonding agent is needed. Therefore, the surface properties of the tooth substrates play an important role in adequate adhesion. Actually, the adhesion of SARC to dentin and several restorative materials are acceptable and comparable to other multi-step resin cements, but the adhesion to enamel seems to be a weak link in regard to their bonding properties. These cements are characterized by the presence of hydrophilic acidic monomers that bind directly to the wet dentin surface [16]. Their ability to adhere to dental structures mainly depends on the monomer infiltration into the tissues and the formation of a resin-infiltrated layer [16], which also depends on the presence of hydroxyapatite to adhere to the dental structures [12,14].

Considering that desensitizers can alter the characteristics of the dentin surface, it could be hypothesized that they have also the potential to alter the SBS of SARCs. A limited number of studies have evaluated the impact of the desensitizers on self-adhesive resin-dentin interface, reporting contradictory results [24–28]. For example, Stawarczyk, et al. [25] and Sailer et al. [24] reported that the application of Gluma Desensitizer had a positive effect on the bond strength of SARCs to dentin. On the other hand, Külünk et al. reported that desensitizing agents containing sodium and calcium fluoride reduced the bond strength of an adhesive resin cement to dentin [18]. The results from the present study showed that both immediate and long-term SBS of a SARC to dentin were unaffected by the prior application of the desensitizers. These results can be explained in part by the mechanism of action of the desensitizers used in this study. Desensitizers act through dentinal tubules occlusion. While Gluma® depends on the protein precipitation on the dentinal tubules [29–31], Soothe® SDI and Nano P® desensitizers act by forming fluoride compounds precipitates, forming an impermeable film that prevents access to external stimuli, sealing the exposed dentinal tubules [32]. In fact, these mechanisms are responsible for the differences found between Gluma® and Soothe® SDI, as it has been proved that fluor could decrease the bond strength of self-adhesive materials [33]. The present study reveals that, irrespectively of the mechanism of action, the desensitizers could not compromise the bond strength of a SARC to dentin [25]. It has been previously demonstrated that, apart from the fact that SARCs demonstrate limited decalcification/diffusion into dentin [12], the cements thixotropic properties (when applied under pressure) are important to enable SARCs to spread across the entire adhered surface and to establish adhesion [34].

In this study, bond strength values were also tested after storing the specimens for six months to verify the long-term performance of tested materials. In this study, irrespectively of the desensitizer used, SBS of the self-adhesive cement to dentin was statistically lower after six months of aging. This reduction can be explained by the higher hydrophilicity and hygroscopic expansion stress that these materials present [14]. The higher hydrophilicity observed for these materials could be due to the presence of acidic monomers within its composition [35]. Moreover, water sorption of the hydrophilic components of these cements could also accelerate the degradation of ester bonds of some of the resin monomer components, which may have an effect on their mechanical properties, dimensional stability, and biocompatibility, thereby inducing a reduction in the SBS [35]. Moreover, hydrolysis of the adhesive resin layer of self-etch materials has been observed in vitro after water storage, the resulted degradation may be caused by areas of imperfect bonding that are more prone to fluid ingress, and this should be considered during restorative material development. [36]. The composition, the degree of double bond conversion, and the length of the polymer network of these SARCs are related to their physical and mechanical properties. Hence, the effects of the presence of water may affect these properties [37]. The study comparing self-cured and dual-mode SARCs showed equal to slightly inferior flexural and compressive strength of abovementioned materials to other resin cements. The dual-cure cements were slightly stronger than the self-cure cements at 24 h, but when retested after 150-day water storage, there was no difference between the two. This is possibly because the dual-curing cement showed a significant reduction in both flexural and compressive strength after aging [38]. In another investigation where the long-term bond between dual-curing cementing agents was evaluated, it was concluded that dual-curing cementing agents achieve higher bond strength values when light activation is used during polymerization than without light activation [39]. In addition, it could be speculated that, due to the acidic nature of these materials, a limited availability of free radicals and poor polymerization of the material could affect its ability to resist the hydrolytic degradation [40].

It should be highlighted that failure mode analysis revealed that 100% of the failures observed were adhesives. Previous study analyzed the fracture surfaces between SARC and dentin, demonstrating that most of the fails were of the adhesive type [41]. It has been previously stated that the failure mode determines the performance of the applied adhesive systems [42], and in the case of self-adhesive systems, the most likely reason for this behavior is that self-adhesive cements are not aggressive enough to etch beyond the smear layer, thereby severely limiting its mechanical interaction with the dentin [34]. The interface between two dissimilar materials, namely the SARC and the dentin, may be affected by several factors, including contaminants from the operatory field, equipment, or adsorbed environmental contaminants, possibly resulting in a failure location. Under these conditions, water may penetrate the restoration either between and/or through materials, reducing the interaction between the cement and the dentin. Moreover, residual stresses from polymerization kinetics may also disrupt an adhesive bond or limit its durability [43]. This may be the reason why SARCs fractured mainly between resin and enamel or dentin surface and the SBS of SARCs was inferior compared to conventional composite resin cements [44].

Changes in the wetting of the dentin surface by the prior application of desensitizers were evaluated by contact angle measurement [45]. Results of the statistical analysis revealed that the water contact angle of dentin was not modified after the application of the different desensitizers. It has been stated that the bond strength between the dentin and the SARC depends on the characteristics and wettability of the adhered surface [46]. Moreover, sealing and bonding characteristics of SARCs mainly depend on their high wettability, which resulted in low microleakage scores at both the cavosurface enamel and dentin surface margins when used as a liner in class II composite restorations [47]. Considering this, the absence of differences in the SBS values observed in this study can be fully explained by this characteristic.

Limitations of the present study include the in vitro design and the fact that only three desensitizers were tested. Further studies are needed to evaluate if these SARCs can adhere to a variety of different substrates, in addition to dentin and enamel, e.g., porcelain and other ceramics, gold, and other metal alloys, as well as indirect composite resins. Moreover, Hardan et al., proved that the use of dentin desensitizer impaired both immediate and aged bond strength [48]. Thus, the effect of the application of these desensitizer agents on demineralized dentin should be evaluated. Additionally, it would be interesting to assess the surface characteristics and the chemical composition after application of different desensitizers (i.e., scanning electron microscopy-energy dispersive X-ray spectroscopy). Moreover, other desensitizing agents and resin cements should be evaluated. Additionally, clinical studies are required to evaluate the performance of these materials in the short and long-term and thus also to evaluate the desensitizing effect and its interaction with SARCs, and in this way to evaluate its limitations and its clinical implications.

5. Conclusions

Within the limitations of the present study, it can be concluded that the application of the different types of desensitizers had no significant influence on the SBS of SARCs to dentin. Therefore, this study suggests that the use of these desensitizers before the cementation of indirect restorations with a self-adhesive cement is reliable.

Author Contributions: Conceptualization, C.P.I., A.E.-H., M.L.-S., R.B. and L.H.; methodology, A.E.-H., C.P.I., C.E.C.-S. and L.H.; software, A.E.-H., M.L.-S., R.B., L.H. and C.E.C.-S.; validation, L.H., R.B., A.S., P.P., E.P., C.E.C.-S., C.P.I. and W.D.; formal analysis, R.B., A.G.M., L.H. and C.E.C.-S.; investigation, P.P., J.E.Z.-C., L.H., R.B., C.E.C.-S. and E.P.; resources, L.H., R.B., A.G.M., A.S. and W.D.; data curation, J.E.Z.-C., L.H., R.B., C.E.C.-S., C.P.I., A.G.M. and E.P.; writing—original draft preparation, A.E.-H., L.H., R.B., E.P., C.P.I., M.L.-S. and C.E.C.-S.; writing—review and editing, L.H. and E.P.; visualization, A.E.-H., L.H., R.B., E.P., C.P.I., M.L.-S., A.G.M. and C.E.C.-S.; supervision, L.H. and C.E.C.-S.; project administration, L.H. All authors have read and agreed to the published version of the manuscript.

Funding: This research received no external funding.

Institutional Review Board Statement: Not applicable.

Informed Consent Statement: Not applicable.

Data Availability Statement: The data presented in this study are available on request from the corresponding author.

Conflicts of Interest: The authors declare no conflict of interest.

References

1. Demirtag, Z.; Uzgur, R.; Turkal, M.; Uzgur, Z.; Colak, H.; Özcan, M. A Survey on Prevalence, Causes and Prevention of Postcementation Hypersensitivity. *Eur. J. Prosthodont. Restor. Dent.* **2016**, *24*, 158–163. [PubMed]
2. Liu, X.-X.; Tenenbaum, H.C.; Wilder, R.S.; Quock, R.; Hewlett, E.R.; Ren, Y.-F. Pathogenesis, Diagnosis and Management of Dentin Hypersensitivity: An Evidence-Based Overview for Dental Practitioners. *BMC Oral Health* **2020**, *20*, 220. [CrossRef] [PubMed]
3. Kim, J.W.; Park, J.-C. Dentin Hypersensitivity and Emerging Concepts for Treatments. *J. Oral Biosci.* **2017**, *59*, 211–217. [CrossRef]
4. Brännström, M. The Hydrodynamic Theory of Dentinal Pain: Sensation in Preparations, Caries, and the Dentinal Crack Syndrome. *J. Endod.* **1986**, *12*, 453–457. [CrossRef]
5. Orsini, G.; Procaccini, M.; Manzoli, L.; Giuliodori, F.; Lorenzini, A.; Putignano, A. A double-blind randomized-controlled trial comparing the desensitizing efficacy of a new dentifrice containing carbonate/hydroxyapatite nanocrystals and a sodium fluoride/potassium nitrate dentifrice. *J. Clin. Periodontol.* **2010**, *37*, 510–517. [CrossRef]
6. Marto, C.M.; Baptista Paula, A.; Nunes, T.; Pimenta, M.; Abrantes, A.M.; Pires, A.S.; Laranjo, M.; Coelho, A.; Donato, H.; Botelho, M.F. Evaluation of the Efficacy of Dentin Hypersensitivity Treatments—A Systematic Review and Follow-up Analysis. *J. Oral Rehabil.* **2019**, *46*, 952–990. [CrossRef]
7. Douglas-de-Oliveira, D.W.; Vitor, G.P.; Silveira, J.O.; Martins, C.C.; Costa, F.O.; Cota, L.O.M. Effect of Dentin Hypersensitivity Treatment on Oral Health Related Quality of Life—A Systematic Review and Meta-Analysis. *J. Dent.* **2018**, *71*, 1–8. [CrossRef]
8. Moraschini, V.; da Costa, L.S.; Dos Santos, G.O. Effectiveness for Dentin Hypersensitivity Treatment of Non-Carious Cervical Lesions: A Meta-Analysis. *Clin. Oral Investig.* **2018**, *22*, 617–631. [CrossRef]
9. Kielbassa, A.M.; Attin, T.; Hellwig, E.; Schade-Brittinger, C. In Vivo Study on the Effectiveness of a Lacquer Containing CaF_2/NaF in Treating Dentine Hypersensitivity. *Clin. Oral Investig.* **1997**, *1*, 95–99. [CrossRef]
10. Yilmaz, H.G.; Kurtulmus-Yilmaz, S.; Cengiz, E. Long-Term Effect of Diode Laser Irradiation Compared to Sodium Fluoride Varnish in the Treatment of Dentine Hypersensitivity in Periodontal Maintenance Patients: A Randomized Controlled Clinical Study. *Photomed. Laser Surg.* **2011**, *29*, 721–725. [CrossRef]
11. Hardan, L.; Devoto, W.; Bourgi, R.; Cuevas-Suárez, C.E.; Lukomska-Szymanska, M.; Fernández-Barrera, M.Á.; Cornejo-Ríos, E.; Monteiro, P.; Zarow, M.; Jakubowicz, N.; et al. Immediate Dentin Sealing for Adhesive Cementation of Indirect Restorations: A Systematic Review and Meta-Analysis. *Gels* **2022**, *8*, 175. [CrossRef] [PubMed]
12. Monticelli, F.; Osorio, R.; Mazzitelli, C.; Ferrari, M.; Toledano, M. Limited Decalcification/Diffusion of Self-Adhesive Cements into Dentin. *J. Dent. Res.* **2008**, *87*, 974–979. [CrossRef] [PubMed]
13. Pedreira, A.P.R.d.V.; D'Alpino, P.H.P.; Pereira, P.N.R.; Chaves, S.B.; Wang, L.; Hilgert, L.; Garcia, F.C.P. Effects of the Application Techniques of Self-Adhesive Resin Cements on the Interfacial Integrity and Bond Strength of Fiber Posts to Dentin. *J. Appl. Oral Sci.* **2016**, *24*, 437–446. [CrossRef]
14. Ferracane, J.L.; Stansbury, J.; Burke, F.J.T. Self-adhesive Resin Cements–Chemistry, Properties and Clinical Considerations. *J. Oral Rehabil.* **2011**, *38*, 295–314. [CrossRef] [PubMed]
15. Gerth, H.U.; Dammaschke, T.; Züchner, H.; Schäfer, E. Chemical Analysis and Bonding Reaction of RelyX Unicem and Bifix Composites—A Comparative Study. *Dent. Mater.* **2006**, *22*, 934–941. [CrossRef]
16. Radovic, I.; Monticelli, F.; Goracci, C.; Vulicevic, Z.R.; Ferrari, M. Self-Adhesive Resin Cements: A Literature Review. *J. Adhes. Dent.* **2008**, *10*, 251–258.
17. *ISO/TS 11405*; Dental Materials—Testing of Adhesion to Tooth Structure. International Organization for Standardization: London, UK, 2003.

18. Külünk, Ş.; Sarac, D.; Külünk, T.; Karakaş, Ö. The Effects of Different Desensitizing Agents on the Shear Bond Strength of Adhesive Resin Cement to Dentin. *J. Esthet. Restor. Dent.* **2011**, *23*, 380–387. [CrossRef]
19. Armstrong, S.; Breschi, L.; Özcan, M.; Pfefferkorn, F.; Ferrari, M.; Van Meerbeek, B. Academy of Dental Materials Guidance on in Vitro Testing of Dental Composite Bonding Effectiveness to Dentin/Enamel Using Micro-Tensile Bond Strength (MTBS) Approach. *Dent. Mater.* **2017**, *33*, 133–143. [CrossRef]
20. Tay, F.R.; Pashley, D.H. Resin Bonding to Cervical Sclerotic Dentin: A Review. *J. Dent.* **2004**, *32*, 173–196. [CrossRef]
21. Tay, F.R.; Nawareg, M.A.; Abuelenain, D.; Pashley, D.H. Cervical Sclerotic Dentin: Resin Bonding. In *Understanding Dental Caries*; Goldberg, M., Ed.; Springer: Berlin/Heidelberg, Germany, 2016; pp. 97–125.
22. Tan, Y.; Gu, M.; Li, W.; Guo, L. Effect of a Filled Adhesive as the Desensitizer on Bond Strength of "Self-Adhesive Cements to" Differently Severity of Fluorosed Dentin. *Microsc. Res. Tech.* **2018**, *81*, 805–815. [CrossRef]
23. Uğur, M.; Altıntaş, S.H. Evaluation of Different Desensitizing Agents Effect on Shear Bond Strength of Adhesive Resin Cement to Dentin. *J. Adhes. Sci. Technol.* **2019**, *33*, 1695–1704. [CrossRef]
24. Sailer, I.; Oendra, A.E.H.; Stawarczyk, B.; Hämmerle, C.H. The Effects of Desensitizing Resin, Resin Sealing, and Provisional Cement on the Bond Strength of Dentin Luted with Self-Adhesive and Conventional Resincements. *J. Prosthet. Dent.* **2012**, *107*, 252–260. [CrossRef]
25. Stawarczyk, B.; Hartmann, R.; Hartmann, L.; Roos, M.; Özcan, M.; Sailer, I.; Hämmerle, C.H. The Effect of Dentin Desensitizer on Shear Bond Strength of Conventional and Self-Adhesive Resin Luting Cements after Aging. *Oper. Dent.* **2011**, *36*, 492–501. [CrossRef]
26. Acar, O.; Tuncer, D.; Yuzugullu, B.; Celik, C. The Effect of Dentin Desensitizers and Nd: YAG Laser Pre-Treatment on Microtensile Bond Strength of Self-Adhesive Resin Cement to Dentin. *J. Adv. Prosthodont.* **2014**, *6*, 88–95. [CrossRef] [PubMed]
27. Dewan, H.; Sayed, M.E.; Alqahtani, N.M.; Alnajai, T.; Qasir, A.; Chohan, H. The Effect of Commercially Available Desensitizers on Bond Strength Following Cementation of Zirconia Crowns Using Self-Adhesive Resin Cement—An in Vitro Study. *Materials* **2022**, *15*, 514. [CrossRef] [PubMed]
28. Huh, J.-B.; Kim, J.-H.; Chung, M.-K.; Lee, H.; Choi, Y.-G.; Shim, J.-S. The Effect of Several Dentin Desensitizers on Shear Bond Strength of Adhesive Resin Luting Cement Using Self-Etching Primer. *J. Dent.* **2008**, *36*, 1025–1032. [CrossRef]
29. Schupbach, P.; Lutz, F.; Finger, W. Closing of Dentinal Tubules by Gluma Desensitizer. *Eur. J. Oral Sci.* **1997**, *105*, 414–421. [CrossRef]
30. Garcia, R.N.; Giannini, M.; Takagaki, T.; Sato, T.; Matsui, N.; Nikaido, T.; Tagami, J. Effect of Dentin Desensitizers on Resin Cement Bond Strengths. *RSBO* **2015**, *12*, 14–22. [CrossRef]
31. Lawaf, S.; Jalalian, E.; Roshan, R.; Azizi, A. Effect of GLUMA Desensitizer on the Retention of Full Metal Crowns Cemented with Rely X U200 Self-Adhesive Cement. *J. Adv. Prosthodont.* **2016**, *8*, 404–410. [CrossRef]
32. Kolker, J.L.; Vargas, M.A.; Armstrong, S.R.; Dawson, D.V. Effect of Desensitizing Agents on Dentin Permeability and Dentin Tubule Occlusion. *J. Adhes. Dent.* **2002**, *4*, 211–222.
33. Nakamoto, A.; Sato, T.; Matsui, N.; Ikeda, M.; Nikaido, T.; Burrow, M.F.; Tagami, J. Effect of Fluoride Mouthrinse and Fluoride Concentration on Bonding of a One-Step Self-Etch Adhesive to Bovine Root Dentin. *J. Oral Sci.* **2019**, *61*, 125–132. [CrossRef] [PubMed]
34. De Munck, J.; Vargas, M.; Van Landuyt, K.; Hikita, K.; Lambrechts, P.; Van Meerbeek, B. Bonding of an Auto-Adhesive Luting Material to Enamel and Dentin. *Dent. Mater.* **2004**, *20*, 963–971. [CrossRef] [PubMed]
35. Ferracane, J.L. Hygroscopic and Hydrolytic Effects in Dental Polymer Networks. *Dent. Mater.* **2006**, *22*, 211–222. [CrossRef] [PubMed]
36. Hashimoto, M. A Review—Micromorphological Evidence of Degradation in Resin-dentin Bonds and Potential Preventional Solutions. *J. Biomed. Mater. Res. Part B Appl. Biomater.* **2010**, *92*, 268–280. [CrossRef]
37. Takenaka, H.; Ouchi, H.; Sai, K.; Kawamoto, R.; Murayama, R.; Kurokawa, H.; Miyazaki, M. Ultrasonic Measurement of the Effects of Light Irradiation and Presence of Water on the Polymerization of Self-adhesive Resin Cement. *Eur. J. Oral Sci.* **2015**, *123*, 369–374. [CrossRef] [PubMed]
38. Piwowarczyk, A.; Lauer, H.-C. Mechanical Properties of Luting Cements after Water Storage. *Oper. Dent. Univ. Wash.* **2003**, *28*, 535–542.
39. Piwowarczyk, A.; Bender, R.; Ottl, P.; Lauer, H.-C. Long-Term Bond between Dual-Polymerizing Cementing Agents and Human Hard Dental Tissue. *Dent. Mater.* **2007**, *23*, 211–217. [CrossRef]
40. Mendes, L.C.; Matos, I.C.; Miranda, M.S.; Benzi, M.R. Dual-Curing, Self-Adhesive Resin Cement: Influence of the Polymerization Modes on the Degree of Conversion and Microhardness. *Mater. Res.* **2010**, *13*, 171–176. [CrossRef]
41. Hikita, K.; Van Meerbeek, B.; De Munck, J.; Ikeda, T.; Van Landuyt, K.; Maida, T.; Lambrechts, P.; Peumans, M. Bonding Effectiveness of Adhesive Luting Agents to Enamel and Dentin. *Dent. Mater.* **2007**, *23*, 71–80. [CrossRef]
42. Mecholsky Jr, J.J. Modes of Failure of Bonding Interfaces in Dentistry. *Fractography Glasses Ceram. VI* **2012**, *230*, 193.
43. Armstrong, S.; Keller, J.; Boyer, D. Mode of Failure in the Dentin-Adhesive Resin–Resin Composite Bonded Joint as Determined by Strength-Based (MTBS) and Fracture-Based (CNSB) Mechanical Testing. *Dent. Mater.* **2001**, *17*, 201–210. [CrossRef]
44. Lührs, A.-K.; Guhr, S.; Günay, H.; Geurtsen, W. Shear Bond Strength of Self-Adhesive Resins Compared to Resin Cements with Etch and Rinse Adhesives to Enamel and Dentin in Vitro. *Clin. Oral Investig.* **2010**, *14*, 193–199. [CrossRef] [PubMed]

45. Wege, H.A.; Aguilar, J.A.; Rodríguez-Valverde, M.Á.; Toledano, M.; Osorio, R.; Cabrerizo-Vílchez, M.Á. Dynamic Contact Angle and Spreading Rate Measurements for the Characterization of the Effect of Dentin Surface Treatments. *J. Colloid Interface Sci.* **2003**, *263*, 162–169. [CrossRef]
46. Asmussen, E.; Peutzfeldt, A.; Sahafi, A. Bonding of Resin Cements to Post Materials: Influence of Surface Energy Characteristics. *J. Adhes. Dent.* **2005**, *7*, 231–234. [PubMed]
47. Al-Saleh, M.; El-Mowafy, O.; Tam, L.; Fenton, A. Microleakage of Posterior Composite Restorations Lined with Self-Adhesive Resin Cements. *Oper. Dent.* **2010**, *35*, 556–563. [CrossRef] [PubMed]
48. Hardan, L.; Bourgi, R.; Kharouf, N.; Mancino, D.; Zarow, M.; Jakubowicz, N.; Haikel, Y.; Cuevas-Suárez, C.E. Bond Strength of Universal Adhesives to Dentin: A Systematic Review and Meta-Analysis. *Polymers* **2021**, *13*, 814. [CrossRef]

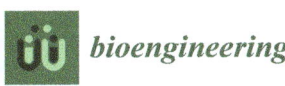

Systematic Review

Treatment of Tooth Wear Using Direct or Indirect Restorations: A Systematic Review of Clinical Studies

Louis Hardan [1], Davide Mancino [2,3,4], Rim Bourgi [1], Carlos Enrique Cuevas-Suárez [5,*], Monika Lukomska-Szymanska [6], Maciej Zarow [7], Natalia Jakubowicz [7], Juan Eliezer Zamarripa-Calderón [5], Laura Kafa [8], Olivier Etienne [2,4,9], François Reitzer [2,3,4], Naji Kharouf [2,3,*] and Youssef Haïkel [2,3,4]

1. Department of Restorative Dentistry, School of Dentistry, Saint-Joseph University, Beirut 11072180, Lebanon; louis.hardan@usj.edu.lb (L.H.); rim.bourgi@net.usj.edu.lb (R.B.)
2. Department of Biomaterials and Bioengineering, INSERM UMR_S 1121, Biomaterials and Bioengineering, 67000 Strasbourg, France; endodontiefrancaise@outlook.com (D.M.); olivier.etienne@unistra.fr (O.E.); f.reitzer@gmail.com (F.R.); youssef.haikel@unistra.fr (Y.H.)
3. Department of Endodontics, Faculty of Dental Medicine, Strasbourg University, 67000 Strasbourg, France
4. Pôle de Médecine et Chrirugie Bucco-Dentaire, Hôpital Civil, Hôpitaux Universitaires de Strasbourg, 67000 Strasbourg, France
5. Dental Materials Laboratory, Academic Area of Dentistry, Autonomous University of Hidalgo State, Circuito Ex Hacienda La Concepción S/N, San Agustín Tlaxiaca 42160, Mexico; eliezerz@uaeh.edu.mx
6. Department of Restorative Dentistry, Medical University of Lodz, 251 Pomorska St., 92-213 Lodz, Poland; monika.lukomska-szymanska@umed.lodz.pl
7. "NZOZ SPS Dentist" Dental Clinic and Postgraduate Course Centre, pl. Inwalidow 7/5, 30-033 Cracow, Poland; dentist@dentist.com.pl (M.Z.); nljakubowicz@gmail.com (N.J.)
8. Department of Oral Medicine, Faculty of Dentistry, Tishreen University, Lattakia 0100, Syria; laurakafa@gmail.com
9. Department of Prosthetic, Faculty of Dental Medicine, Strasbourg University, 67000 Strasbourg, France
* Correspondence: cecuevas@uaeh.edu.mx (C.E.C.-S.); dentistenajikharouf@gmail.com (N.K.); Tel.: +52-177172000 (C.E.C.-S.); +33-66752-2841 (N.K.)

Abstract: Tooth wear is considered a well-developed issue in daily clinical practice; however, there is no standard protocol for treatment. The aim of this manuscript was to systematically review the literature to evaluate the clinical outcomes of direct or indirect restorations for treating tooth wear. A literature search was conducted through the PubMed MedLine, Scopus, ISI Web of Science, Scielo, and EMBASE databases up to 29 April 2022. Clinical studies evaluating the clinical performance of direct or indirect restorations for treating tooth wear for a minimum follow-up of 6 months were included in the review. A total of 2776 records were obtained from the search databases. After full-text reading, 16 studies were included in the qualitative analysis. Considering the high heterogenicity of the studies included, a meta-analysis could not be performed. All studies included the rehabilitation of anterior and posterior teeth with extensive wear, using both indirect and direct restorations for a maximum follow-up of 10 years. Restoration materials included ceramo-metal crowns, full gold crowns, lithium disilicate ceramic, zirconia, polymer infiltrated ceramic networks, and resin composites. Most of the reports assessed the survival rate of the restorations and the clinical features using the United States Public Health Service (USPHS) Evaluation System criteria. Contradictory discoveries were perceived concerning the type of restoration with better clinical performance. Considering the current literature available, there is no evidence in the superiority of any restoration technique to ensure the highest clinical performance for treating tooth wear.

Keywords: crowns; fixed prosthodontics; resin composite; survival

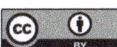

1. Introduction

Currently, tooth wear, defined as a simple loss of dental substance, is considered a well-developed issue in daily clinical practice [1,2]. Progressive tooth wear with large zones of exposed dentinal surface is a restorative drawback for older patients who want to maintain their remaining dental structure. Usually, conventional restorative techniques for these patients include costly dental laboratory-fabricated crowns and fixed prostheses as a full-mouth rehabilitation [3].

In general, tooth wear, an irreversible non-carious loss of tooth structure, is an effect of diverse mechanisms, such as a dissolution by means of acidic substances of hard tissues (erosion), an interaction with exogenous materials (abrasion), or tooth-to-tooth contact (attrition) [4]. These mechanisms of tooth wear frequently act chronologically or in synchrony, which can enhance extreme tooth wear at a somewhat young age [5]. This circumstance creates plentiful problems, such as changes in vertical dimension of occlusion with possible functional deficiency, increased tooth hypersensitivity, pulp involvement, and perhaps diminished esthetic appearance [6]. Essentially, several factors, such as pain, speech, chewing ability, taste, and esthetics could affect aspects of patient quality of life [7]. The multiple factors of tooth wear and its associated restorative process are difficult for dental practitioners, as a multifaceted holistic rehabilitation program is needed that addresses changes in the occlusal surface [8].

Several approaches have been designated in the literature to rehabilitate a worn dentition by means of direct composite restorations [9–14], indirect restorations of lithium disilicate [15], composite resin [16], polymer infiltrated ceramic networks [17,18], and combined techniques [19–21]. However, the accessible clinical recommendations for any restorative method of worn dentition were quite limited, and a systematic review was not available on which techniques and materials are favored [22]. Most of the studies used direct or indirect resin composites to restore specifically worn anterior teeth and had stated failure rates of nearly 10% [16,23,24]. It is worth mentioning that failure rate, defined as the frequency at which a restoration fails, is exceptionally high when treating dental wear.

Preventive procedures and measures for advocating and examining tooth wear need to be in place before the initiation of any restorative procedure [12,25]. Worn dentition must be treated with a reversible, adhesive, additive method whenever achievable [26]. Nevertheless, patients frequently seek solutions when tooth wear has progressed significantly [27], and, in certain circumstances, prosthetic rehabilitation might be required.

The multifactorial assessment regarding severe tooth wear must be established based on its severity as well as the patient's needs [28]. This assessment is not regularly done because the remaining tooth structure and the impact of persistent mechanical and chemical processes influences the performance of the restoration [7,29,30]. Because using composite resin could lead to a fracture and amplify the long lasting costs [16,31], a full crown persists as the chosen treatment [31], and metal–ceramic restorations are the average treatment for fixed partial dentures and crowns [32]. The drawback of metal–ceramic restorations is the grayish discoloration at the gingival margin. High-strength ceramic constituents such as lithium disilicate and zirconia have been developed and become popular due to their biocompatibility [33,34]. Compared to multilayer restorations, monolithic restorations are thinner, need less reduction of the tooth surface [35], and do not chip [36].

So far, there is no standard protocol for the treatment of individuals with tooth wear. Thus, the aim of this paper was to systematically review the literature to evaluate the clinical outcomes of direct or indirect restorations for treating tooth wear.

2. Materials and Methods

This review was implemented in agreement with the PRISMA 2020 instructions [37]. The registration protocol was carried out in Open Science Framework with the registration number 0000-0002-2759-8984. The following PICOS framework was used: population, dental substrate; intervention, indirect restorations; control, direct restorations; outcomes, Federation Dentaire Internationale (FDI) or United States Public Health Service (USPHS) criteria; and study design, clinical trials. The research question was: "What is the best treatment for treating tooth wear: direct or indirect restorations?"

2.1. Literature Search

A literature search was directed through the PubMed MedLine, Scopus, ISI Web of Science, Scielo, and EMBASE databases up to 29 April 2022. The search strategy performed in PubMed, which was adjusted for the other databases, is summarized in Table 1. The researchers manually patterned the list of references of each manuscript for the search of additional manuscripts. After the search, the papers were entered into Mendeley Desktop 1.17.11 software (Glyph & Cog, LLC, London, UK) to remove duplicates and then exported to the Rayyan web platform.

Table 1. Search strategy used in PubMed.

#1	Tooth Wear OR Tooth erosion OR Tooth attrition OR Dental Wear
#2	Restoration OR Direct Restoration OR Composite OR Resin Composite OR Composite Resin OR Dental Composite OR Resin Based Composite OR Composite Dental Resin OR Fillings OR Indirect Restoration OR Partial Restorations OR Posterior Partial Crowns OR Full-Coverage Restoration OR Ceramic OR Bonded OR Partial Preparations OR Indirect Bonded Restorations OR Porcelain OR Ceramic Veneer OR Overlay OR Inlay OR Onlay
#3	Clinical Trials OR Controlled Clinical Trial OR Retrospective Studies OR Randomized Controlled Trial OR Randomized Controlled Trials OR Prospective Clinical Trial OR Retrospective Study OR Prospective Studies OR Prospective Study OR Clinical Trial OR Randomized Clinical Trial OR Random Allocation OR Double-Blind Method OR Single-Blind Method OR Clinical Trial OR Clinical Trials OR Follow-up Studies OR Prospective Studies OR Cross-over Studies
#4	#1 and #2 and #3

2.2. Study Selection

Two investigators (L.H. and R.B.) evaluated the abstracts and titles of all the articles using the blind mode on the Rayyan platform. Studies for full-text review were chosen based on the following eligibility criteria: (1) clinical studies assessing the clinical performance of direct or indirect restorations for treating tooth wear; (2) included a follow-up for at least 6 months; and (3) available in the English language. In vitro reports, case series, reviews, pilot studies, and case reports were omitted. Full versions of any possible reports were examined. Papers that had insufficient data in the abstract and title to offer a clear judgment were considered for full-text evaluation. The inter-examiner agreement was measured using the kappa coefficient. Any variations in the decision-making procedure in regard to the appropriateness of the accepted manuscripts was agreed and decided upon through the accord of a third author (C.E.C.-S.). Only texts that fulfilled all of the eligibility norms were incorporated for assessment.

2.3. Data Extraction

The information of interest from the papers selected was tabulated using a standardized sheet in a Microsoft Office Excel 2019 spreadsheet (Microsoft Corporation, Redmond, WA, USA). These data included type of clinical trial, number of the participants, reasons for tooth wear, restoration techniques used, follow-up, clinical criteria for evaluation, and main conclusion (Table 2).

2.4. Quality Assessment

The methodological quality of each included articles was individually evaluated by two reviewers (R.B. and L.H.) based on the Cochrane guidelines for the description of the subsequent parameters: selection bias (sequence generation and allocation concealment), performance and detection bias (blinding of operators or participants and personnel), bias due to incomplete data, reporting bias (selective reporting, unclear withdrawals, missing outcomes), and other bias (including industry sponsorship bias). A proposed judgement about the risk of bias arising from each domain was generated by an algorithm based on answers to the signaling questions. The aforementioned algorithm and the guidance on how to use it is available elsewhere [38]. Through risk of bias evaluation, any inconsistencies between the investigators were decided by a third reviewer (C.E.C.-S.).

3. Results

A total of 2776 records were obtained from the search databases. After removing the duplicates, the total amount of manuscripts found was 2443 publications for the primary examination. Of these, 2419 papers were excluded after reviewing the titles and abstracts, leaving 24 articles to be selected for full-text review. The inter-examiner agreement was excellent (kappa coefficient = 0.87). Of these, eight studies were excluded [12,14,39–44]. Exclusion reasons are shown in the PRISMA flow diagram of the review (Figure 1), which resulted in a total of 16 articles for the qualitative analysis [3,13,16,18,20,21,23,45–53]. Considering the high heterogeneity of the studies included, a meta-analysis could not be performed.

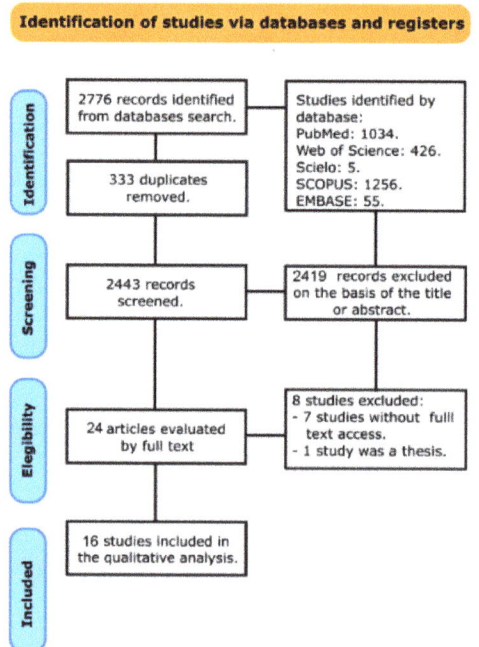

Figure 1. Flowchart according to the PRISMA statement.

The features of the manuscripts included in this review are summarized in Table 2. This review identified randomized clinical trials and observational studies. The maximum follow-up observed in the included studies was 10 years. All studies included the rehabilitation of anterior or posterior teeth with extensive wear using both indirect and direct restorations. Tooth wear was described to be mainly due to the presence of gastroesophageal reflux, excessive ingestion of acidic beverages, tooth grinding, abrasive restorative materials, vigorous labor, or exercise.

Restoration materials included ceramo-metal crowns, full gold crowns, lithium disilicate ceramic, zirconia, polymer infiltrated ceramic networks, and resin composites. The last were used as both indirect and direct techniques. Most of the studies evaluated the survival rate of the restorations and the clinical characteristics using the USPHS Evaluation System criteria.

Studying the methodological quality assessment parameters, most of the studies included were counted as having a high risk of bias (Table 3), as most of them failed to avoid performance and detection bias, reporting bias, and other bias.

Table 2. Qualitative analysis of the studies included.

Author and Year	Type of Clinical Trial	Number of Participants	Reason for Tooth Wear	Restoration Techniques Used	Follow-Up	Clinical Criteria for Evaluation	Main Conclusion
Bartlett 2006 [16]	Randomized clinical study	16 patients with severe tooth wear 13 controls without evidence of tooth wear	Mixture of bruxism and erosion	Direct or indirect microfilled resin composite restorations	3-year period	United States Public Health Service Evaluation System (USPHS) criteria	Using direct and indirect resin composites for fixing worn posterior teeth is contraindicated
Burian 2021 [49]	In-vivo study	Complex rehabilitations with deviations in vertical dimension of occlusion (VDO) 12 patients with severe tooth wear underwent prosthetic rehabilitation, restoring the VDO	Not described	Lithium disilicate ceramic (LS2) Experimental CAD/CAM polymer (COMP)	3-year period	Geomagic Qualify software (2 January 2012, Geomagic Inc., Morrisville, NC, USA) was used to compare resulting baseline and follow-up STL datasets.	LS2 presented less wear, yet tooth preparation was needed. Clinicians should balance well between required preparation invasiveness and long-term occlusal stability in patients with worn dentitions
Crins 2021 [48]	Randomized controlled trial	49 patients	Grinding/clenching and Gastro-Oesophageal Reflux Disease	Direct composite restorations (DRC) with micro-hybrid composite restorations (Clearfil AP-X, Kuraray) and nano-hybrid composite restorations (IPS Empress Direct, Ivoclar Vivadent) for buccal veneers indirect composite restorations with indirect palatal veneer restorations (Clearfil Estenia C&B, cemented with Panavia F, Kuraray)	3-year period	Functional (debond, fracture, adaptation, anatomy), Biological (caries, endodontic treatment) Esthetic conditions	Composite restorations showed superior behavior compared to the indirect composite restorations, when used in the molar region
Gresnigt 2019 [47]	Randomized split-mouth clinical trial	11 patients	Not described	48 indirect resin composite (Estenia) and ceramic laminate veneers (IPS Empress Esthetic)	10 years	USPHS criteria	Anterior ceramic laminate veneers might be favored over indirect composite laminate veneers
Hammoudi 2020 [46]	Randomized clinical trial	62 participants with extensive tooth wear	Mechanical (bruxism or engaged in vigorous labor or exercise), and chemical factors	713 lithium disilicate (LD) and translucent zirconia (TZ) crowns	65 months	USPHS criteria	The use of high-strength ceramic materials, as well as consistent adhesive bonding, are probably the key factors in the long-term success of ceramic crowns in participants with extensive tooth wear independent of the specific etiology

Table 2. Cont.

Author and Year	Type of Clinical Trial	Number of Participants	Reason for Tooth Wear	Restoration Techniques Used	Follow-Up	Clinical Criteria for Evaluation	Main Conclusion
Hemmings 2000 [23]	Clinical study	16 patients	Not described	52 restorations composed of Durafill composite and Scotchbond Multipurpose dentine adhesive system 52 Herculite XRV composite and Optibond dentine bonding agent	30 months	Loss Fracture Marginal discoloration Loss of marginal integrity Noticeable wear Pain or sensitivity Endodontic failure Esthetic failure	Direct composite restorations may be a treatment option for localized anterior tooth wear
Katsoulis 2011 [45]	Observational study	42 patients	High daily consumption of tough and acidic food, reflux problems, bulimia combined with clenching and grinding	48 full prosthodontic rehabilitation	3 years	Complete oral examination Photos Functional and cast analysis General health conditions and behavioral aspects	The rehabilitation of partially edentulous patients with severe tooth wear is a complex task, and more information regarding treatment protocols, prosthetic indications and treatment outcome is needed
da Rocha Scalzer Lopes 2021 [50]	Retrospective study with cross-sectional design	43 individuals	Not described	112 single crowns	120 months	Analysis parameters of morphological variations in tooth wear are indicated	Ceramic systems can be considered as alternatives of restorative material, even in individuals with clinical features evocative of chronic tooth wear
Mehta 2021 [52]	Prospective trial	34 participants	Chemical (erosion) and mechanical wear (bruxism) signs	Direct restorations using a micro-hybrid (Clearfil AP-X; Kuraray, Japan) and a nanohybrid (IPS Empress Direct; Ivoclar Vivadent, Schaan, Liechtenstein) composite	1 month and 1-, 3-, and 5-years, post-treatment	Presence or absence of any symptoms of pain, difficulty with phonetics and/or mastication, challenges with the adaption to the new VDO, or any TMJ-related concerns	Premolar restorations exposed lesser risks of failure compared to the molar restorations
Mehta 2021 (b) [51]	Prospective trial	34 participants	Chemical (erosion) and mechanical wear (bruxism) signs	Direct restorations using a micro-hybrid (Clearfil AP-X; Kuraray, Japan) and a nanohybrid (IPS Empress Direct; Ivoclar Vivadent, Schaan, Liechtenstein) composite	5.5 years	Presence or absence of any symptoms of pain, difficulty with phonetics and/or mastication, challenges with the adaption to the new VDO, or any TMJ-related concerns	Molar restorations, posterior mandibular restorations and the anterior restorations requiring two further sessions for completion, were associated with significantly higher risks for failure

Table 2. Cont.

Author and Year	Type of Clinical Trial	Number of Participants	Reason for Tooth Wear	Restoration Techniques Used	Follow-Up	Clinical Criteria for Evaluation	Main Conclusion
Milosevic 2016 [13]	Prospective trial	164 patients	Not described	Nano-particle hybrid composite material (Spectrum®; Dentsply, Weybridge, UK)	8 years	Failure of the restoration	The assessed failure rate in the first year was 5.4%. Time to failure was significantly greater in older subjects and when a deficiency of posterior support was present. Bruxism and an increase in the Occlusal Vertical Dimension were not associated with failure
Oudkerk 2020 [18]	Prospective trial	7 patients	Chemical (erosion) and mechanical wear (bruxism)	PICN blocks (Vita Enamic HT, Vita Zahnfabrik, Germany; Ceramill Motion 2, Amann Girrbach)	One month, six months, 1 year and 2 years	World Dental Federation	PICN restorations displayed elevated survival and success rates after two years
Redman 2003 [20]	Retrospective	31 subjects	Primarily erosion, Primarily attrition, Combined erosion/attrition	Microfilled (Durafill), hybrid (Herculite—97 direct and 18 indirect) composites, and 73 indirect 'ceromer' (Artglass)	5 years	Modified United States Public Health Services criteria	Placement of resin-based composite restorations to treat localised anterior tooth wear has worthy short to medium term survival
Smales 2007 [3]	Retrospective	25 patients	Tooth grinding, gastric and dietary acids, and abrasive restorative materials	Resin-based composites (RBC), indirect ceramo-metal crowns (CMCs), and full gold crowns		Survival rate	RBCs usually failed from fractures, and CMCs from complete losses. RBC failures were usually replaced or repaired, while CMC failures often required root canal therapies or extractions
Taubock 2021 [53]	Prospective trial	13 patients	Erosion-induced tooth wear and no signs of temporomandibular disorders	Microhybrid (first cohort; n = 59) or nanofilled (second cohort; n = 105) composite restorations	11 years	USPHS criteria	Direct composite restorations employed at an amplified vertical dimension of occlusion display suitable clinical long-term performance in patients presenting severe tooth wear
Vailati 2013 [21]	Prospective	12 patients	Presence of gastroesophageal reflux, excessive ingestion of acidic beverages	Direct and Indirect composite restorations (Miris, Coltène/Whaledent) and feldspathic ceramic veneers (Creation CC, Willi Geller International)	6 years	Modified United States Public Health Services criteria	Restoring compromised maxillary anterior teeth by means of veneers prevents excessive tooth structure removal and loss of tooth vitality

Table 3. Risk of bias for clinical trials.

Study and Year	Selection Bias	Performance and Detection Bias	Bias Due to Incomplete Data	Reporting Bias	Other Bias
Bartlett 2006 [16]	Low risk	High risk	Low risk	High risk	High risk
Burian 2021 [49]	Low risk	High risk	High risk	High risk	High risk
Crins 2021 [48]	Low risk	Low risk	Low risk	High risk	High risk
Gresnigt 2019 [47]	Low risk	Low risk	Low risk	High risk	High risk
Hammoudi 2020 [46]	Low risk	Low risk	Low risk	Low risk	High risk
Hemmings 2000 [23]	Low risk	High risk	High risk	High risk	Low risk
Katsoulis 2011 [45]	High risk	High risk	High risk	High risk	Low risk
da Rocha Scalzer Lopes 2021 [50]	High risk	High risk	High risk	High risk	Low risk
Mehta 2021 [52]	Low risk	Low risk	High risk	High risk	Low risk
Mehta 2021 (b) [51]	Low risk	High risk	High risk	High risk	Low risk
Milosevic 2016 [13]	High risk	High risk	High risk	High risk	Low risk
Oudkerk 2020 [18]	High risk	High risk	Low risk	High risk	Low risk
Redman 2003 [20]	High risk	High risk	Low risk	High risk	Low risk
Smales 2007 [3]	High risk	High risk	High risk	High risk	High risk
Taubóck 2021 [53]	High risk	High risk	Low risk	High risk	High risk
Vailati 2013 [21]	High risk	High risk	Low risk	Low risk	High risk

4. Discussion

This systematic review was focused towards examining the optimal treatment of tooth wear. This study included randomized clinical trials and observational studies for a maximum follow-up of 10 years. All the manuscripts included the rehabilitation of anterior and posterior teeth with extensive wear, using both indirect and direct restorations, with direct resin composite being the most common restorative treatment used. According to preceding reports, these materials seem to show acceptable fracture resistance and simulated wear rates [53–56]. In addition, they have shown suitable long-term achievement in other reports [53,55]. However, failure rates of approximately 10% were reported previously when comparing both materials after a mean follow-up of 30 months [23].

A previous systematic review performed in 2014 focused on the analysis of the steps that are recommended for treatment procedures when treating tooth wear, including diagnostic waxing, occlusal positioning, vertical dimension increase, restoration, and follow-up [8]. The present review is focused on the type of material (ceramic or resin-based) and the technique (direct or indirect) used for the treatment of tooth wear.

In addition, another important factor to be noted is that the etiology of the tooth wear for the studies included in this review could be divided mainly into two types: chemical and mechanical. Although none of the studies offered a comparison in the outcomes of the restorations according to the specific etiology, it should be recognized that different restorative materials do not have the same performance under different pH and mechanical challenges [57].

In the same way, it is worth mentioning that treating tooth wear in anterior teeth represents different challenges than treating tooth wear of posterior teeth. Further, different materials are indicated for both mouth regions, which is a comparison that is not presented in any of the manuscripts in this review.

Most of the researchers used the resin composites in both indirect and direct techniques. Restoring worn teeth by means of resin composites was advocated as a conservative and non-invasive procedure [3,23]. Further, resin composite restorations were inexpensive, provided an overall suitable esthetic appearance, and focused on additive instead of subtractive strategies [3,13,20,23]. However, most of the manuscripts on the restoration of worn teeth did not report long-term results of these restorative materials [20,23]. Preceding studies investigated the finding of resin composite and suggest that treating worn posterior teeth with these materials is contraindicated. This could be because of the brittle physical properties of the microfilled dental resin composites or the high loading forces on these restorations from either bruxing actions or increased vertical dimensions [16].

Another material found in this systematic review was ceramo-metal crowns. This material is seen as the standard of distinction for follow-up examination of clinical studies, and its performance was comparable to the metal-free systems (In-Ceram Alumina and feldspathic ceramic) [50,58]. With the development of adhesive dentistry, metal-free ceramic materials were established in response to the rising concern of biocompatibility and aesthetics [59]. Initially metal-free ceramics were characterized by conventional feldspathic ceramics and, subsequently, by reinforced ceramic systems [60].

Metal-free ceramic crowns display appropriate intrinsic characteristics such as color stability, compressive and abrasion resistance, chemical stability, coefficient of thermal expansion similar to that of the dental structures, radiopacity, and excellent potential to mimic the appearance of natural teeth as the chief materials in restorative dentistry [61]. Nevertheless, their inelastic feature can permit devastating fractures when the applied stresses touch the resistance of the material [62]. It should be emphasized that ceramic based materials such as feldspathic all-ceramic, metal-ceramic with a core in gold electropositive alloy, and In-Ceram Alumina can be considered as alternatives for treating individuals with tooth wear [50].

It is important to define the full gold crown used as an indirect single crown to treat advanced tooth wear in the elderly. A previous report examined the effect of this material and demonstrated lower proportions of failures when compared to direct resin-based composites and indirect ceramo-metal crowns. Most of these failures happened in anterior restorations, and this was observed at 10-year follow-up. Moreover, accumulative survival estimates were 62.0% for all direct restorations and 74.5% for all indirect restorations, including full gold crowns. This study showed no statistically noteworthy alteration between the survival of direct and indirect restorations and highlighted the importance of conducting large, long-term, controlled clinical trials to confirm these findings [3].

The present study demonstrated the use of lithium disilicate ceramic and zirconia crowns for treating patients with widespread tooth wear. One should bear in mind that metal–ceramic crowns are considered to be the standard treatment, as shown previously for crowns and fixed partial dentures [32]. However, this material has some drawbacks, including grayish discoloration at the gingival margin [63]. That is why materials with high strength, such as lithium disilicate and zirconia, have become widespread due to their appearance and biocompatibility [33,34]. Through a 6-year surveillance period, the use of both lithium disilicate and zirconia crowns showed promising survival rates of 99.7% when restoring extensive tooth wear. Normally, when 1 mm thick ceramic was inserted, bulk fracture did not happen (some zones in certain crowns were only 0.6 mm thick). Therefore, for patients with little remaining tooth tissue and extensive tooth wear, the use of minimally invasive high-strength ceramic crowns with cement seems to be helpful, regardless of the precise etiology. Nevertheless, zirconia crowns were rated by a blinded examiner as less esthetic than lithium disilicate crowns, knowing that no differences were found between both materials [46].

Knowing that tooth wear holds challenges for dental clinicians, novel solutions are needed for minimal invasive dentistry. This could be possible by using computer aided design (CAD)—computer aided manufacturer (CAM) technology. Polymer infiltrated ceramic with beneficial characters have been manufactured in the market [49]. These CAD—CAM polymers, launched under industrial standards, exhibit higher mechanical assets compared to those of direct polymers and have even been contemplated as a substitute to glass–ceramic [64–66]. Numerous benefits of CAD—CAM composites have been previously witnessed in diverse in vitro studies: high fatigue resistance, proper optical property, and an antagonistic friendly behavior [66,67]. Therefore, they were realized in distinctive fields of prosthetic dentistry [68,69]. Particularly in complex cases of worn dentition, the use of CAD—CAM-fabricated polymer allow for biomimetic methodologies and minimally invasive dentistry [68].

CAD—CAM polymers display important superior wear rates, with a mean vertical loss during the first year of 186 μm and 342 μm in premolar and molar regions, respectively.

However, it should be noted that a full occlusal load had to be absorbed by these restorations. Consequently, use of an occlusal splint might be suggested for reducing the wear progression [49].

It should be highlighted that a 5-year recall showed no statistically significant differences between direct and indirect resin composites, and the authors recommended that these materials were preferable to those observed in other restorative materials [70]. Unfortunately, restoring severely worn posterior teeth involves alternatives such as more extensive prosthodontic techniques, comprising possibly elective endodontics and crown lengthening. Further research in this area is needed to investigate the optimal treatment of patients with tooth wear.

Most of the papers evaluated the survival rate of the restorations and the clinical characteristics using the United States Public Health Service Evaluation System criteria, as this criterion has gained considerable acceptability in clinical trials involving dental materials [21,53].

From this systematic review, clinical proof was evaluated with regard to compare the direct and indirect materials used in the treatment of worn teeth. The outcomes of this study should be carefully considered in clinical practice, as worn dentition could be caused by several factors, and defining the standard treatment option could not be done. Some of the studies lacked a sufficient time period, whereas other studies tested only indirect restorations without comparison to direct restorations. Thus, further inspection should focus on randomized controlled clinical trials, with the drive of reaching a better understanding of the performance of different materials in the clinical success of tooth wear in terms of novel materials and broad analysis. It is also recommended that research should focus on more consistent methods in an effort to lessen the heterogeneity among manuscripts on this topic and also to establish the ideal protocol for restoring tooth wear.

5. Conclusions

Contradictory discoveries were perceived concerning the type of restoration with better clinical performance. Considering the current literature available, there is no evidence in the superiority of any restoration technique to ensure the highest clinical performance for treating tooth wear. Further well designed randomized clinical trials are required in order to establish an optimal restoration technique protocol for the restoration of tooth wear.

Author Contributions: Conceptualization, L.H., R.B. and C.E.C.-S.; methodology, L.H., R.B. and C.E.C.-S.; software, N.K., L.H., R.B., D.M. and M.L.-S.; validation, L.H., R.B., N.K., C.E.C.-S., M.L.-S., L.K. and Y.H.; formal analysis, L.H., R.B., N.K. and C.E.C.-S.; investigation, J.E.Z.-C., O.E., Y.H., N.K., L.H., R.B., M.Z. and C.E.C.-S.; resources, F.R., M.Z., N.J., D.M., N.K., R.B., L.H., Y.H. and M.L.-S.; data curation, J.E.Z.-C., L.H., R.B. and C.E.C.-S.; writing—original draft preparation, L.H., R.B., C.E.C.-S., N.K., D.M. and Y.H.; writing—review and editing, D.M., L.H., N.K., C.E.C.-S., R.B., Y.H. and M.L.-S.; visualization, Y.H., L.K., N.J., N.K. and R.B.; supervision, L.H.; project administration, L.H. All authors have read and agreed to the published version of the manuscript.

Funding: This research received no external funding.

Institutional Review Board Statement: Not applicable.

Informed Consent Statement: Not applicable.

Data Availability Statement: The data that support the findings of this study are available from the first author (L.H.) upon reasonable request.

Acknowledgments: Authors Louis Hardan and Rim Bourgi would like to recognize the Saint-Joseph University of Beirut, Lebanon. Moreover, the referees would also recognize the Medical University of Lodz, the University of Hidalgo State, Mexico, and the University of Strasbourg for accompanying this research.

Conflicts of Interest: The authors declare no conflict of interest.

References

1. Salas, M.; Nascimento, G.; Huysmans, M.; Demarco, F. Estimated Prevalence of Erosive Tooth Wear in Permanent Teeth of Children and Adolescents: An Epidemiological Systematic Review and Meta-Regression Analysis. *J. Dent.* **2015**, *43*, 42–50. [CrossRef] [PubMed]
2. Van't Spijker, A.; Rodriguez, J.M.; Kreulen, C.M.; Bronkhorst, E.M.; Bartlett, D.W.; Creugers, N. Prevalence of Tooth Wear in Adults. *Int. J. Prosthodont.* **2009**, *22*, 35–42. [PubMed]
3. Smales, R.J.; Berekally, T.L. Long-Term Survival of Direct and Indirect Restorations Placed for the Treatment of Advanced Tooth Wear. *Eur. J. Prosthodont. Restor. Dent.* **2007**, *15*, 2–6. [PubMed]
4. Shellis, R.P.; Addy, M. The Interactions between Attrition, Abrasion and Erosion in Tooth Wear. *Erosive Tooth Wear* **2014**, *25*, 32–45.
5. Addy, M.; Shellis, R. Interaction between Attrition, Abrasion and Erosion in Tooth Wear. *Dent. Eros.* **2006**, *20*, 17–31.
6. Wetselaar, P.; Wetselaar-Glas, M.J.; Katzer, L.D.; Ahlers, M.O. Diagnosing Tooth Wear, a New Taxonomy Based on the Revised Version of the Tooth Wear Evaluation System (TWES 2.0). *J. Oral Rehabil.* **2020**, *47*, 703–712. [CrossRef]
7. Li, M.H.; Bernabé, E. Tooth Wear and Quality of Life among Adults in the United Kingdom. *J. Dent.* **2016**, *55*, 48–53. [CrossRef]
8. Muts, E.-J.; van Pelt, H.; Edelhoff, D.; Krejci, I.; Cune, M. Tooth Wear: A Systematic Review of Treatment Options. *J. Prosthet. Dent.* **2014**, *112*, 752–759. [CrossRef]
9. Al-Khayatt, A.; Ray-Chaudhuri, A.; Poyser, N.; Briggs, P.; Porter, R.; Kelleher, M.; Eliyas, S. Direct Composite Restorations for the Worn Mandibular Anterior Dentition: A 7-year Follow-up of a Prospective Randomised Controlled Split-mouth Clinical Trial. *J. Oral Rehabil.* **2013**, *40*, 389–401. [CrossRef]
10. Attin, T.; Filli, T.; Imfeld, C.; Schmidlin, P.R. Composite Vertical Bite Reconstructions in Eroded Dentitions after 5·5 Years: A Case Series. *J. Oral Rehabil.* **2012**, *39*, 73–79. [CrossRef]
11. Hamburger, J.T.; Opdam, N.J.; Bronkhorst, E.M.; Kreulen, C.M.; Roeters, J.J.; Huysmans, M.-C. Clinical Performance of Direct Composite Restorations for Treatment of Severe Tooth Wear. *J. Adhes. Dent.* **2011**, *13*, 585–593. [PubMed]
12. Loomans, B.; Kreulen, C.; Huijs-Visser, H.; Sterenborg, B.; Bronkhorst, E.; Huysmans, M.; Opdam, N. Clinical Performance of Full Rehabilitations with Direct Composite in Severe Tooth Wear Patients: 3.5 Years Results. *J. Dent.* **2018**, *70*, 97–103. [CrossRef] [PubMed]
13. Milosevic, A.; Burnside, G. The Survival of Direct Composite Restorations in the Management of Severe Tooth Wear Including Attrition and Erosion: A Prospective 8-Year Study. *J. Dent.* **2016**, *44*, 13–19. [CrossRef] [PubMed]
14. Poyser, N.; Briggs, P.; Chana, H.; Kelleher, M.; Porter, R.; Patel, M. The Evaluation of Direct Composite Restorations for the Worn Mandibular Anterior Dentition–Clinical Performance and Patient Satisfaction. *J. Oral Rehabil.* **2007**, *34*, 361–376. [CrossRef] [PubMed]
15. Edelhoff, D.; Güth, J.; Erdelt, K.; Brix, O.; Liebermann, A. Clinical Performance of Occlusal Onlays Made of Lithium Disilicate Ceramic in Patients with Severe Tooth Wear up to 11 Years. *Dent. Mater.* **2019**, *35*, 1319–1330. [CrossRef]
16. Bartlett, D.; Sundaram, G. An up to 3-Year Randomized Clinical Study Comparing Indirect and Direct Resin Composites Used to Restore Worn Posterior Teeth. *Int. J. Prosthodont.* **2006**, *19*, 613–617.
17. Mainjot, A.K.J. The One Step-No Prep Technique: A Straightforward and Minimally Invasive Approach for Full-mouth Rehabilitation of Worn Dentition Using Polymer-infiltrated Ceramic Network (PICN) CAD-CAM Prostheses. *J. Esthet. Restor. Dent.* **2020**, *32*, 141–149. [CrossRef] [PubMed]
18. Oudkerk, J.; Eldafrawy, M.; Bekaert, S.; Grenade, C.; Vanheusden, A.; Mainjot, A. The One-Step No-Prep Approach for Full-Mouth Rehabilitation of Worn Dentition Using PICN CAD-CAM Restorations: 2-Yr Results of a Prospective Clinical Study. *J. Dent.* **2020**, *92*, 103245. [CrossRef]
19. Mainjot, A.K.J.; Charavet, C. Orthodontic-assisted One Step-no Prep Technique: A Straightforward and Minimally-invasive Approach for Localized Tooth Wear Treatment Using Polymer-infiltrated Ceramic Network CAD-CAM Prostheses. *J. Esthet. Restor. Dent.* **2020**, *32*, 645–661. [CrossRef]
20. Redman, C.; Hemmings, K.; Good, J. The Survival and Clinical Performance of Resin–Based Composite Restorations Used to Treat Localised Anterior Tooth Wear. *Br. Dent. J.* **2003**, *194*, 566–572. [CrossRef]
21. Vailati, F.; Gruetter, L.; Belser, U.C. Adhesively Restored Anterior Maxillary Dentitions Affected by Severe Erosion: Up to 6-Year Results of a Prospective Clinical Study. *Eur. J. Esthet. Dent.* **2013**, *8*, 506–530. [PubMed]
22. Mesko, M.E.; Sarkis-Onofre, R.; Cenci, M.S.; Opdam, N.J.; Loomans, B.; Pereira-Cenci, T. Rehabilitation of Severely Worn Teeth: A Systematic Review. *J. Dent.* **2016**, *48*, 9–15. [CrossRef] [PubMed]
23. Hemmings, K.W.; Darbar, U.R.; Vaughan, S. Tooth Wear Treated with Direct Composite Restorations at an Increased Vertical Dimension: Results at 30 Months. *J. Prosthet. Dent.* **2000**, *83*, 287–293. [CrossRef]
24. Gow, A.M.; Hemmings, K.W. The Treatment of Localised Anterior Tooth Wear with Indirect Artglass Restorations at an Increased Occlusal Vertical Dimension. Results after Two Years. *Eur. J. Prosthodont. Restor. Dent.* **2002**, *10*, 101–105.
25. Elderton, R. Clinical Studies Concerning Re-Restoration of Teeth. *Adv. Dent. Res.* **1990**, *4*, 4–9. [CrossRef]
26. Mehta, S.; Banerji, S.; Millar, B.; Suarez-Feito, J.-M. Current Concepts on the Management of Tooth Wear: Part 2. Active Restorative Care 1: The Management of Localised Tooth Wear. *Br. Dent. J.* **2012**, *212*, 73–82. [CrossRef]
27. Lussi, A.; Hellwig, E.; Zero, D.; Jaeggi, T. Erosive Tooth Wear: Diagnosis, Risk Factors and Prevention. *Am. J. Dent.* **2006**, *19*, 319.
28. Loomans, B.; Opdam, N.; Attin, T.; Bartlett, D.; Edelhoff, D.; Frankenberger, R.; Benic, G.; Ramseyer, S.; Wetselaar, P.; Sterenborg, B. Severe Tooth Wear: European Consensus Statement on Management Guidelines. *J. Adhes. Dent.* **2017**, *19*, 111–119.

29. Van de Sande, F.; Opdam, N.; Da Rosa Rodolpho, P.; Correa, M.; Demarco, F.; Cenci, M. Patient Risk Factors' Influence on Survival of Posterior Composites. *J. Dent. Res.* **2013**, *92*, S78–S83. [CrossRef]
30. Mehta, S.B.; Banerji, S.; Millar, B.J.; Suarez-Feito, J.-M. Current Concepts on the Management of Tooth Wear: Part 4. An Overview of the Restorative Techniques and Dental Materials Commonly Applied for the Management of Tooth Wear. *Br. Dent. J.* **2012**, *212*, 169–177. [CrossRef]
31. Varma, S.; Preiskel, A.; Bartlett, D. The Management of Tooth Wear with Crowns and Indirect Restorations. *Br. Dent. J.* **2018**, *224*, 343–347. [CrossRef] [PubMed]
32. Anusavice, K.J. Standardizing Failure, Success, and Survival Decisions in Clinical Studies of Ceramic and Metal–Ceramic Fixed Dental Prostheses. *Dent. Mater.* **2012**, *28*, 102–111. [CrossRef] [PubMed]
33. Denry, I.; Kelly, J.R. State of the Art of Zirconia for Dental Applications. *Dent. Mater.* **2008**, *24*, 299–307. [CrossRef]
34. Warreth, A.; Elkareimi, Y. All-Ceramic Restorations: A Review of the Literature. *Saudi Dent. J.* **2020**, *32*, 365–372. [CrossRef]
35. Zhang, Y.; Lawn, B. Novel Zirconia Materials in Dentistry. *J. Dent. Res.* **2018**, *97*, 140–147. [CrossRef]
36. Weigl, P.; Sander, A.; Wu, Y.; Felber, R.; Lauer, H.-C.; Rosentritt, M. In-Vitro Performance and Fracture Strength of Thin Monolithic Zirconia Crowns. *J. Adv. Prosthodont.* **2018**, *10*, 79–84. [CrossRef]
37. Page, M.J.; McKenzie, J.E.; Bossuyt, P.M.; Boutron, I.; Hoffmann, T.C.; Mulrow, C.D.; Shamseer, L.; Tetzlaff, J.M.; Akl, E.A.; Brennan, S.E. The PRISMA 2020 Statement: An Updated Guideline for Reporting Systematic Reviews. *Int. J. Surg.* **2021**, *88*, 105906. [CrossRef] [PubMed]
38. Sterne, J.A.; Savović, J.; Page, M.J.; Elbers, R.G.; Blencowe, N.S.; Boutron, I.; Cates, C.J.; Cheng, H.-Y.; Corbett, M.S.; Eldridge, S.M. RoB 2: A Revised Tool for Assessing Risk of Bias in Randomised Trials. *BMJ* **2019**, *366*, l4898. [CrossRef]
39. Aljawad, A.; Rees, J.S. Retrospective Study of the Survival and Patient Satisfaction with Composite Dahl Restorations in the Management of Localised Anterior Tooth Wear. *Eur. J. Prosthodont. Restor. Dent.* **2016**, *24*, 222–229.
40. Bartlett, D.; Sundaram, G.; Moazzez, R. Trial of protective effect of fissure sealants, in vivo, on the palatal surfaces of anterior teeth, in patients suffering from erosion. *J. Dent.* **2011**, *39*, 26–29. [CrossRef]
41. Hamburger, J.T. *Treatment of Severe Tooth Wear: A Minimally Invasive Approach*; [Sl: Sn]; Radboud University: Nijmegen, The Netherlands, 2015; ISBN 90-90-28731-0.
42. Walls, A. The Use of Adhesively Retained All-Porcelain Veneers during the Management of Fractured and Worn Anterior Teeth: Part 2. Clinical Results after 5 Years of Follow-Up. *Br. Dent. J.* **1995**, *178*, 337–340. [CrossRef] [PubMed]
43. Walls, A. The Use of Adhesively Retained All-Porcelain Veneers during the Management of Fractured and Worn Anterior Teeth: Part 1. Clinical Technique. *Br. Dent. J.* **1995**, *178*, 333–336. [CrossRef] [PubMed]
44. Woodley, N.; Griffiths, B.; Hemmings, K. Retrospective Audit of Patients with Advanced Toothwear Restored with Removable Partial Dentures. *Eur. J. Prosthodont. Restor. Dent.* **1996**, *4*, 185–191. [PubMed]
45. Katsoulis, J.; Nikitovic, S.G.; Spreng, S.; Neuhaus, K.; Mericske-Stern, R. Prosthetic Rehabilitation and Treatment Outcome of Partially Edentulous Patients with Severe Tooth Wear: 3-Years Results. *J. Dent.* **2011**, *39*, 662–671. [CrossRef]
46. Hammoudi, W.; Trulsson, M.; Svensson, P.; Smedberg, J.-I. Long-Term Results of a Randomized Clinical Trial of 2 Types of Ceramic Crowns in Participants with Extensive Tooth Wear. *J. Prosthet. Dent.* **2020**, *127*, 248–257. [CrossRef]
47. Gresnigt, M.; Cune, M.; Jansen, K.; Van der Made, S.; Özcan, M. Randomized Clinical Trial on Indirect Resin Composite and Ceramic Laminate Veneers: Up to 10-Year Findings. *J. Dent.* **2019**, *86*, 102–109. [CrossRef]
48. Crins, L.; Opdam, N.; Kreulen, C.; Bronkhorst, E.; Sterenborg, B.; Huysmans, M.; Loomans, B. Randomized Controlled Trial on the Performance of Direct and Indirect Composite Restorations in Patients with Severe Tooth Wear. *Dent. Mater.* **2021**, *37*, 1645–1654. [CrossRef]
49. Burian, G.; Erdelt, K.; Schweiger, J.; Keul, C.; Edelhoff, D.; Güth, J.-F. In-Vivo-Wear in Composite and Ceramic Full Mouth Rehabilitations over 3 Years. *Sci. Rep.* **2021**, *11*, 14056. [CrossRef]
50. da Rocha Scalzer Lopes, G.; de Faria Viana, A.A.; Diniz, V.; de Matos, J.D.; Andrade, V.C.; Bottino, M.A.; Nishioka, R.S.; Chiarelli, F.M.; Feitosa, A.C.R.; Guerra, S.M.G. Incidence of Fracture in Single Ceramic Crowns in Patients with Chronic Tooth Wear: A Clinical Follow-up. *Int. J. Odontostomatol.* **2021**, *15*, 102–110. [CrossRef]
51. Mehta, S.B.; Lima, V.P.; Bronkhorst, E.M.; Crins, L.; Bronkhorst, H.; Opdam, N.J.; Huysmans, M.-C.D.; Loomans, B.A. Clinical Performance of Direct Composite Resin Restorations in a Full Mouth Rehabilitation for Patients with Severe Tooth Wear: 5.5-Year Results. *J. Dent.* **2021**, *112*, 103743. [CrossRef]
52. Mehta, S.B.; Bronkhorst, E.M.; Lima, V.P.; Crins, L.; Bronkhorst, H.; Opdam, N.J.; Huysmans, M.-C.D.; Loomans, B.A. The Effect of Pre-Treatment Levels of Tooth Wear and the Applied Increase in the Vertical Dimension of Occlusion (VDO) on the Survival of Direct Resin Composite Restorations. *J. Dent.* **2021**, *111*, 103712. [CrossRef]
53. Tauböck, T.T.; Schmidlin, P.R.; Attin, T. Vertical Bite Rehabilitation of Severely Worn Dentitions with Direct Composite Restorations: Clinical Performance up to 11 Years. *J. Clin. Med.* **2021**, *10*, 1732. [CrossRef]
54. Alhadainy, H.A.; Abdalla, A.I. 2-Year Clinical Evaluation of Dentin Bonding Systems. *Am. J. Dent.* **1996**, *9*, 77–79.
55. Clelland, N.L.; Villarroel, S.C.; Knobloch, L.A.; Seghi, R.R. Simulated Oral Wear of Packable Composites. *Oper. Dent.* **2003**, *28*, 830–837.
56. Knobloch, L.A.; Kerby, R.E.; Seghi, R.; Berlin, J.S.; Clelland, N. Fracture Toughness of Packable and Conventional Composite Materials. *J. Prosthet. Dent.* **2002**, *88*, 307–313. [CrossRef]

57. Lima, V.P.; Machado, J.B.; Zhang, Y.; Loomans, B.A.; Moraes, R.R. Laboratory methods to simulate the mechanical degradation of resin composite restorations. *Dent. Mater.* **2022**, *38*, 214–229. [CrossRef]
58. Raposo, L.H.A.; Neiva, N.A.; da Silva, G.R.; Carlo, H.L.; da Mota, A.S.; do Prado, C.J.; Soares, C.J. Ceramic Restoration Repair: Report of Two Cases. *J. Appl. Oral Sci.* **2009**, *17*, 140–144. [CrossRef]
59. Campos, T.; Ramos, N.; Machado, J.; Bottino, M.; Souza, R.; Melo, R. A New Silica-Infiltrated Y-TZP Obtained by the Sol-Gel Method. *J. Dent.* **2016**, *48*, 55–61. [CrossRef]
60. de Matos, J.D.M.; Nakano, L.J.N.; Bottino, M.A.; de Jesus, R.H.; Maciel, L.C. Current Considerations for Dental Ceramics and Their Respective Union Systems. *Rev. Bras. Odontol.* **2020**, *77*, e1768. [CrossRef]
61. Erpenstein, H.; Borchard, R.; Kerschbaum, T. Long-Term Clinical Results of Galvano-Ceramic and Glass-Ceramic Individual Crowns. *J. Prosthet. Dent.* **2000**, *83*, 530–534. [CrossRef]
62. Cehreli, M.C.; Kökat, A.M.; Ozpay, C.; Karasoy, D.; Akca, K. A Randomized Controlled Clinical Trial of Feldspathic versus Glass-Infiltrated Alumina All-Ceramic Crowns: A 3-Year Follow-Up. *Int. J. Prosthodont.* **2011**, *24*, 77–84. [PubMed]
63. Wall, J.G.; Cipra, D.L. Alternative Crown Systems: Is the Metal-Ceramic Crown Always the Restoration of Choice? *Dent. Clin. N. Am.* **1992**, *36*, 765–782. [CrossRef]
64. Mainjot, A.K.; Dupont, N.M.; Oudkerk, J.C.; Dewael, T.Y.; Sadoun, M.J. From Artisanal to CAD-CAM Blocks: State of the Art of Indirect Composites. *J. Dent. Res.* **2016**, *95*, 487–495. [CrossRef] [PubMed]
65. Alt, V.; Hannig, M.; Wöstmann, B.; Balkenhol, M. Fracture Strength of Temporary Fixed Partial Dentures: CAD/CAM versus Directly Fabricated Restorations. *Dent. Mater.* **2011**, *27*, 339–347. [CrossRef] [PubMed]
66. Stawarczyk, B.; Liebermann, A.; Eichberger, M.; Güth, J.-F. Evaluation of Mechanical and Optical Behavior of Current Esthetic Dental Restorative CAD/CAM Composites. *J. Mech. Behav. Biomed. Mater.* **2016**, *55*, 1–11. [CrossRef]
67. Magne, P.; Schlichting, L.H.; Maia, H.P.; Baratieri, L.N. In Vitro Fatigue Resistance of CAD/CAM Composite Resin and Ceramic Posterior Occlusal Veneers. *J. Prosthet. Dent.* **2010**, *104*, 149–157. [CrossRef]
68. Güth, J.; Edelhoff, D.; Goldberg, J.; Magne, P. CAD/CAM Polymer vs Direct Composite Resin Core Buildups for Endodontically Treated Molars without Ferrule. *Oper. Dent.* **2016**, *41*, 53–63. [CrossRef]
69. Yilmaz, B. CAD-CAM High-Density Polymer Implant-Supported Fixed Diagnostic Prostheses. *J. Prosthet. Dent.* **2018**, *119*, 688–692. [CrossRef]
70. Wassell, R.; Walls, A.; McCabe, J. Direct Composite Inlays versus Conventional Composite Restorations: 5-Year Follow-Up. *J. Dent.* **2000**, *20*, 375–302. [CrossRef]

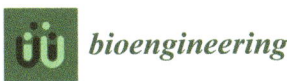

Article

Adhesion of Resin to Lithium Disilicate with Different Surface Treatments before and after Salivary Contamination—An In-Vitro Study

Ryan Harouny [1,2], Louis Hardan [1], Elie Harouny [1], Cynthia Kassis [1], Rim Bourgi [1], Monika Lukomska-Szymanska [3], Naji Kharouf [4,5], Vincent Ball [4,5,*] and Carlos Khairallah [1]

1. Department of Restorative Dentistry, School of Dentistry, Saint-Joseph University, Beirut 1107 2180, Lebanon; ryaneliott.harouny@net.usj.edu.lb (R.H.); louis.hardan@usj.edu.lb (L.H.); elie.harouny@usj.edu.lb (E.H.); cynthia.kassis@usj.edu.lb (C.K.); rim.bourgi@net.usj.edu.lb (R.B.); carlos.khairallah@usj.edu.lb (C.K.)
2. Craniofacial Research Laboratory, Division of Biomaterials, School of Dentistry, Saint-Joseph University, Beirut 1107 2180, Lebanon
3. Department of General Dentistry, Medical University of Lodz, 251 Pomorska St., 92-213 Lodz, Poland; monika.lukomska-szymanska@umed.lodz.pl
4. Department of Endodontics, Faculty of Dental Medicine, Strasbourg University, 67000 Strasbourg, France; dentistenajikharouf@gmail.com
5. Department of Biomaterials and Bioengineering, INSERM UMR_S 1121, Strasbourg University, 67000 Strasbourg, France
* Correspondence: vball@unistra.fr

Abstract: The salivary contamination occurring at the try-in procedures of lithium disilicate (LDS) can jeopardize their bond strength. Various laboratory reports have concluded that applying 37% phosphoric acid (H_3PO_4) could be considered as a predictable way of removing salivary contaminants. An experimental method that consists of sealing the intaglio of the ceramic restorations with a layer of cured adhesive could allow consequent time saving for dental practitioners. It is, besides, necessary to establish an optimal decontamination protocol. Hence, this study aimed to determine the most efficient surface treatment, before and after salivary contamination, by comparing the adhesion between resin and LDS. In order to do so, five groups of ten specimens ($n = 10$) each underwent the different types of surface treatments before bonding, followed by 2500 cycles in the thermocycler. A shear bond strength (SBS) test was then conducted on a universal testing machine (YLE GmbH Waldstraße Bad König, Germany), followed by a fracture-type analysis on an optical microscope (Olympus BX53, Shinjuku, Tokyo, Japan). Statistical analysis was set with a level of significance of $\alpha = 0.05$. The surface treatment significantly affected the SBS results. The decontamination with HF (12.59 ± 2.71 MPa) and H_3PO_4 (13.11 ± 1.03 MPa) obtained the highest values, silanizing only before contamination obtained intermediate values (11.74 ± 3.49 MPa), and silanizing both before and after the salivary contamination (10.41 ± 2.75 MPa) along with applying a bonding agent before contamination (9.65 ± 1.99 MPa) resulted in the lowest values. In conclusion, H_3PO_4 proved to be efficient, thus, allowing the practitioner to avoid the clinical use of HF; it can, therefore, be considered as a valid alternative. Presilanization and resilanization of specimens, along with applying a bonding agent before contamination, did not yield satisfying results.

Keywords: decontamination; lithium disilicate; resin; saliva; shear bond strength

Citation: Harouny, R.; Hardan, L.; Harouny, E.; Kassis, C.; Bourgi, R.; Lukomska-Szymanska, M.; Kharouf, N.; Ball, V.; Khairallah, C. Adhesion of Resin to Lithium Disilicate with Different Surface Treatments before and after Salivary Contamination—An In-Vitro Study. *Bioengineering* **2022**, *9*, 286. https://doi.org/10.3390/bioengineering9070286

Academic Editors: Chengfei Zhang and Liang Luo

Received: 31 May 2022
Accepted: 23 June 2022
Published: 29 June 2022

Publisher's Note: MDPI stays neutral with regard to jurisdictional claims in published maps and institutional affiliations.

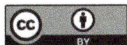

Copyright: © 2022 by the authors. Licensee MDPI, Basel, Switzerland. This article is an open access article distributed under the terms and conditions of the Creative Commons Attribution (CC BY) license (https://creativecommons.org/licenses/by/4.0/).

1. Introduction

All-ceramic restorations, including lithium disilicate (LDS), are increasingly preferred by both patients and practitioners [1]. With their esthetic advantage and their satisfying durability, they represent a good alternative to conventional ceramo-metallic crowns [2,3]. An important step for this success is proper bonding [4], which includes etching the intaglio with HF and then applying a silane agent. Furthermore, it is essential to find the best way to clean the prosthetic intaglio of the saliva after the intra-oral try-in, since this thin film is known to reduce the bond strength [5,6]. Numerous techniques have been proposed and tested, such as cleaning with ethanol, isopropanol, sodium hypochlorite, water spray, or putting the restoration in an ultrasonic bath, but the results were not satisfying [5,7–9]. Although the standard method is to conduct the try-in of the restoration in the mouth before applying the HF and silane agent, the etching of the restoration is sometimes undergone at the dental laboratory [9]. This is either done to make it easier for the practitioner or because chairside use of HF is prohibited in some countries due to its potential hazardous effects [10–14]. It is, therefore, necessary to have an efficient alternative to HF in order to clean the intaglio after the try-in. This could be made possible by using phosphoric acid (H_3PO_4), which is considered an interesting cleaning method due to its low cost and availability in every practitioner's clinic. It yields the same findings as non-salivary contaminated LDS specimens according to a previous study [15], or slightly or significantly lower bond strength according to other studies [5,9,16]. This disparity of results made the inclusion of H_3PO_4 in this study interesting.

Aside from the cleaning methods applied after the try-in, it also seems valuable to evaluate the influence of the intaglio's pretreatment on the bond strength obtained after contamination and cleaning.

Silanizing the specimens after the HF etching and before their contamination yielded a significant increase in the bond strength obtained compared to specimens without pre-silanization and treated with the same decontamination method. Nevertheless, only a few studies took this parameter into account. It is worth noting that this technique goes against the manufacturer's recommendations, which warns of eventual harm to the silane layer [7,17].

Moreover, the need to resilanize the specimens, which were pre-silanized before contamination, should be evaluated. This parameter was, therefore, included in this study.

Lastly, an experimental method, which is already used in some countries, could help to avoid the step of HF etching in dental practice while still protecting the etched prosthetic intaglio and the silane layer by applying and polymerizing an adhesive layer on the intaglio after the etching and the silanization, but before the try-in. After trying the restoration in the mouth, the intaglio would simply be cleaned with ethanol and the adhesive surface simply reactivated by a new adhesive layer. However, only one study describing this method is available [17]. It was consequently included in this manuscript, with an additional innovation, by applying this method on a more frequently used material, LDS, on which it had not been tested before. LDS was chosen for being a dental biomaterial well known by practitioners, as they frequently use it when high aesthetic is requested by the patient. LDS has a high translucency when compared to the opacity shown by zirconia, and it also presents high mechanical properties and good long-term survival rates [18–20].

Hence, the main objective of this study was to evaluate the effect of different pretreatments and cleaning methods following contamination by saliva on the adhesion of resin to LDS after ageing. The null hypothesis was that the surface treatment before and after the contamination would not have a significant influence on the bond strength of resin to LDS between the different groups.

2. Materials and Methods

2.1. Specimen Preparation

LDS blocks (n = 50) were used after the approval of the Institutional Review Board of Saint-Joseph University (FMD-SF30; ref.#USJ-2020-163).

Type, brand, composition, lot number, and manufacturer of the materials used in this study are listed in Table 1.

Table 1. Specifications of the materials used in the study.

Material	Brand	Lot	Composition	Manufacturer
Glass-based ceramic	IPS e.max CAD LT A1 shade	Y30837	SiO_2, LiO_2, K_2O, P_2O_5, ZrO_2, ZnO, other oxides, coloring oxides	IvoclarVivadent, Schaan, Liechtenstein
Ceramic etchant	Porcelain Etch	BGTV7	9% buffered hydrofluoric acid	Ultradent, Schaan, Liechtenstein
Ceramic primer	Porcelain Primer	1900001117	Pre-hydrolyzed silane primer with alcohol and acetone	Bisco, Schaumburg, IL, USA
Etching gel	DentoEtch	DE-4.12	37% phosphoric acid	Itena, Avenue Foch, Paris, France
Bonding agent	Adper Single Bond 2	NA61948	Bis-GMA, HEMA, dimethacrylates, ethanol, water, photoinitiators, methacrylate functional copolymer of polyacrylic and polyitaconic acids, and silica nanofiller	3M ESPE, St. Paul, MN, USA
Flowable composite	Filtek Z350 XT, Flowable Restorative, A1 shade	NA37278	Bis-GMA, TEGDMA, procrylatresins; ytterbium trifluoride, silica, zirconia/silica cluster fillers	3M ESPE, St. Paul, MN, USA

Silicon dioxide (SiO_2), Lithium superoxide (LiO_2), Potassium oxide (K_2O), Phosphorus pentoxide (P_2O_5), Zirconium dioxide (ZrO_2), Zinc oxide (ZnO), Bisphenol A-glycidyl methacrylate (Bis-GMA), Hydroxyethylmethacrylate (HEMA), Triethylenglycol-di-methacrylate (TEGDMA).

LDS blocks were cut before crystallization with a low-speed precision cutting machine (Exakt 30, EXAKT Vertriebs GmbH, Norderstedt, Gemany) to obtain 50 specimens with the following dimensions: 5 mm length, 5 mm width, and 3 mm height. The specimens were then crystallized according to the manufacturer's instructions and embedded in acrylic resin (Novacryl, Tricodent LTD, Victoria Road, Burgess Hill, England), then poured in Ultradent's plastic mold. The exposed bonding surface was polished with 600 µm grit silicon carbide paper under irrigation for one minute to obtain a flat surface. The specimens were thereafter placed in an ultrasonic bath with distilled water for five minutes and subsequently dried with an air syringe. They were then randomly divided into five groups of ten specimens each, according to the surface treatment to be performed.

All specimens were treated by a single operator and with saliva freshly collected the same day. Figure 1 shows the surface treatment methods executed in the different groups.

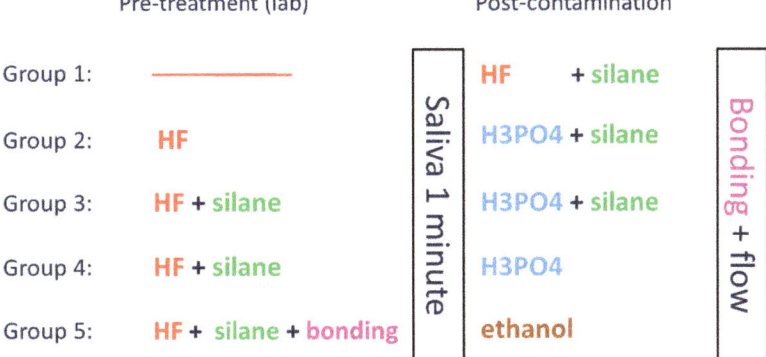

Figure 1. Surface treatment methods of the different groups (hydrofluoric acid (HF); phosphoric acid (H_3PO_4)).

2.2. Bonding of the Specimens

After surface treatment, all the specimens received a layer of adhesive resin (Adper Single Bond 2, 3M ESPE) spread with a gentle air stream for 15 s to evaporate the solvent [21,22] and to obtain a homogeneous thickness, then polymerized for 20 s (Woodpecker 1000–1200 mW/cm^2). A polyethylene cylindrical mold with an internal diameter of 2.38 mm and a height of 2.15 mm (Bonding Jig, Ultradent Products, Inc., South Jordan, UT, USA) [23,24] was then placed on the surface of the specimens covered with the adhesive, and flowable composite (Filtek Z350 XT Flowable Restorative, A1 Shade, 3M ESPE) was injected in it from the bottom to the top, with the tip of the syringe kept inside the material to avoid the incorporation of air bubbles. The flowable resin was then polymerized for 40 s with the same light-curing device [8,9].

The bonded specimens were washed with an air-water spray and kept for 24 h in distilled water at 37 °C, in an incubator, to allow complete polymerization of the resin [25].

2.3. Bond Strength Test and Failure Analysis

After thermocycling (2500 cycles, 5–55 °C, dwell time: 45 s, transition time: 15 s), the shear bond strength (SBS) tests for all the specimens were performed on a universal testing machine (YLE GmbH Waldstraße Bad König, Germany) with a knife-edge blade placed perpendicularly and touching only the bonding interface, at a crosshead speed of 1 mm/min until fracture occurred, according to ISO/TS 11405:2015 [26]. The SBS was then calculated according to the following formula: R = F/A (R being the bond strength in MPa, F the failure force in Newtons, and A the bonding area in mm^2).

After debonding, the type of fracture was determined under x10 magnification with an optical microscope (Olympus BX53, Shinjuku, Tokyo, Japan) and classified as follows:

(a) Either adhesive: between the ceramic and the resin; no remnant of composite resin on the ceramic surface; (b) either cohesive: within the composite resin; resin remnants can be seen on most of the ceramic surface; (c) either mixed (combination of adhesive and cohesive failure): remnants can be seen on parts of the ceramic, while other parts have no remnant.

2.4. Statistical Analysis

IBM SPSS Statistics version 26.0 was used to analyze the data. The level of significance was set at -p-value $\leq$ 0.05. The primary outcome measurement was the SBS (MPa). Kolmogorov–Smirnov tests were used to assess the normality of the distribution of the variables. Levene's test was used to assess the homogeneity of variances between groups. One-way analysis of variance (ANOVA) followed by Tukey (HSD) post-hoc tests were used to compare mean bond strength between groups. Fisher Exact tests were used to compare the type of fracture among groups.

3. Results

3.1. Shear Bond Strength Results

The SBS was significantly different between the five groups (-p-value = 0.019; ANOVA). The highest mean SBS was obtained by groups 1 (12.59 ± 2.71 MPa) and 2 (13.11 ± 1.03 MPa) (Figure 2). Group 4 showed intermediate values (11.74 ± 3.49 MPa) while the lowest results were obtained in groups 5 (9.65 ± 1.99 MPa) and 3 (10.41 ± 2.75 MPa). The SBS values obtained are listed in Table 2, along with the mean, the standard deviation, the 95% confidence interval, and the minimal and maximal value.

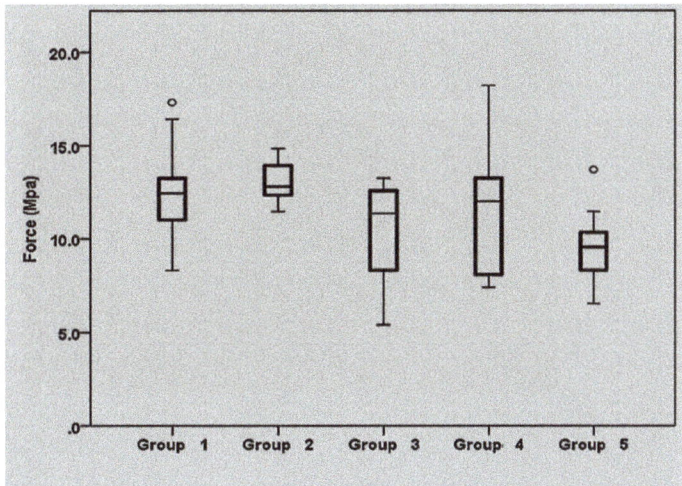

Figure 2. Mean shear bond strength of the different groups. Surface treatment: Group 1: Cleaning with HF after contamination; Group 2: cleaning with H_3PO_4 after contamination; Group 3: Silanization before and after contamination; Group 4: Silanization only before contamination; Group 5: Sealing of the ceramic with adhesive. °: Extreme outliers: the outliers are points that stay out of the interval.

Table 2. Shear bond strength values. Groups with the same letter are not significantly different ($p > 0.05$).

	N	Mean	Standard Deviation	95% Confidence Interval		Minimum	Maximum
				Lowerbound	Upperbound		
Group 1	10	12.59 [a]	2.71	10.65	14.53	8.32	17.31
Group 2	10	13.11 [a]	1.03	12.37	13.84	11.47	14.84
Group 3	10	10.41 [b]	2.75	8.44	12.38	5.40	13.26
Group 4	10	11.74 [a,b]	3.49	9.24	14.23	7.42	18.21
Group 5	10	9.65 [b]	1.99	8.22	11.07	6.52	13.71

3.2. Comparison of the Types of Fracture

Cuts obtained with an optical microscope (Olympus BX53, Shinjuku, Tokyo, Japan) (x10) show the aspect of adhesive and mixed fractures (Figures 3 and 4).

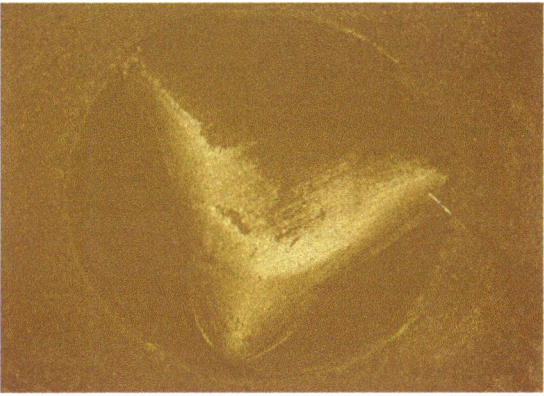

Figure 3. Representative image (optical microscope x10) of a mixed failure.

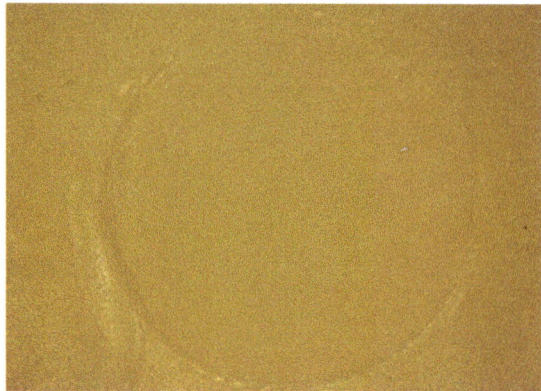

Figure 4. Representative image (optical microscope x10) of an adhesive failure.

Figure 5 shows the distribution of the types of fractures among the groups tested.

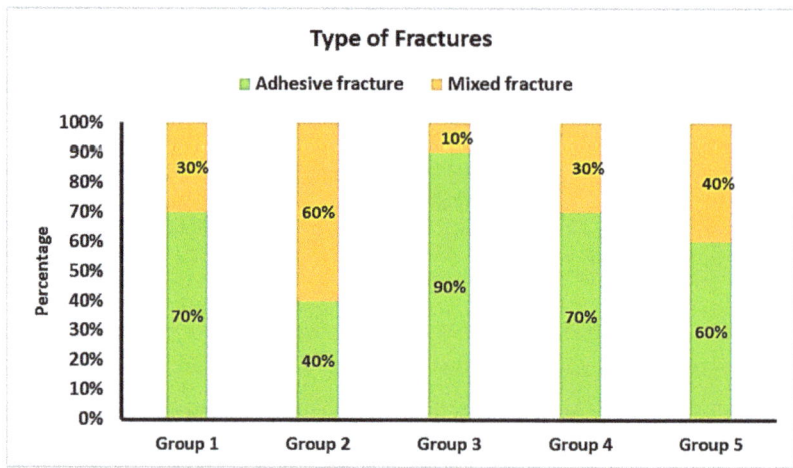

Figure 5. Distribution of the types of fractures in the different groups.

4. Discussion

This study was conducted to establish the most efficient surface treatment before and after salivary contamination of LDS specimens, in order to ensure an optimal bond strength of resin to ceramic after artificial aging. According to the results obtained, the mean SBS was significantly different depending on the surface treatment. Therefore, the null hypothesis tested in this study was rejected.

Many contaminants can impair the bonding of ceramic restorations, such as blood, silicone, dental stone, or isolation medium. However, saliva remains the most relevant from a clinical point of view. The adhesion of saliva to restorations and to the surface of the teeth leads to the formation of a thin pellicle that reaches a thickness of 10 to 20 nm within a few minutes [6]. This layer is not eliminated by water rinsing [16] and has a negative influence on the wettability and surface free energy of the substrate [9]. An inefficient decontamination could cause an important decrease in bond strength values, as shown in numerous studies, and saliva should, therefore, be correctly eliminated in order to achieve a long-lasting adhesion [9,27,28].

The specimens in groups 1 and 2 showed the best results. Group 1, where the ceramic was etched with HF after contamination, was the control group, since it represents the typical situation of a practitioner decontaminating ceramic restorations after the try-in following the universally accepted protocol. The specimens in group 2 were decontaminated with H_3PO_4. The high values obtained with the first method correspond with those obtained in other studies [9,15,16,27–29], where values after HF decontamination were similar to the control (uncontaminated) group. The results of the second method were more controversial in the literature; they were identical to the control group on LDS [15], on feldspathic ceramic [30], and on zirconia [31], like in this study, unlike other studies, where it was either fair [5,16] or unsatisfying [28]. Although it is not entirely clear how phosphoric acid helps in removing saliva, it is suggested that it perhaps penetrates the salivary film and then etches the surface of the ceramic below it, liberating the saliva from the surface [6].

Specimens in groups 3 and 4 received a layer of silane before contamination. Abboush et al. and Marfenko et al. reported that this would increase the bond strength [17,30], while Alfaro et al. did not obtain better results with this method [16].

Group 4, silanized only before contamination, yielded intermediate values, which were significantly lower than those in groups 1 and 2. This could be due to the fact that the silane layer was put in one week prior to contamination, decontamination, and bonding, to simulate the time of delivery from the laboratory. The mechanical application of saliva with a microbrush and the eventual degradation by H_3PO_4 could be added as factors that could have harmed the silane layer, therefore, decreasing the values obtained. Marfenko et al. questioned the stability of the silane layer after a mechanical action, although their study addressed mechanical cleaning with Ivoclean [17].

Group 3, however, in which silanization was performed before and after contamination, showed values significantly lower than those in group 4, and statistically similar to those in group 5. This could be explained by the negative impact of the application of thick or multiple silane layers, which could interact with one another and interfere with the bonding of the resin to the ceramic [7]. It is, therefore, possible that the application of a second layer of silane could have affected the bonding more than the application of H_3PO_4 on the first layer of silane, since H_3PO_4 acted chemically, not mechanically, which yielded significantly higher values in group 4 compared to group 3. However, these results are in contradiction with those of other studies [7,17,30], which did not show a deleterious impact to reapplying silane after decontamination. Further research is, therefore, deemed necessary to clarify the effect of such a procedure.

Group 5, which represented the experimental method of this study, with the sealing of the ceramic with a bonding agent before contamination, obtained the lowest values, unlike the study of Bomicke et al. [27], which showed that after thermocycling, values are significantly higher than those in the uncontaminated group. Numerous factors that differ between these two studies could explain the heterogeneity of the results: the material on which the bonding was applied (LDS compared to lithium silicate reinforced with zirconia), the bonding agent, the bond strength test setting (SBS test compared to tensile bond strength test), the method used for artificial aging (2500 thermal cycles versus 6 months of storage in distilled water), and the diameter of the composite resin (2.38 mm versus 3.3 mm). It is important to note that in the study of Bomicke et al., pre-polymerized "core build-up" composite resin cylinders were bonded to the ceramic with a resin cement, which differs from the application of the flowable resin on the ceramic topped with a layer of polymerized adhesive, as was performed in this study. To our knowledge, these two studies are the only ones that evaluated this method and further research is, therefore, necessary to make a conclusion about its efficiency.

Yet, the quality of the bonding should not only be evaluated by bond strength values. The type of fracture (adhesive, cohesive, mixed), determined with a microscope, is also an indicator of the bonding mechanism [15,32]. A higher incidence of adhesive fractures indicates a lower quality of bonding in one group of specimens when compared to others.

The specimens in group 2, which had the highest mean SBS value (13.11 ± 1.03 MPa), showed the most mixed fractures (60%), while the specimens in group 3, which had significantly lower mean SBS values (10.41 ± 2.75 MPa), showed only 10% mixed fractures. However, the difference in the type of fracture rate was not statistically significant, which does not allow any conclusion. This is probably due to the relatively small number of specimens, which is one of the limitations of the study. Nevertheless, it can be stated that the significant overall proportion of mixed failures is due to the testing method, namely the macroshear bond strength test. In fact, a wider bonding interface probably contains more defects [33,34], which raises the prevalence of cohesive and mixed failures when compared to the microtensile bond strength test. The latter, indeed, allows for a higher precision because of a more homogeneous distribution of the forces on the bonded interface [35–39], and it can, therefore, be considered as another limitation of this study.

Even so, the SBS test was chosen for its easy use, and it is important to mention that shear forces outweigh tensile forces on ceramic veneers. Studying this parameter would then be more interesting for this type of restoration where the absence of mechanical retention makes bonding an essential element for its longevity [40]. Moreover, when compared to a microtensile bond strength test, it helps avoiding pre-testing failures since it does not need to be cut before testing, which would be problematic with a brittle material, such as ceramic [6,17].

This research did not include a group of specimens without saliva contamination, since it has already been proved that etching with HF allows one to obtain the same bond strength values as before contamination [9,15,28], so these two groups would lead to identical values.

Similar to Lapinska et al. [9], this study used a flowable composite resin instead of a resin cement, for two reasons. Firstly, the principal aim of the study was not to evaluate the resistance of resin itself but the surface treatment of LDS and its influence on the bond strength values. Secondly, these two types of materials share the same physical and chemical properties because of their resin matrix and their comparable filler content. It is, consequently, possible to use one instead of the other in some circumstances.

Further, all the specimens underwent thermocycling, since the long-term values are the most relevant to the practitioner. This was also the case in several studies [6,17,28], where all the specimens were subjected to thermocycling, which was considered more suitable than water storage [25,41] to simulate the aging of the restorations and their bonding to resin.

Although decontamination with H_3PO_4 prevents the chairside use of HF, it does not change the fact that the protocol of decontamination and bonding after the try-in is time-consuming. Future studies on LDS and with a higher number of specimens should be undertaken, along with the method evaluated by Bomicke et al. [27], which is the sealing of the ceramic before contamination, because any efficient method that can save chairside time would be advantageous for both the practitioner and the patient.

5. Conclusions

According to the results obtained in this study, it can be concluded that H_3PO_4 is as efficient in removing saliva contamination from the surface of LDS as HF. On the other hand, the silanization only before contamination lessened bond strength when compared to the specimens that were not silanized prior to contamination. Resilanizing of pre-silanized specimens that were cleaned with H_3PO_4 did not improve bonding to LDS. The experimental method consisting of sealing the intaglio with a layer of cured adhesive did not prove its efficiency. Therefore, none of the pre-treatment methods tested allowed superior bond strength of resin to LDS.

Author Contributions: Conceptualization, R.H., E.H., C.K. (Carlos Khairallah) and L.H.; methodology, R.H.; software, R.H. and R.B.; validation, R.H., E.H., V.B., C.K. (Cynthia Kassis), R.B. and L.H.; formal analysis, R.H.; investigation, R.H. and R.B.; resources, E.H., V.B., C.K. (Carlos Khairallah), M.L.-S., N.K. and L.H.; data curation, R.H. and C.K. (Carlos Khairallah); writing—original draft preparation,

R.H., E.H., C.K. (Cynthia Kassis), M.L.-S., V.B., R.B. and L.H.; writing—review and editing, R.H., E.H., C.K. (Carlos Khairallah), R.B. and L.H.; visualization, R.H., E.H., C.K. (Cynthia Kassis), R.B. and L.H.; supervision, C.K. (Carlos Khairallah) and L.H.; project administration, C.K. (Carlos Khairallah) and L.H. All authors have read and agreed to the published version of the manuscript.

Funding: This research received no external funding.

Informed Consent Statement: Not applicable.

Acknowledgments: The authors would like to acknowledge the Saint-Joseph University of Beirut. A special thank you to the team of the laboratories of Biomaterials and Histology, located in the Innovation and Sports' Campus (Beirut, Lebanon).

Conflicts of Interest: The authors declare no conflict of interest.

References

1. Nasr, E.; Makhlouf, A.C.; Zebouni, E.; Makzoumé, J. All-ceramic Computer-aided Design and Computer-aided Manufacturing Restorations: Evolution of Structures and Criteria for Clinical Application. *J. Contemp. Dent. Pract.* **2019**, *20*, 516–523. [PubMed]
2. Tian, T.; Tsoi, J.K.-H.; Matinlinna, J.P.; Burrow, M.F. Aspects of bonding between resin luting cements and glass ceramic materials. *Dent. Mater.* **2014**, *30*, 147–162. [CrossRef] [PubMed]
3. Sailer, I.; Makarov, N.A.; Thoma, D.S.; Zwahlen, M.; Pjetursson, B.E. All-ceramic or metal-ceramic tooth-supported fixed dental prostheses (FDPs)? A systematic review of the survival and complication rates. Part I: Single crowns (SCs). *Dent. Mater.* **2015**, *31*, 603–623. [CrossRef]
4. Puppin-Rontani, J.; Sundfeld, D.; Costa, A.R.; Correr, A.B.; Puppin-Rontani, R.M.; Borges, G.A.; Sinhoreti, M.; Correr-Sobrinho, L. Effect of Hydrofluoric Acid Concentration and Etching Time on Bond Strength to Lithium Disilicate Glass Ceramic. *Oper. Dent.* **2017**, *42*, 606–615. [CrossRef] [PubMed]
5. Borges, A.L.S.; Posritong, S.; Özcan, M.; Campos, F.; Melo, R.; Bottino, M.C. Can Cleansing Regimens Effectively Eliminate Saliva Contamination from Lithium Disilicate Ceramic Surface? *Eur. J. Prosthodont. Restor. Dent.* **2017**, *25*, 9–14.
6. Koc-Dundar, B.; Özcan, M. Effect of clinical and laboratory contamination media on the adhesion of luting cement to direct and indirect resin composite materials. *J. Adhes. Sci. Technol.* **2017**, *31*, 1251–1263. [CrossRef]
7. Nikolaus, F.; Wolkewitz, M.; Hahn, P. Bond strength of composite resin to glass ceramic after saliva contamination. *Clin. Oral Investig.* **2013**, *17*, 751–755. [CrossRef]
8. Aladağ, A.; Elter, B.; Çömlekoğlu, E.; Kanat, B.; Sonugelen, M.; Kesercioğlu, A.; Özcan, M. Effect of different cleaning regimens on the adhesion of resin to saliva-contaminated ceramics. *J. Prosthodont.* **2015**, *24*, 136–145. [CrossRef]
9. Lapinska, B.; Rogowski, J.; Nowak, J.; Nissan, J.; Sokolowski, J.; Lukomska-Szymanska, M. Effect of Surface Cleaning Regimen on Glass Ceramic Bond Strength. *Molecules* **2019**, *24*, 389. [CrossRef]
10. Lopes, G.; Ballarin, A. Hydrofluoric Acid—Simple Things You May Do Not Know about Something You Are So Habituated to Use. *Odovtos Int. J. Dent. Sci.* **2015**, *1*, 15–23.
11. Ozcan, M.; Allahbeickaraghi, A.; Dündar, M. Possible hazardous effects of hydrofluoric acid and recommendations for treatment approach: A review. *Clin. Oral Investig.* **2012**, *16*, 15–23. [CrossRef] [PubMed]
12. Bajraktarova-Valjakova, E.; Korunoska-Stevkovska, V.; Georgieva, S.; Ivanovski, K.; Bajraktarova-Misevska, C.; Mijoska, A.; Grozdanov, A. Hydrofluoric Acid: Burns and Systemic Toxicity, Protective Measures, Immediate and Hospital Medical Treatment. *Maced. J. Med. Sci.* **2018**, *6*, 2257–2269. [CrossRef]
13. Schwerin, D.L.; Hatcher, J.D. Hydrofluoric Acid Burns. In *StatPearls*; StatPearls Publishing: Treasure Island, FL, USA, 2021.
14. Yoshida, K. Influence of cleaning methods on the bond strength of resin cement to saliva-contaminated lithium disilicate ceramic. *Clin. Oral Investig.* **2020**, *24*, 2091–2097. [CrossRef] [PubMed]
15. Klosa, K.; Wolfart, S.; Lehmann, F.; Wenz, H.-J.; Kern, M. The effect of storage conditions, contamination modes and cleaning procedures on the resin bond strength to lithium disilicate ceramic. *J. Adhes. Dent.* **2009**, *11*, 127–135. [PubMed]
16. Alfaro, M.J.; Meyers, E.J.; Ashcraft-Olmscheid, D.; Vandewalle, K.S. Effect of a new salivary-contaminant removal method on bond strength. *Gen. Dent.* **2016**, *64*, 51–54. [PubMed]
17. Marfenko, S.; Özcan, M.; Attin, T.; Tauböck, T.T. Treatment of surface contamination of lithium disilicate ceramic before adhesive luting. *Am. J. Dent.* **2020**, *33*, 33–38. [PubMed]
18. Zarone, F.; Di Mauro, M.I.; Ausiello, P.; Ruggiero, G.; Sorrentino, R. Current status on lithium disilicate and zirconia: A narrative review. *BMC Oral Health* **2019**, *19*, 134. [CrossRef]
19. Aziz, A.; El-Mowafy, O.; Paredes, S. Clinical outcomes of lithium disilicate glass-ceramic crowns fabricated with CAD/CAM technology: A systematic review. *Dent. Med. Probl.* **2020**, *57*, 197–206. [CrossRef]
20. Maroulakos, G.; Thompson, G.A.; Kontogiorgos, E.D. Effect of cement type on the clinical performance and complications of zirconia and lithium disilicate tooth-supported crowns: A systematic review. Report of the Committee on Research in Fixed Prosthodontics of the American Academy of Fixed Prosthodontics. *J. Prosthet. Dent.* **2019**, *121*, 754–765. [CrossRef]
21. Hardan, L.; Bourgi, R.; Kharouf, N.; Mancino, D.; Zarow, M.; Jakubowicz, N.; Haikel, Y.; Cuevas-Suárez, C.-E. Reinforced Universal Adhesive by Ribose Crosslinker: A Novel Strategy in Adhesive Dentistry. *Polymers* **2021**, *13*, 704.

22. Kharouf, N.; Eid, A.; Hardan, L.; Bourgi, R.; Arntz, Y.; Jmal, H.; Foschi, F.; Sauro, S.; Ball, V.; Haikel, Y.; et al. Antibacterial and bonding properties of universal adhesive dental polymers doped with pyrogallol. *Polymers* **2021**, *13*, 1538. [CrossRef] [PubMed]
23. Irmak, Ö.; Yaman, B.C.; Orhan, E.O.; Kılıçarslan, M.A.; Mante, F.K.; Ozer, F. Influence of cleaning methods on bond strength to saliva contaminated zirconia. *J. Esthet. Restor. Dent.* **2018**, *30*, 551–556. [CrossRef] [PubMed]
24. Veríssimo, A.H.; Moura, D.M.D.; Tribst, J.P.M.; Araújo, A.M.M.d.; Leite, F.P.P.; Souza, R.d.A.E. Effect of hydrofluoric acid concentration and etching time on resin-bond strength to different glass ceramics. *Braz. Oral Res.* **2019**, *33*, e041. [CrossRef] [PubMed]
25. Blumer, L.; Schmidli, F.; Weiger, R.; Fischer, J. A systematic approach to standardize artificial aging of resin composite cements. *Dent. Mater.* **2015**, *31*, 855–863. [CrossRef]
26. *ISO/TS 11405:2015*; Dentistry-Testing of Adhesion to Tooth Structure. International Organizazion for Standardization: Geneva, Switzerland, 2015.
27. Bömicke, W.; Rammelsberg, P.; Krisam, J.; Rues, S. The Effects of Surface Conditioning and Aging on the Bond Strength Between Composite Cement and Zirconia-reinforced Lithium-Silicate Glass-Ceramics. *J. Adhes. Dent.* **2019**, *21*, 567–576.
28. Alnassar, T.; Vohra, F.; Abualsaud, H.; Al-Thobity, A.M.; Flinton, R. Efficacy of novel cleansing agent for the decontamination of lithium disilicate ceramics: A shear bond strength study. *J. Adhes. Sci. Technol.* **2017**, *31*, 202–210. [CrossRef]
29. Lyann, S.K.; Takagaki, T.; Nikaido, T.; Wada, T.; Uo, M.; Ikeda, M.; Sadr, A.; Tagami, J. Efficacy of Various Surface Treatments on the Bonding Performance of Saliva-contaminated Lithium-Disilicate Ceramics. *J. Adhes. Dent.* **2019**, *21*, 51–58.
30. Aboush, Y.E. Removing saliva contamination from porcelain veneers before bonding. *J. Prosthet. Dent.* **1998**, *80*, 649–653. [CrossRef]
31. Zhang, S.; Kocjan, A.; Lehmann, F.; Kosmac, T.; Kern, M. Influence of contamination on resin bond strength to nano-structured alumina-coated zirconia ceramic. *Eur. J. Oral Sci.* **2010**, *118*, 396–403. [CrossRef]
32. Della Bona, A.; Anusavice, K.J.; Mecholsky, J.J. Failure analysis of resin composite bonded to ceramic. *Dent. Mater.* **2003**, *19*, 693–699. [CrossRef]
33. Sano, H.; Shono, T.; Sonoda, H.; Takatsu, T.; Ciucchi, B.; Carvalho, R.; Pashley, D.H. Relationship between surface area for adhesion and tensile bond strength–evaluation of a micro-tensile bond test. *Dent. Mater.* **1994**, *10*, 236–240. [CrossRef]
34. Sano, H.; Chowdhury, A.F.M.A.; Saikaew, P.; Matsumoto, M.; Hoshika, S.; Yamauti, M. The microtensile bond strength test: Its historical background and application to bond testing. *Jpn. Dent. Sci. Rev.* **2020**, *56*, 24–31. [CrossRef] [PubMed]
35. Sirisha, K.; Rambabu, T.; Shankar, Y.R.; Ravikumar, P. Validity of bond strength tests: A critical review: Part I. *J. Conserv. Dent.* **2014**, *17*, 305–311. [CrossRef] [PubMed]
36. Sirisha, K.; Rambabu, T.; Ravishankar, Y.; Ravikumar, P. Validity of bond strength tests: A critical review-Part II. *J. Conserv. Dent.* **2014**, *17*, 420–426. [CrossRef]
37. Inoue, S.; Vargas, M.A.; Abe, Y.; Yoshida, Y.; Lambrechts, P.; Vanherle, G.; Sano, H.; Van Meerbeek, B. Microtensile bond strength of eleven contemporary adhesives to dentin. *J. Adhes. Dent.* **2001**, *3*, 237–245. [PubMed]
38. Braga, R.R.; Meira, J.B.C.; Boaro, L.C.C.; Xavier, T.A. Adhesion to tooth structure: A critical review of 'macro' test methods. *Dent. Mater.* **2010**, *26*, 38–49. [CrossRef] [PubMed]
39. Della Bona, A.; van Noort, R. Shear vs. tensile bond strength of resin composite bonded to ceramic. *J. Dent. Res.* **1995**, *74*, 1591–1596. [CrossRef]
40. Klosa, K.; Warnecke, H.; Kern, M. Effectiveness of protecting a zirconia bonding surface against contaminations using a newly developed protective lacquer. *Dent. Mater.* **2014**, *30*, 785–792. [CrossRef]
41. Wegner, S.M.; Gerdes, W.; Kern, M. Effect of different artificial aging conditions on ceramic-composite bond strength. *Int. J. Prosthodont.* **2002**, *15*, 267–272.

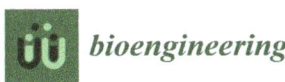

Article

Effectiveness of the REvision System and Sonic Irrigation in the Removal of Root Canal Filling Material from Oval Canals: An In Vitro Study

Marc Krikor Kaloustian [1], Claire El Hachem [2], Carla Zogheib [1], Walid Nehme [1], Louis Hardan [3], Pamela Rached [4], Naji Kharouf [4,5,*], Youssef Haikel [4,5,6] and Davide Mancino [4,5,6]

1. Department of Endodontics, Faculty of Dentistry, Saint Joseph University, Beirut 1107 2180, Lebanon; mkaloustian75@gmail.com (M.K.K.); zogheibcarla@gmail.com (C.Z.); walidnehmeendo@gmail.com (W.N.)
2. Department of Pediatric Dentistry, Faculty of Dentistry, Saint Joseph University, Beirut 1107 2180, Lebanon; claire.elhachem@gmail.com
3. Department of Restorative Dentistry, School of Dentistry, Saint-Joseph University, Beirut 1107 2180, Lebanon; louis.hardan@usj.edu.lb
4. Department of Biomaterials and Bioengineering, INSERM UMR_S 1121, Strasbourg University, 67000 Strasbourg, France; pamelarached98@gmail.com (P.R.); youssef.haikel@unistra.fr (Y.H.); mancino@unistra.fr (D.M.)
5. Department of Endodontics, Faculty of Dental Medicine, Strasbourg University, 67000 Strasbourg, France
6. Pôle de Médecine et Chirurgie Bucco-Dentaire, Hôpital Civil, Hôpitaux Universitaires, 67000 Strasbourg, France
* Correspondence: dentistenajikharouf@gmail.com; Tel.:+33-66752-2841

Citation: Kaloustian, M.K.; Hachem, C.E.; Zogheib, C.; Nehme, W.; Hardan, L.; Rached, P.; Kharouf, N.; Haikel, Y.; Mancino, D. Effectiveness of the REvision System and Sonic Irrigation in the Removal of Root Canal Filling Material from Oval Canals: An In Vitro Study. *Bioengineering* 2022, 9, 260. https://doi.org/10.3390/bioengineering9060260

Academic Editors: Dietmar W. Hutmacher and Abhay Pandit

Received: 17 May 2022
Accepted: 17 June 2022
Published: 19 June 2022

Publisher's Note: MDPI stays neutral with regard to jurisdictional claims in published maps and institutional affiliations.

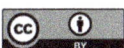

Copyright: © 2022 by the authors. Licensee MDPI, Basel, Switzerland. This article is an open access article distributed under the terms and conditions of the Creative Commons Attribution (CC BY) license (https://creativecommons.org/licenses/by/4.0/).

Abstract: This study aimed to evaluate the effectiveness of the Endostar REvision system (Poldent, Warsaw, Poland) in the removal of filling materials from oval root canals using sonic irrigation as an additional cleaning method. Thirty human-extracted mandibular premolars with oval canals were prepared using the ProTaper Universal system (Dentsply Maillefer, Ballaigues, Switzerland) up to instrument F1 (20/.07), and then filled by the continuous wave vertical compaction technique using pulp canal sealer EWT (Sybron Dental Specialties, Orange, CA, USA). The teeth were randomly divided into two groups (n = 15) according to the instrumentation system and the additional cleaning method, as follows: REvision (30/.08, 25/.06) with EQ-S sonic activation (Meta Biomed, Chungcheongbuk-do, Korea), REvision (30/.08, 25/.06) without additional activation. All specimens were sectioned longitudinally at 3 and 7 mm from the apex, and analyzed using digital microscopy (KEYENCE, Osaka, Japan) to measure the total area of the residual obturation materials, followed by SEM analysis. The data on the percentage of remaining filling material were analyzed by Kruskal–Wallis one-way Analysis of Variance on ranks. None of the retreatment protocols completely removed the filling material from the root canals (p > 0.05); the retreatment technique using sonic activation showed statistically less residual filling materials than the retreatment technique using irrigants without activation at the coronal third (p < 0.05), whilst no significant difference was found between both tested groups at the apical and middle thirds (p > 0.05). The REvision system showed promising results in the removal of filling materials from oval canals.

Keywords: retreatment procedure; filling materials removal; revision system; sonic activation; oval-shaped canal

1. Introduction

Restoring the periradicular and periapical regions is the main aim of nonsurgical root canal retreatment [1]. Around 46% of endodontic treatments are nonsurgical secondary treatments [2]. In addition, the long-term success of nonsurgical endodontic retreatment relies on the complete removal of the existing filling materials, debris, organic tissues, and microorganisms through proper cleaning, reshaping, and refilling of the root canal system [3]. The removal of the filling materials from the root canal system, especially in a curved-oval canal, presents a real challenge [4,5].

Nickel–titanium (Ni–Ti) instruments are recommended with the combination of different irrigants for facilitating the removal of old filling materials [6–8]. Some manufacturers have even developed instrumentation systems specifically designed for filling material removal, such as Mtwo Retreatment (VDW, Munich, Germany), ProTaper Universal Retreatment (Dentsply Maillefer, Ballaigues, Switzerland), and HyFlex Remover (Coltene Micromega). Until now, there is no validated system that ensures the complete removal of filling materials, including gutta-percha and sealer, from the root canal system [9]. The authors explain this by pointing out the unpredictable root canal anatomy and its variations, and the fact that there are regions unattained by instrumentation, especially when dealing with premolars [10].

The Endostar REvision system (Poldent, Warsaw, Poland) is a newly marketed heat retreatment system consisting of three blue files, the 30/.08, 25/.06, and 20/.04, characterized by a modified S-shaped cross-section with two cutting edges. The system has undergone a heat treatment process provided by particularly advanced technology, Azure HT technology, that offers extreme flexibility and great resistance to fracture [11]. So far, the effectiveness of REvision in the removal of filling materials from oval canals has not yet been evaluated.

Moreover, it was suggested in the literature that one should use supplementary approaches to enhance the removal of filling materials, since none of the proposed systems were able to render the root canal completely free of remnants [12,13]. Passive ultrasonic irrigation [3], sonic activation [12], Self-Adjusting File (SAF) instruments (ReDent, Ra'anana, Israel) [14], and an XP-endo Finisher (FKG Dentaire, La Chaux-de-Fonds, Switzerland) [1] were recommended.

The EQ S (Meta Biomed, Chungcheongbuk-do, Korea) sonic activation system is a cordless device with two speeds, a multidirectional movement, and tips in three different sizes (15/.02, 25/.02, and 35/.02) that can be used at 13000 and 8000 cycles per minute, producing a 133/217 Hz frequency [14]. This device demonstrated higher smear layer removal than other commercial devices, especially at the apical third [15].

All studies have agreed that predictable removal of all the materials from the root canal system is impossible. The use of sonic activation in retreatment was recommended by some authors [16], while others did not find sonic activation useful in filling material removal [12]. The combined use of a retreatment system and sonic activation did not render the canal free of residual materials [5]. Therefore, researchers continue to find more effective techniques, instruments, and devices to promote the complete removal of root canal filling materials [9,17]. The combined use of sonic irrigation and the REvision system is a novel methodology in filling material removal.

The objective of this study was to evaluate the effectiveness of a novel Ni–Ti system, the REvision sequence, in removing filling materials from oval canals with and without the use of the EQ-S sonic irrigation. The null hypothesis was that there is no difference in the effectiveness of the REvision system in filling material removal with or without the additional usage of the EQ-S device.

2. Materials and Methods

2.1. Sample Selection

After approval by the institutional ethics committee of Saint Joseph University, Beirut, Lebanon (USJ-2017-55), 85 lower premolars, extracted for reasons unrelated to the study, were cleaned using an ultrasonic insert (1S, Satelec Acteon Group, Mérignac, France) and stored in 0.1% formocresol. Teeth were inspected under an operating microscope (Zeiss Extaro 300, Oberkochen, Germany) at x25 magnification to eliminate teeth with cracks or advanced external resorption. Mesiodistal and vestibulolingual X-rays were taken (Sopix, Satelec Acteon Group, Merignac, France) to discard teeth with treated canals, pulpal calcification, or internal resorption. Cone beam computed tomography (Newtom VGI,

Verona, Italy) (CBCT) was performed, and only teeth with mature apices and a single oval canal with a moderate curvature of 15 to 22 degrees according to the Schneider technique, were included in the study [18–20]. Finally, 30 mandibular premolars were selected. Access cavity was prepared using an 856 diamond bur (Komet Italia SRL, Milan, Italy) with a high-speed handpiece under running water under an operating microscope, and a size #10 k-file (Dentsply Sirona, Ballaigues, Switzerland) was introduced to verify patency. This study followed the CRIS guidelines for in vitro studies, as discussed in the 2014 concept note [21].

2.2. Root Canal Initial Shaping and Filling

The crowns of the teeth were sectioned with a diamond disc (Kerr Dental, Bioggio, Switzerland) to standardize the root length at 15 mm. A size #15 K-file (Dentsply Sirona, Ballaigues, Switzerland) was inserted to establish the working length (WL) by reducing 1 mm from the apical foramen, and it was verified with a digital radiograph (Sopix, Satelec Acteon Group, Merignac, France). All the canals were prepared with the ProTaper Gold (Dentsply Sirona, Ballaigues, Switzerland). After this, glide path Proglider Sx, S1, S2, and F1 files were manipulated in an in/out and brushing motion with an amplitude of 3 mm to the WL, according to the manufacturer's instructions. To preserve apical patency, a size #10 K-file was introduced after each file. Subsequently, 3 mL of 6% sodium hypochlorite (NaOCl) was flushed using a 30-gauge NaviTip needle (Ultradent, South Jordan, UT, USA) to irrigate each canal. The smear layer was dissolved with 3 mL of 17% EDTA, followed by a final rinse with 5 mL of distilled water and 3 mL of 6% sodium hypochlorite. A new sequence was used to shape each canal. At the end of the shaping procedure, sterile size F1 absorbent points (Dentsply Sirona, Ballaigues, Switzerland) were used to dry the canals, which were filled with F1 gutta-percha (GP) points (Dentsply Sirona, Ballaigues, Switzerland) and pulp canal sealer EWT (Sybron Dental Specialties, Orange, CA, USA), using the continuous wave vertical compaction technique with a fine (F) 06 plugger (Sybron Dental Specialties, Orange, CA, USA). Using the Obtura II with a 23 G tip (Obtura Spartan Endodontics, Algonquin, IL, USA), GP was injected into the canal orifice. A buccolingual and a distomesial digital radiograph was taken to validate the quality of the filling in terms of length and density. None of the teeth exhibited a poor quality of obturation; therefore, none were discarded. The access cavities were sealed with a temporary restoration material (Cavit, 3M ESPE, Seefeld, Germany). Teeth were then incubated at 37 °C for 14 days with full saturated humidity to allow the final setting [22].

2.3. Nonsurgical Root Canal Secondary Treatment

After removing the temporary material using a round 856 diamond bur (Komet Italia SRL, Milan, Italy), the teeth were retreated using the REvision heat retreatment sequence. At the coronal third, 30/.08 instrument (Figure 1) was used; then, the 25/.06 instrument (Figure 1) was used at the middle and apical thirds. The files were manipulated using an Optimum Torque Reverse motor (OTR, patented by J. Morita Corp., Tokyo, Japan). The samples were then randomly divided using an online software at www.randomizer.org (accessed on 17 May 2022) to obtain two equal and balanced groups ($n = 15$) according to the following irrigation protocol:

Group 1: 12 mL of 6% NaOCl with a 30-G NaviTip needle was used and the canals were dried with F2 Paper points (Dentsply Sirona). Afterward, 3 mL of 17% EDTA was applied inside the canal for 1 min, followed by a final wash with 3 mL of 6% NaOCl.

Group 2: 12 mL of 6% NaOCl with a 30-G NaviTip needle was used. Sonic activation was then applied using the EQ-S cordless sonic endo irrigator coupled with the 25/02 tip at 13,000 cycles/min (217 Hz) [15], with 3 mm amplitude in-and-out movements without approaching the canal walls. Subsequently, 3 mL of 6% NaOCl irrigation, followed by 20 s of activation was repeated three times at 1 mm from the WL. F2 paper points (Dentsply Sirona) were used to dry the canals, and then 3 mL of 17% EDTA was applied, followed by 1 min of activation, and a final rinse with 3 mL of 6% NaOCl.

When the filling material was no longer apparent on the instrument or the canal walls under a ×16 operating microscope, the retreatment procedure was deemed complete.

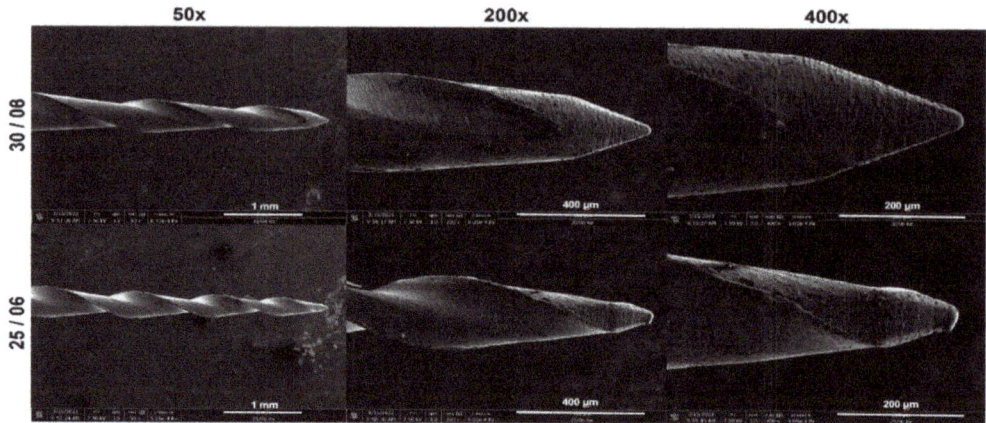

Figure 1. Scanning electron microscopy images demonstrating the Endostar REvision instrument (30/08 and 25/06).

2.4. Sectioning and Digital Microscopy Analysis

After retreatment procedures, two sections were positioned perpendicularly to the longitudinal axis of each tooth root, at 3 and 7 mm from the apex, with a diamond disc (Kerr Dental, Bioggio, Switzerland) to obtain three parts corresponding to the coronal, middle, and apical thirds. After that, to analyze the internal dentinal walls of the root canal, the specimens were sectioned by cutting two shallow longitudinal grooves (approximately 0.6 mm) in the buccolingual direction by means of a carbide bur (ref #329, KG Sorensen, São Paulo, Brazil) with a water-cooled, high-speed handpiece. The grooves were formed following the canal curvature and did not penetrate the canal. A chisel and mallet were used to split each sample. Both specimen halves were first observed using a digital microscope (KEYENCE, Osaka, Japan). One image was taken for each specimen using a 100× magnification. The micrographs at 100× magnification, showing the canal wall surface of both groups at the coronal, middle, and apical thirds, were coded for blinded analysis by an experienced examiner independent of the experiment, using the VHX-5000 communication software (KEYENCE, Osaka, Japan) to measure the total area of the residual obturation materials (gutta-percha and sealer) (Figure 2). The residual filling material percentages after retreatment were calculated by dividing the area of the residual materials measured during the analysis by the total area of the root canal of each specimen.

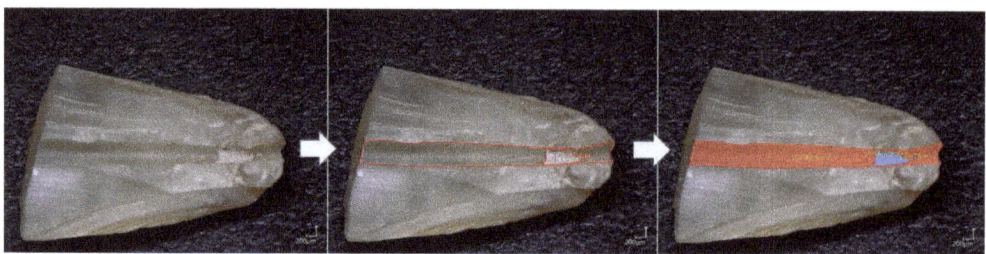

Figure 2. Methodology of residual materials area measurements using VHX-5000 software.

2.5. Scanning Electron Microscope Observations (SEM)

To better distinguish dentinal walls and filling material remnants, five samples were selected from each group and further analyzed using a scanning electron microscope to verify the regions observed using the digital microscope. The specimens were dehydrated in a graded series of ethanol solutions and sputter-coated with a gold–palladium alloy (20/80 weight %) using a Hummer JR sputtering device (Technics, Rocklin, CA, USA). A Quanta 250 FEG scanning electron microscope (SEM) (FEI Company, Eindhoven, The Netherlands) with an electron acceleration voltage of 10 kV at a magnification of ×100 to ×4000 was used to analyze the prepared samples. The obtained images from SEM were considered an extra tool to help the examiner be more meticulous in measuring the total area of the residual obturation materials, which exhibit different colors under the digital microscope (Figure 3).

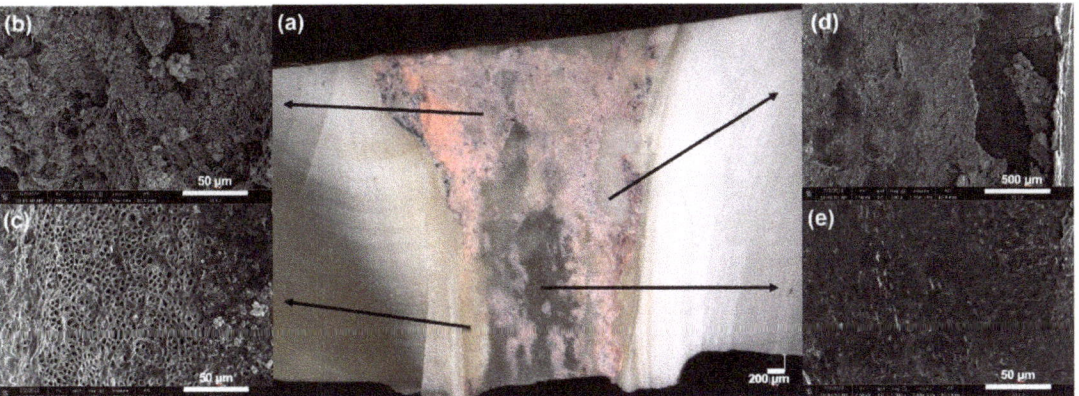

Figure 3. Scanning electron microscope micrographs showing the different observed colors and structures of the root canal and residual materials, which were detected under a digital microscope. (**a**) Digital microscope image; (**b**) residual materials (gutta-percha/sealer); (**c**) dentinal wall with open tubules; (**d**) residual materials–dentin interface; (**e**) dentinal walls with closed tubules.

2.6. Statistical Analysis

Sigma Plot software (11.2, Systat Software, Inc., San Jose, CA, USA) was used for data analysis, with a significance level of $\alpha = 0.05$. The normality of data distribution within both groups was tested using the Shapiro–Wilk test. The normality was not verified, thus, Kruskal–Wallis one-way Analysis of Variance on ranks including multiple comparison procedures (Tukey Test) was applied to determine whether significant differences existed between the different retreatment techniques for the removal of filling materials at apical, middle, and coronal thirds.

3. Results

The retreatment technique using activation for the endodontic irrigants showed statistically less residual filling materials than the retreatment technique using irrigants without activation at the coronal third ($p < 0.05$), whilst no significant difference was found between both tested groups at the apical and middle thirds ($p > 0.05$) (Table 1).

Table 1. Residual material percentages after both retreatment techniques with or without activation of endodontic irrigants. Different superscripted letters indicate significant differences between the different groups ($p < 0.05$).

	Apical	Middle	Coronal	Statistical Analysis ($p < 0.05$)
Activation (%)	9.59 ± 12.40	4.57 ± 8.56 [a]	8.939.05 [a]	$p = 0.021$
Without activation (%)	14.02 ± 20.14	8.66 ± 13.71 [b]	19.17 ± 22.60 [b]	$p = 0.0040$
Statistical analysis ($p < 0.05$)	No ($p = 0.253$)	No ($p = 0.386$)	Yes ($p = 0.036$)	

The results of digital microscope analysis for materials removal after both final irrigation protocols are summarized in Figure 4. No statistically significant difference was found between apical–coronal and apical–middle thirds for both groups ($p > 0.05$). The middle third of each group, with and without activation, had significantly less residual obturation materials than the coronal third, ($p = 0.021$ and $p = 0.04$, respectively) (Table 1).

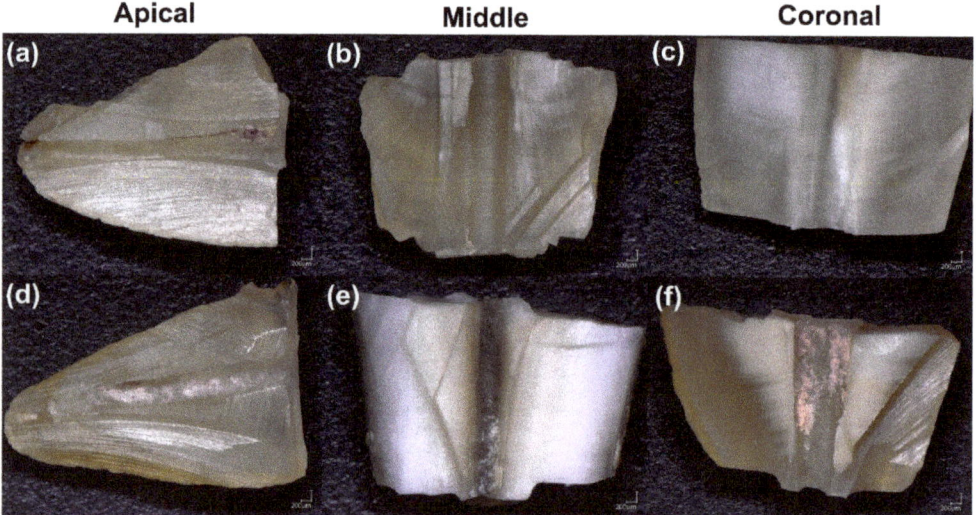

Figure 4. Digital microscope images demonstrate the effectiveness of the retreatment technique with irrigant activation (**a**–**c**) and without irrigant activation (**d**–**f**) in the apical, middle, and coronal thirds of the root canal.

4. Discussion

Oval-shaped canals are frequently associated with insufficient preparation and cleaning during initial and secondary root canal treatment [23]. There is a discrepancy between buccolingual and mesiodistal dimensions resulting in untouched recessed areas that harbor residues of filling material, bacteria, and debris, which increases the risk of persistent infection [24,25]. Incomplete removal of filling material may hinder the prognosis of root canal secondary treatment [10]. This study aimed to determine the effectiveness of the REvision retreatment system in the removal of filling materials from oval canals with and without sonic irrigation (SI) activation as an additional cleaning method.

The results show that the REvision system alone, and coupled with SI, failed to remove 100% of the filling material from the root canals, corroborating the findings of previous studies [17,26]. However, the REvision system showed interesting results in removing filling materials without sonic activation, with 14.02% remnants in the apical third, 8.66% in the middle third, and 19.17% in the coronal third. This may be credited to the cutting efficiency of the Endostar Azure instruments with an S-shaped section [11], and to their metallurgic properties that combine the enhanced flexibility and controlled memory of martensitic files with the stiffness and hardness of austenitic files. This may also be attributed to anatomical variations. When compared with mesial canals of mandibular molars with the presence of a filled isthmus, or lower incisors with a high degree of flatness, mandibular premolars are less flattened, which favors a greater contact area of the instrument against the canal walls and, therefore, better cleaning without the need for additional methods, making the agitation of the irrigating solutions a minor factor in obtaining improved cleaning [12]. The lack of improvement in the debris score after using a supplementary cleaning method was probably also because of the high bond strength of the pulp canal sealer EWT to root dentin [27]. In recent years, the introduction of Bioceramic sealers, such as EndoSequence BC Sealer (BC Sealer, Brasseler USA, Savannah, GA, USA) and Bio-C Sealer (Angelus, Londrína, PR, Brazil), has drastically impacted the endodontic fields [28]. These sealers offer great advantages, including biocompatibility, the ability to set in humidity, and to form a chemical bond with the tooth structure, achieving an excellent hermetic seal [29]. However, a major drawback of Bioceramic sealers is their retreatability in the case of apical periodontitis [30]. The quality of evidence is low regarding the efficiency of available instrumentation in entirely removing a Bioceramic sealer [31,32]. Very few studies have evaluated the capacity of heat-treated files such as the REvision system in Bioceramic retreatment. Al Meida et al. concluded that Reciproc Blue file (VDW, Munich, Germany) did not induce dentinal defects when removing a Bioceramic sealer. Some authors suggested the use of ultrasonics, XP Endo Finisher, and Photon-initiated photoacoustic streaming (PIPS) to raise the efficiency of sealer removal, whereas the use of sonic irrigation has not yet been evaluated in the retreatability of a Bioceramic sealer [30,33]. It would be interesting to conduct a series of in vitro and clinical randomized studies to develop a feasible and reproducible protocol for bioceramic retreatment.

The results of this study suggest that the REvision retreatment system associated with sonic irrigation using EQ-S could enhance the removal of filling materials from the coronal third compared to removal by the REvision retreatment system associated with irrigation by needles ($p < 0.05$). This result may be attributed to the root canal preparation size (F1), which allowed sufficient debris transportation coronally. Moreover, no significant difference was found between the two groups for the middle and apical thirds ($p > 0.05$). Therefore, the null hypothesis must be partially rejected. This was also observed in the study of Rodriguez et al., in which there was no significant difference in the efficiency of sonic activation in canal thirds when compared with Passive Ultrasonic Activation (PUI), and in the study of Martins et al., where the EndoActivator (Dentsply Tulsa Dental Specialties, Tulsa, OK) performed similarly for all of the root canal levels evaluated, and did not improve the removal of filling material significantly [34,35]. This was also observed in the clinical study of Grischke et al., where the performance of the EndoActivator was reasonably heterogeneous with measured values of residues all over the canal [36].

No significant difference was found between the middle and apical thirds in both groups ($p > 0.05$). The study of Park et al. confirmed that the use of EDDY (VDW, Munich, Germany) sonic activation was beneficial for removing smear layers in apical regions in retreatment cases [8]. Interestingly, in the same tested group (for both groups), a significantly higher percentage of residual materials was observed at the coronal third compared to the middle third ($p < 0.05$). This was also concluded in the study of Zuolo et al., with no significant difference among the retreatment systems in the coronal third, and a lower residual filling material volume in the middle third, and in the study of Masiero et al., where most of the residual filling material was retained in the coronal third [24,37].

The effectiveness of EQ-S sonic activation is attributed to acoustic streaming within the irrigant, generated by the oscillating tip. Such streaming fields produce hydrodynamic shear stress along the endosonic files and mainly at the tip [38,39]. Even when the tip is constrained, streaming still occurs along the whole length of the file [40]; a polyamide tip in the case of EQ-S. The effect of activation is dependent on the frequency of the instrument inside the root canal and the amplitude of the swinging instrument [41]. Thus, activation might occur at lower frequencies; for example, the EQ-S irrigator operating at 217 Hz. In the literature, sonic activation was proved to be helpful in retreatment [8,16,22]. Özyürek and Demiryüek found the EndoActivator less effective than the XP-endo Finisher, whereas Grischke et al. and Martins et al. stipulated in their studies that there was no difference between the EndoActivator and PUI [12,22,36]. Differences in root canal morphology, type of filling material, and retreatment techniques could explain the contradictory results.

Various techniques have been advocated to evaluate the residual filling materials left in the root canal after retreatment, including radiographic imaging [42], clearing techniques, sectioning, and microscopic evaluation [43,44]. Recently, micro-CT imaging with high resolution has been praised in numerous studies because it is a noninvasive technique that allows accurate quantification measurements at different stages of the treatment, the specimen thus serving as its control [1,45]. However, micro-CT usage can lead to artifacts in the reconstructed images, such as beam-hardening, complicating the interpretation of the image [46]. In this study, we opted for digital microscopy followed by SEM analysis for some samples. This methodology can provide direct topographical and morphological data on the filling materials, especially the presence of sealer on the surface of the root canal walls and in dentinal tubules [44,47]. Moreover, a numerical optical microscope with composition images taken at a magnification of $\times 100$ could be a reliable alternative to the suboptimal micro-CT axial sections resolution [44,47,48]. The teeth were sectioned with a diamond saw, and then split into two halves without touching the canal. This method was used to avoid the alteration of our results due to the debris created during sectioning procedures. Moreover, the use of SEM allowed the identification of the gutta-percha, sealer, the dentinal walls with open or closed tubules, and the residual materials–dentin areas. This could be particularly interesting for educational purposes and clinical improvement, as it allows one to visualize unprepared areas of the canals, debris, and smear layer persistence in the dental tubules.

The limitations of this study relate to its invasive methodology, consisting of sectioning the teeth, and the reduced sample size. In addition, during the sample preparation for the optical analysis, different steps could affect the results, including the use of a diamond disc and the preparation of grooves, which could generate some supplementary debris. Further in vitro study using other activation techniques and devices, such as ultrasonic and mechanical activation, should be performed. Further in vivo studies are needed to confirm the results regarding the effectiveness of the REvision system in filling material removal from oval canals with or without the additional usage of sonic irrigation.

5. Conclusions

The results of this study suggest that the REvision retreatment system associated with sonic irrigation using EQ-S could enhance the removal of filling materials from the coronal third compared to removal by the REvision retreatment system associated with irrigation by needles. No statistically significant difference was found between the middle and apical thirds in both groups. None of the techniques removed the root canal filling materials entirely from the oval canal of mandibular premolars. The combination of EQ-S sonic irrigation and REvision retreatment system seemed to increase the removal of filling material from the coronal third, whilst no significant difference was observed for the middle and apical thirds. Moreover, when no additional cleaning method was applied, the REvision system alone showed interesting results that merit further investigations. Additional studies could eventually evaluate the use of extended irrigation time or the use of other irrigation techniques in different anatomical situations to attain a safe and reliable removal of old filling materials from the root canal system.

Author Contributions: Conceptualization, M.K.K. and W.N.; methodology, M.K.K., P.R., C.E.H.; software, N.K.; validation, N.K., D.M., L.H. and Y.H.; data curation, N.K.; writing—original draft preparation, M.K.K.; writing—review and editing, N.K. and C.E.H.; supervision, W.N., C.Z., D.M. and N.K.; project administration, M.K.K. and N.K. All authors have read and agreed to the published version of the manuscript.

Funding: This research received no external funding.

Institutional Review Board Statement: This in vitro study was approved by the institutional ethics committee of Saint Joseph University, Beirut, Lebanon (USJ-2017-55).

Informed Consent Statement: Not applicable.

Data Availability Statement: Not applicable.

Conflicts of Interest: The authors declare no conflict of interest.

References

1. Crozeta, B.M.; Silva-Sousa, Y.T.C.; Leoni, G.B.; Mazzi-Chaves, J.F.; Fantinato, T.; Baratto-Filho, F.; Sousa-Neto, M.D. Micro-Computed Tomography Study of Filling Material Removal from Oval-shaped Canals by Using Rotary, Reciprocating, and Adaptive Motion Systems. *J. Endod.* **2016**, *42*, 793–797. [CrossRef] [PubMed]
2. Lin, S.; Sabbah, W.; Sedgley, C.M.; Whitten, B. A survey for endodontists in today's economy: Exploring the current state of endodontics as a profession and the relationship between endodontists and their referral base. *J. Endod.* **2015**, *41*, 325–332. [CrossRef] [PubMed]
3. Crozeta, B.M.; Chaves de Souza, L.; Correa Silva-Sousa, Y.T.; Sousa-Neto, M.D.; Jaramillo, D.E.; Silva, R.M. Evaluation of Passive Ultrasonic Irrigation and GentleWave System as Adjuvants in Endodontic Retreatment. *J. Endod.* **2020**, *46*, 1279–1285. [CrossRef] [PubMed]
4. Kfir, A.; Tsesis, I.; Yakirevich, E.; Matalon, S.; Abramovitz, I. The efficacy of five techniques for removing root filling material: Microscopic versus radiographic evaluation. *Int. Endod. J.* **2012**, *45*, 35–41. [CrossRef] [PubMed]
5. Jiang, S.; Zou, T.; Li, D.; Chang, J.W.W.; Huang, X.; Zhang, C. Effectiveness of Sonic, Ultrasonic, and Photon Induced Photoacoustic Streaming Activation of NaOCl on Filling Material Removal Following Retreatment in Oval Canal Anatomy. *Photomed. Laser Surg.* **2016**, *34*, 3–10. [CrossRef] [PubMed]
6. Pirani, C.; Pelliccioni, G.A.; Marchionni, S.; Montebugnoli, L.; Piana, G.; Prati, C. Effectiveness of three different retreatment techniques in canals filled with compacted gutta-percha or Thermafil: A scanning electron microscope study. *J. Endod.* **2009**, *35*, 1433–1440. [CrossRef]
7. Mollo, A.; Botti, G.; Prinicipi Goldoni, N.; Randellini, E.; Paragliola, R.; Chazine, M.; Ounsi, H.F.; Grandini, S. Efficacy of two Ni-Ti systems and hand files for removing gutta-percha from root canals. *Int. Endod. J.* **2012**, *45*, 1–6. [CrossRef]
8. Park, S.Y.; Kang, M.K.; Choi, H.W.; Shon, W.-J. Comparative Analysis of Root Canal Filling Debris and Smear Layer Removal Efficacy Using Various Root Canal Activation Systems during Endodontic Retreatment. *Medicina* **2020**, *56*, 615. [CrossRef] [PubMed]
9. Duncan, H.F.; Chong, B.S. Removal of root filling materials. *Endod. Top.* **2008**, *19*, 33–57. [CrossRef]
10. Gorni, F.G.M.; Gagliani, M.M. The outcome of endodontic retreatment: A 2-yr follow-up. *J. Endod.* **2004**, *30*, 1–4. [CrossRef]
11. Rebeiz, J.; Claire, E.H.; El Osta, N.; Habib, M.; Rebeiz, T.; Zogheib, C.; Kaloustian, M. Shaping ability of a new heat-treated NiTi system in continuous rotation or reciprocation in artificial curved canals. *Odontology* **2021**, *109*, 792–801. [CrossRef] [PubMed]
12. Martins, M.P.; Duarte, M.A.H.; Cavenago, B.C.; Kato, A.S.; da Silveira Bueno, C.E. Effectiveness of the ProTaper Next and Reciproc Systems in Removing Root Canal Filling Material with Sonic or Ultrasonic Irrigation: A Micro-computed Tomographic Study. *J. Endod.* **2017**, *43*, 467–471. [CrossRef] [PubMed]
13. Bago, I.; Suk, M.; Katić, M.; Gabrić, D.; Anić, I. Comparison of the effectiveness of various rotary and reciprocating systems with different surface treatments to remove gutta-percha and an epoxy resin-based sealer from straight root canals. *Int. Endod. J.* **2019**, *52*, 105–113. [CrossRef]
14. Solomonov, M.; Paqué, F.; Kaya, S.; Adigüzel, O.; Kfir, A.; Yiğit-Özer, S. Self-adjusting files in retreatment: A high-resolution micro-computed tomography study. *J. Endod.* **2012**, *38*, 1283–1287. [CrossRef] [PubMed]
15. Kharouf, N.; Pedullà, E.; La Rosa, G.R.M.; Bukiet, F.; Sauro, S.; Haikel, Y.; Mancino, D. In Vitro Evaluation of Different Irrigation Protocols on Intracanal Smear Layer Removal in Teeth with or without Pre-Endodontic Proximal Wall Restoration. *J. Clin. Med.* **2020**, *9*, 3325. [CrossRef]
16. Kaloustian, M.K.; Nehme, W.; El Hachem, C.; Zogheib, C.; Ghosn, N.; Mallet, J.P.; Diemer, F.; Naaman, A. Evaluation of two shaping systems and two sonic irrigation devices in removing root canal filling material from distal roots of mandibular molars assessed by micro CT. *Int. Endod. J.* **2019**, *52*, 1635–1644. [CrossRef]
17. Taşdemir, T.; Er, K.; Yildirim, T.; Celik, D. Efficacy of three rotary NiTi instruments in removing gutta-percha from root canals. *Int. Endod. J.* **2008**, *41*, 191–196. [CrossRef] [PubMed]

18. Schneider, S.W. A comparison of canal preparations in straight and curved root canals. *Oral Surg. Oral Med. Oral Pathol.* **1971**, *32*, 271–275. [CrossRef]
19. Schirrmeister, J.F.; Wrbas, K.-T.; Meyer, K.M.; Altenburger, M.J.; Hellwig, E. Efficacy of different rotary instruments for gutta-percha removal in root canal retreatment. *J. Endod.* **2006**, *32*, 469–472. [CrossRef] [PubMed]
20. de Oliveira, D.P.; Barbizam, J.V.B.; Trope, M.; Teixeira, F.B. Comparison between gutta-percha and resilon removal using two different techniques in endodontic retreatment. *J. Endod.* **2006**, *32*, 362–364. [CrossRef]
21. Krithikadatta, J.; Gopikrishna, V.; Datta, M. CRIS Guidelines (Checklist for Reporting In-vitro Studies): A concept note on the need for standardized guidelines for improving quality and transparency in reporting in-vitro studies in experimental dental research. *J. Conserv. Dent. JCD* **2014**, *17*, 301–304. [CrossRef] [PubMed]
22. Özyürek, T.; Demiryürek, E.Ö. Comparison of the Effectiveness of Different Techniques for Supportive Removal of Root Canal Filling Material. *Eur. Endod. J.* **2016**, *1*, 6. [CrossRef]
23. Ricucci, D.; Siqueira, J.F. Fate of the tissue in lateral canals and apical ramifications in response to pathologic conditions and treatment procedures. *J. Endod.* **2010**, *36*, 1–15. [CrossRef] [PubMed]
24. Masiero, A.V.; Barletta, F.B. Effectiveness of different techniques for removing gutta-percha during retreatment. *Int. Endod. J.* **2005**, *38*, 2–7. [CrossRef]
25. Vieira, A.R.; Siqueira, J.F.; Ricucci, D.; Lopes, W.S.P. Dentinal tubule infection as the cause of recurrent disease and late endodontic treatment failure: A case report. *J. Endod.* **2012**, *38*, 250–254. [CrossRef] [PubMed]
26. Bernardes, R.A.; Duarte, M.a.H.; Vivan, R.R.; Alcalde, M.P.; Vasconcelos, B.C.; Bramante, C.M. Comparison of three retreatment techniques with ultrasonic activation in flattened canals using micro-computed tomography and scanning electron microscopy. *Int. Endod. J.* **2016**, *49*, 890–897. [CrossRef]
27. da Silva Machado, A.P.; Câncio Couto de Souza, A.C.; Lima Gonçalves, T.; Franco Marques, A.A.; da Fonseca Roberti Garcia, L.; Antunes Bortoluzzi, E.; Acris de Carvalho, F.M. Does the ultrasonic activation of sealer hinder the root canal retreatment? *Clin. Oral Investig.* **2021**, *25*, 4401–4406. [CrossRef]
28. Raura, N.; Garg, A.; Arora, A.; Roma, M. Nanoparticle technology and its implications in endodontics: A review. *Biomater. Res.* **2020**, *24*, 21. [CrossRef]
29. Camilleri, J.; Atmeh, A.; Li, X.; Meschi, N. Present status and future directions: Hydraulic materials for endodontic use. *Int. Endod. J.* **2022**, *55* (Suppl. 3), 710–777. [CrossRef]
30. Zhekov, K.I.; Stefanova, V.P. Retreatability of Bioceramic Endodontic Sealers: A Review. *Folia Med.* **2020**, *62*, 258–264. [CrossRef] [PubMed]
31. Hess, D.; Solomon, E.; Spears, R.; He, J. Retreatability of a bioceramic root canal sealing material. *J. Endod.* **2011**, *37*, 1547–1549. [CrossRef]
32. Arul, B.; Varghese, A.; Mishra, A.; Elango, S.; Padmanaban, S.; Natanasabapathy, V. Retrievability of bioceramic-based sealers in comparison with epoxy resin-based sealer assessed using microcomputed tomography: A systematic review of laboratory-based studies. *J. Conserv. Dent. JCD* **2021**, *24*, 421–434. [CrossRef] [PubMed]
33. Sinsareekul, C.; Hiran-us, S. Comparison of the efficacy of three different supplementary cleaning protocols in root-filled teeth with a bioceramic sealer after retreatment—a micro-computed tomographic study. *Clin. Oral Investig.* **2022**, *26*, 3515–3521. [CrossRef] [PubMed]
34. Rodrigues, C.T.; Duarte, M.A.H.; Guimarães, B.M.; Vivan, R.R.; Bernardineli, N. Comparison of two methods of irrigant agitation in the removal of residual filling material in retreatment. *Braz. Oral Res.* **2017**, *31*, e113. [CrossRef]
35. Machado, A.G.; Guilherme, B.P.S.; Provenzano, J.C.; Marceliano-Alves, M.F.; Gonçalves, L.S.; Siqueira, J.F.; Neves, M.A.S. Effects of preparation with the Self-Adjusting File, TRUShape and XP-endo Shaper systems, and a supplementary step with XP-endo Finisher R on filling material removal during retreatment of mandibular molar canals. *Int. Endod. J.* **2019**, *52*, 709–715. [CrossRef] [PubMed]
36. Grischke, J.; Müller-Heine, A.; Hülsmann, M. The effect of four different irrigation systems in the removal of a root canal sealer. *Clin. Oral Investig.* **2014**, *18*, 1845–1851. [CrossRef]
37. de Siqueira Zuolo, A.; Zuolo, M.L.; da Silveira Bueno, C.E.; Chu, R.; Cunha, R.S. Evaluation of the Efficacy of TRUShape and Reciproc File Systems in the Removal of Root Filling Material: An Ex Vivo Micro–Computed Tomographic Study. *J. Endod.* **2016**, *42*, 315–319. [CrossRef] [PubMed]
38. Ahmad, M.; Pitt Ford, T.J.; Crum, L.A. Ultrasonic debridement of root canals: Acoustic streaming and its possible role. *J. Endod.* **1987**, *13*, 490–499. [CrossRef]
39. Walmsley, A.D.; Williams, A.R. Effects of constraint on the oscillatory pattern of endosonic files. *J. Endod.* **1989**, *15*, 189–194. [CrossRef]
40. Lumley, P.J.; Walmsley, A.D.; Laird, W.R. Streaming patterns produced around endosonic files. *Int. Endod. J.* **1991**, *24*, 290–297. [CrossRef]
41. Lumley, P.J.; Blunt, L.; Walmsley, A.D.; Marquis, P.M. Analysis of the surface cut by sonic files. *Endod. Dent. Traumatol.* **1996**, *12*, 240–245. [CrossRef] [PubMed]
42. Baxter, S.; Schöler, C.; Dullin, C.; Hülsmann, M. Sensitivity of conventional radiographs and cone-beam computed tomography in detecting the remaining root-canal filling material. *J. Oral Sci.* **2020**, *62*, 271–274. [CrossRef] [PubMed]

43. Raj, P.K.T.; Mudrakola, D.P.; Baby, D.; Govindankutty, R.K.; Davis, D.; Sasikumar, T.P.; Ealla, K.K.R. Evaluation of Effectiveness of Two Different Endodontic Retreatment Systems in Removal of Gutta-percha: An in vitro Study. *J. Contemp. Dent. Pract.* **2018**, *19*, 726–731. [PubMed]
44. Mancino, D.; Kharouf, N.; Cabiddu, M.; Bukiet, F.; Haïkel, Y. Microscopic and chemical evaluation of the filling quality of five obturation techniques in oval-shaped root canals. *Clin. Oral Investig.* **2021**, *25*, 3757–3765. [CrossRef] [PubMed]
45. Amoroso-Silva, P.; Alcalde, M.P.; Hungaro Duarte, M.A.; De-Deus, G.; Ordinola-Zapata, R.; Freire, L.G.; Cavenago, B.C.; De Moraes, I.G. Effect of finishing instrumentation using NiTi hand files on volume, surface area and uninstrumented surfaces in C-shaped root canal systems. *Int. Endod. J.* **2017**, *50*, 604–611. [CrossRef] [PubMed]
46. De-Deus, G.; Belladonna, F.G.; Cavalcante, D.M.; Simões-Carvalho, M.; Silva, E.J.N.L.; Carvalhal, J.C.A.; Zamolyi, R.Q.; Lopes, R.T.; Versiani, M.A.; Dummer, P.M.H.; et al. Contrast-enhanced micro-CT to assess dental pulp tissue debridement in root canals of extracted teeth: A series of cascading experiments towards method validation. *Int. Endod. J.* **2021**, *54*, 279–293. [CrossRef]
47. Kharouf, N.; Arntz, Y.; Eid, A.; Zghal, J.; Sauro, S.; Haikel, Y.; Mancino, D. Physicochemical and Antibacterial Properties of Novel, Premixed Calcium Silicate-Based Sealer Compared to Powder–Liquid Bioceramic Sealer. *J. Clin. Med.* **2020**, *9*, 3096. [CrossRef]
48. Mancino, D.; Kharouf, N.; Hemmerlé, J.; Haïkel, Y. Microscopic and Chemical Assessments of the Filling Ability in Oval-Shaped Root Canals Using Two Different Carrier-Based Filling Techniques. *Eur. J. Dent.* **2019**, *13*, 166–171. [CrossRef]

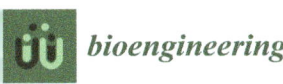

Case Report

Implant Periapical Lesion: Clinical and Histological Analysis of Two Case Reports Carried Out with Two Different Approaches

Roberto Luongo [1], Fabio Faustini [2], Alessandro Vantaggiato [3], Giuseppe Bianco [4], Tonino Traini [5], Antonio Scarano [4], Eugenio Pedullà [6] and Calogero Bugea [3,*]

1. Independent Researcher, 70121 Bari, Italy; rl66@nyu.edu
2. Independent Researcher, 29020 Piacenza, Italy; info@dentalfaustini.it
3. Independent Researcher, 73100 Lecce, Italy; alessandrovantaggiato@gmail.com
4. Department of Medical, Oral and Biotechnological Sciences, University of "G. D'Annunzio" of Chieti-Pescara, 66100 Chieti, Italy; gb373@nyu.edu (G.B.); ascarano@unich.it (A.S.)
5. Department of Innovative Technologies in Medicine & Dentistry, University of "G. D'Annunzio" of Chieti-Pescara, 66100 Chieti, Italy; t.traini@unich.it
6. Department of General Surgery and Surgical-Medical Specialties, University of Catania, 95100 Catania, Italy; eugenio.pedulla@unict.it
* Correspondence: calogerobugea@yahoo.it

Abstract: Periapical implantitis (IPL) is an increasingly frequent complication of dental implants. The causes of this condition are not yet entirely clear, although a bacterial component is certainly part of the etiology. In this case series study, two approaches will be described: because of persistent IPL symptoms, a patient had the implant removed and underwent histological analysis after week 6 from implantation. The histomorphometric examination revealed a 35% bone-implant contact area involving the coronal two-thirds of the implant. The apical portion of the fixture on the other hand was affected by an inflammatory process detectable on radiography as a radiolucent area. The presence of a probable root fragment, detectable as an imprecise radiopaque mass in the zone where the implant was later placed, confirms the probable bacterial etiology of this case of IPL. On the other hand, in case number 2, the presence of IPL around the fixture was solved by surgically removing the implant apical third as well as the adjacent tooth apex. It may be concluded from our histological examination that removal of the apical portion of the fixture should be considered an effective treatment for IPL since the remaining implant segment remains optimally osseointegrated and capable of continuing its function as a prosthetic abutment. Careful attention, however, is required at the implantation planning stage to identify in advance any sources of infection in the edentulous area of interest which might compromise the final outcome.

Keywords: implant periapical lesion; implant failure; peri-implantitis; endodontic surgery; complication

1. Introduction

Although the predictability of endosseous implants is well supported in studies, the possibility of failure in the long and short term still exists [1]. Implant failures have been defined as a host tissue inadequacy in stabilizing or maintaining osseointegration. Correlated with the time of onset, such failures may be classified as early or late depending on whether they occur before or after occlusal loading. Implant failures may be due to iatrogenic causes associated with a less-than-optimal surgical technique, bacterial causes secondary to contamination of the implant site during or after insertion of the fixture, possible systemic comorbidities, and excessive occlusal loading [1–5].

The clinical signs of early failure of an implant are local inflammation of the peri-implant hard and soft tissue, defined above as "peri-implantitis", and sometimes accompanied by secretion of purulent exudate, bleeding, and probing depth more than 3 mm. Histological findings from the peri-implant area include the presence of an inflammatory cellular infiltrate, epithelial proliferation, bacteria, and ultimately areas of osseous necrosis [1]. Radiographically, however, a radiolucent zone is detectable in the peri-implantitis affected area around the fixture, resembling an osseous crater at the crestal level that extends in the apical direction. Peri-implantitis and periodontitis may trigger interactions between host immune defense mechanism and bacteria that eventually lead to implant failures.

The most common type of peri-implantitis generally involves the more coronal part of the implant and only later tends to spread in the apical direction, sometimes leaving the apical portion of the fixture still firmly integrated in the crestal bone [6].

It may happen occasionally that peri-implantitis will develop apically in the same manner as a periapical lesion of a dental structure, i.e., without involvement of the coronal crest bone. This particular condition has been defined as implant periapical lesion (IPL), apical peri-implantitis, retrograde peri-implantitis, or endodontic implant pathology. It should be considered a distinct form relative to the more common form of peri-implantitis, which involves the coronal portion of the fixture [7,8].

A retrospective study of approximately 3800 implants found an IPL incidence of 0.26%. In another study, Quirynen reported an IPL incidence of 1.6% in the maxilla and 2.7% in the mandible [9,10].

The best evidence-supported etiology of IPL is diffusion of pathogenic bacteria from infected dental remnants present in the bone around the tip of the implant, or implant-adjacent dental structures with endodontic periapical lesions [9,10]. Depending on the sources releasing the peri-implant infection, the IPL may be divided into Type 1, when diffusion proceeds from the fixture to the adjacent dental structure and Type 2, when the structure is affected first by an inflammatory process diffusing to the nearby implant [11].

This article describes two cases of IPL, which were treated with two different approaches: a surgical removal of the entire affected fixture and a surgical removal of just the apical third of the implant as well as the adjacent tooth apex.

2. Case Report n.1

A 45-year-old patient in good general health, non-smoker, with partial edentulism in the right mandible, presented to our service for rehabilitation of the missing structures with implant-supported prostheses.

On presentation, the patient was already edentulous in the area of the right mandibular second premolar and the first and second molar for more than 10 years. Before developing an adequate treatment plan, we ordered a pantomograph (Figure 1), after which CT was needed because of the close proximity of the alveolar canal.

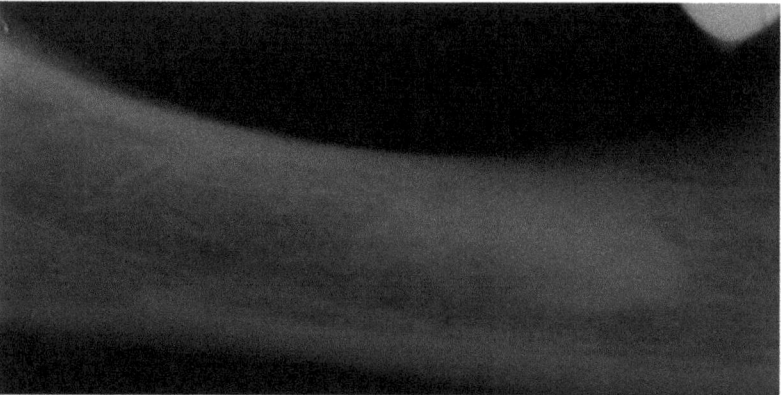

Figure 1. Preoperative intraoral radiograph of the edentulous area.

The CT scan demonstrated the presence of a small area of radiopacity of the bony structure at teeth 46–47, the nature of which could not be defined (Figure 2). The patient treatment plan proposed rehabilitation with a 3-unit fixed partial denture supported on 2 implants at #45 and #47. The patient was administered antibiotic therapy from day 1 of the intervention: the regimen was 1 g amoxicillin/clavulanic acid (Augmentin; Glaxo SmithKline, Verona, Italy), 1 g q12 h for 6 days postoperatively for a total of 7 days of treatment. Following local/regional anesthesia with mepivacaine 2% and adrenaline 1:100,000 (Scandonest, Septodont, Saint-Maur des Fossés, France), a full-thickness flap was raised from tooth 44 to 47. Trunk anesthesia was not performed so as to preserve the sensitivity of the alveolar nerve during the subsequent osteotomies, thereby avoiding injury of the vascular-neural bundle. Later, two osteotomies were prepared free-handed at teeth 45 and 47 with the aid of a surgical template. Lastly, two cylindrical Biomet 3i (Palm Beach Gardens, FL, USA) implants were placed, one with 4 mm diameter × 10 mm length at #45 and the other of the expanded platform (Xp) type, i.e., an implant diameter of 4 mm and a platform with 5 mm diameter × 10 mm length at #47. In view of the high primary stability obtained, it was decided to place the healing screws directly on the fixtures according to the procedure for one-stage implants (Figure 3A). Lastly, 4/0 interrupted silk sutures were placed for flap closure. On completion of the surgical procedure, follow-up intraoral radiography was performed to confirm correct implant placement.

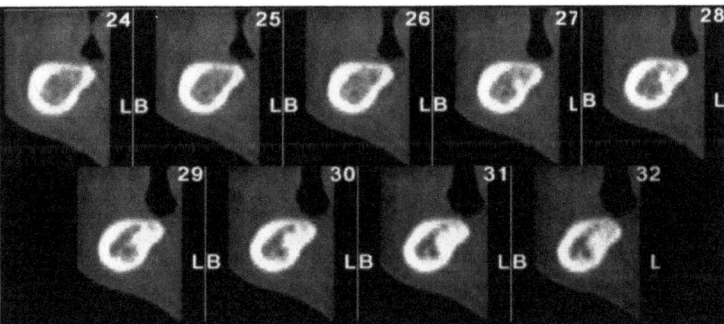

Figure 2. Preoperative CT scan of #45–47 region: an ill-defined radiopacity is visible, which could be due to the presence of a root fragment left in the alveolus at the time of extraction of #46.

Several hours after the intervention and on subsequent days, the patient spontaneously reported continuous pain of a pulsating type, similar to pulpits pain, close to the right mandibular molar area. The authors made the diagnosis of IPL after intraoral radiographic examination. The IPL was relieved only through administration of an analgesic (nimesulide 100 mg—Aulin, Roche, Milan, Italy), but no neurosensory changes were reported for the right mandible.

The IPL symptoms lasted for more than a month from the date of the intervention, during which intraoral radiographs were taken to detect possible abnormalities in loading of the peri-implant hard tissue. The implant at tooth 47 did not present any bleeding or probing depth more than 3 mm, but an intraoral radiograph showed an area of radiolucency close to the apical segment of the fixture (Figure 3B). Because of the persistence of IPL symptoms, it was decided (with the patient's consent) on week 6 after the implantation to remove the implant at tooth 47 (Figure 3C). After antibiotic therapy with 1 g Augmentin twice daily, starting on preoperative day 1 and continuing for 6 days afterwards, the area was infiltrated with local/regional anesthesia using mepivacaine 2% and adrenaline 1:100,000 and we prepared a muco-periosteal flap to expose the crest at teeth 46–47. Although abnormal loading of the peri-implant crestal bone was not found (Figure 3D), we drilled the implant with a 6 mm diameter trephine bur at #47 (Figure 3E,F). Then, we placed another implant at #46 (Biomet 3i, Palm Beach Gardens, FL, USA, 4 mm diameter, 10 mm length), free-handed using a one-stage procedure which required the immediate insertion of a healing screw on the same day. Lastly, we removed the granulation tissue present and packed the drilling site with a collagen sponge (Hemocollagene, Septodont, Saint-Maur des Fossés, France). The flaps were sutured with 4/0 silk interrupted sutures (Figure 4A–C). After the intervention, the patient did not report IPL symptoms, nor were there any signs of local inflammation.

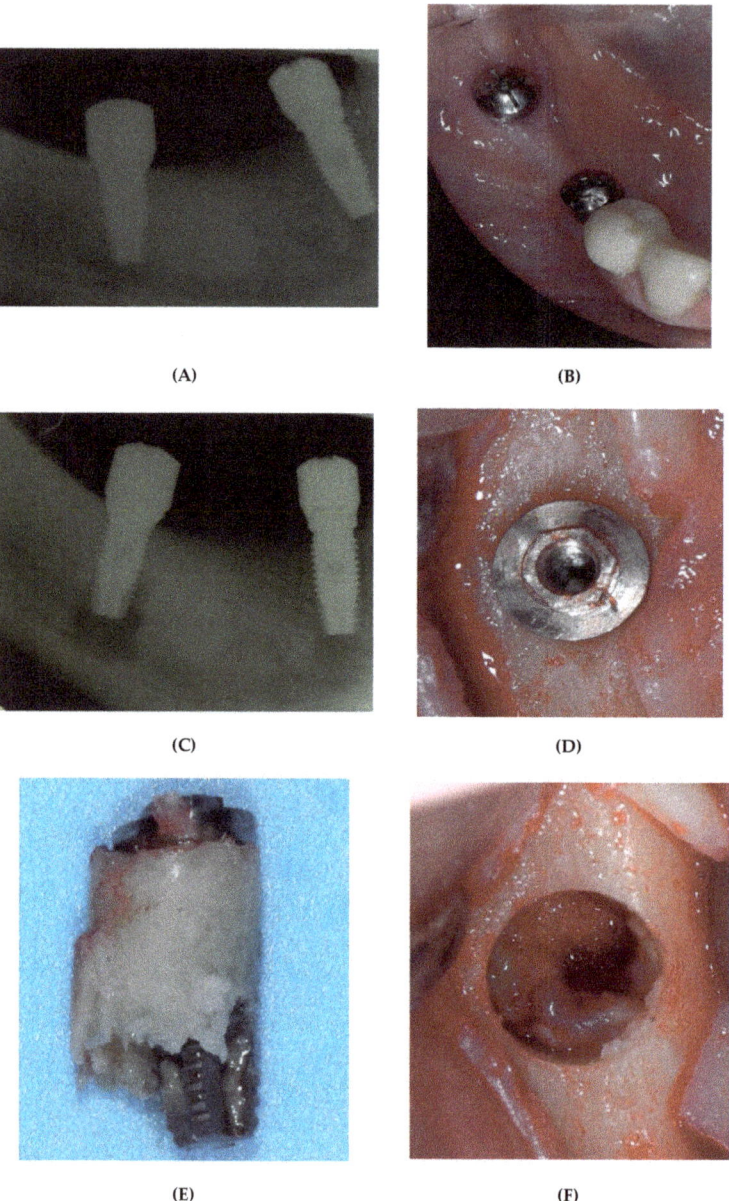

Figure 3. (**A**) Postoperative intraoral radiograph showing the position of the implants at #45 and #47. (**B**) Intraoral radiograph taken one month after the intervention. An area of radiolucency is visible at the apex of the implant at #47. (**C**) Clinical image 6 weeks after the implantation: there are no visible

clinical signs of inflammation in the oral mucosa. (**D**) Clinical image of the implant at #47 after a mucoperiosteal flap was raised. The implant appears perfectly integrated and does not seem to have undergone crestal resorption. (**E**) The implant shortly after removal. The apical portion of the implant is not in contact with the bone. (**F**) Bony crest at #47 after removal of the implant. Note the presence of granulation tissue at the bottom of the cavity.

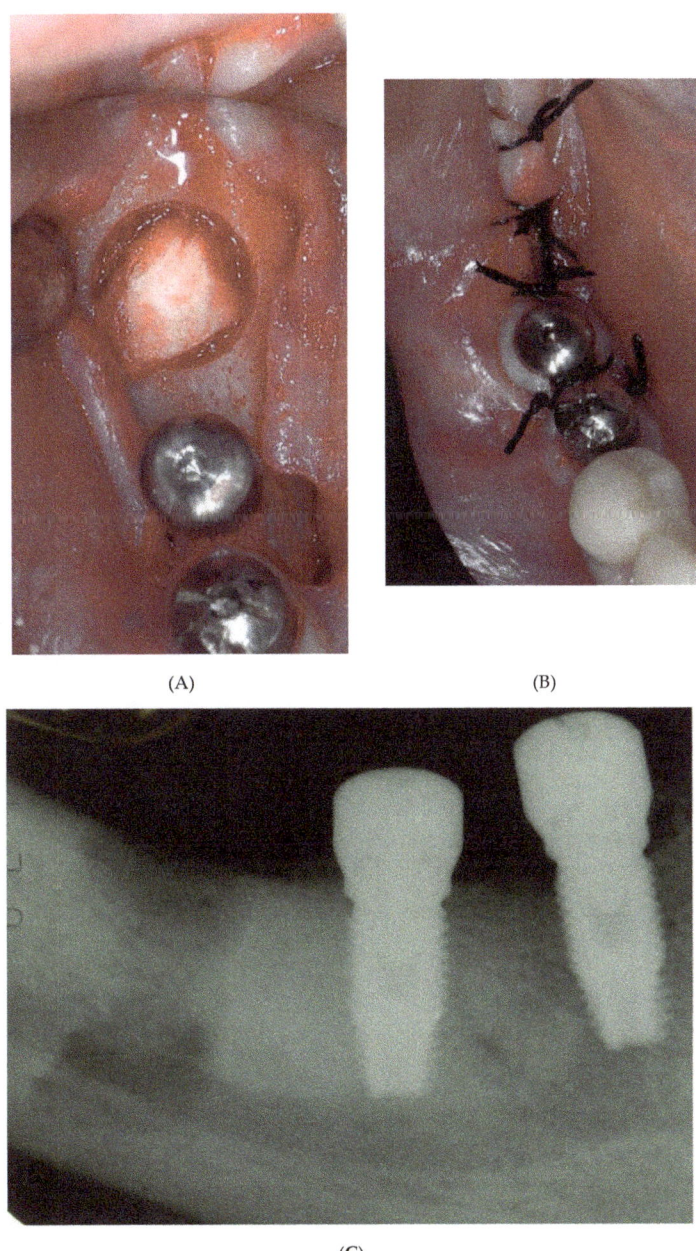

Figure 4. *Cont.*

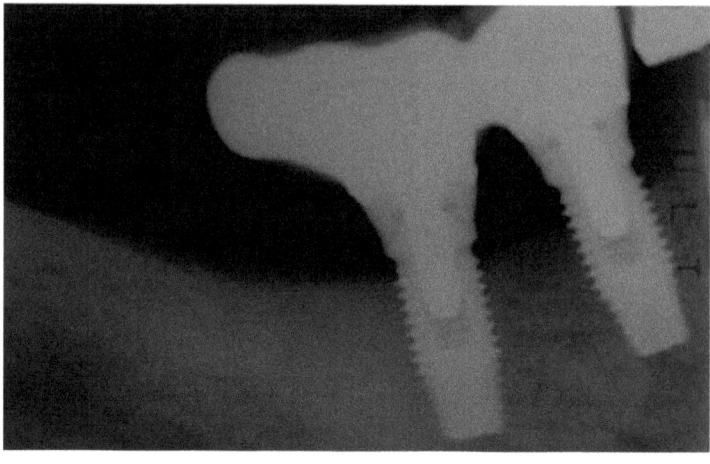

(D)

Figure 4. (**A**) Same area after packing with a collagen sponge and insertion of an implant at #46. (**B**) Clinical image after insertion of a healing screw in the implant at #46 and initial closure with 4/0 interrupted silk sutures. (**C**) Postoperative intraoral radiograph of area #45–#47. (**D**) Radiograph one year after the definitive prosthetic restoration.

After approximately three months from the intervention, in which no complications were observed, we proceeded to mount prostheses on the implants at teeth 45 and 46, which consisted in a two-unit fixed partial denture supported on 2 implants at #45 and #46 (Figure 4D).

2.1. Histological Preparation

The drilled implant was preserved in buffered formalin 10%, dehydrated in a progressive series of washings with alcohol, and embedded in glycol methacrylic resin in preparation for histological analysis (Technovit 7200 VCL, Kulzer, Wehreim, Germany). After polymerization, the implant was sectioned along its longitudinal axis with a high-speed diamond disk (Precise System, Assing, Rome, Italy). Sections of approximately 46 μm thickness were obtained and then stained with basic fuchsin and toluidine blue. A second staining procedure was performed with von Kossa and basic fuchsin to evaluate the level of bone mineralization.

2.2. Histological Analysis

The histological analysis shows adequate osseointegration in the coronal aspect, with a BIC of approximately 35%, while the apical portion of the implant is totally free of bone. (Figure 5).

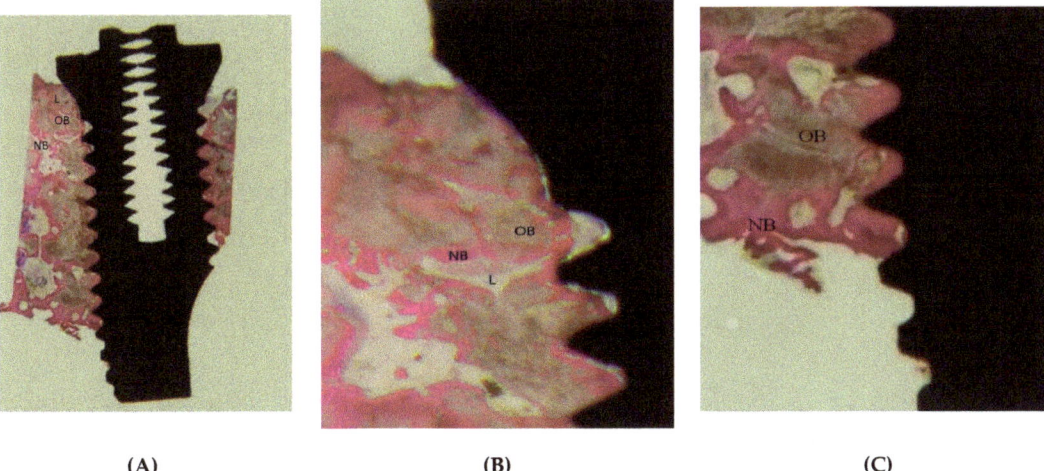

Figure 5. (**A**) In the coronal segment of the implant the old bone (OB) is in contact with the trabeculae of new bone (NB), interspersed with bony lacunae (L). The detachment of the first three threads of the implant from the bone seems to be due to a histological preparation artifact (basic fuchsin, 15× magnification). (**B**) Direct contact of the old bone (OB) and new bone (NB) with the implant thread in the apical portion of the implant (basic fuchsin, 15× magnification), L = lacunae. (**C**) Histological view of the removed implant. Only the middle and coronal segments of the implant are in contact with bone (1.5× magnification).

3. Case Report n. 2

In September 2020, a 52-year-old patient came to our attention with pain and swelling in the upper right premolar area. The fixture showed no clinical signs of peri-implantitis and no mobility but the whole area was sensitive upon percussion. Upon radiographic examination, a radiolucent area involving the implant apical third as well as the root apex of tooth number 5 was observed (Figure 6A). The root canal treatment seemed to be correctly performed as the obturation material was thoroughly compacted, lateral accessory canals were present and filled. The tooth was restored with a metallic post and core and a prosthetic crown. A surgical approach was chosen to remove the infected apexes of both the fixture and tooth number 5.

Antibiotic therapy was administered: 1 g amoxicillin/clavulanic acid (Augmentin; GlaxoSmithKline, Verona, Italy) every 12 h for 6 days.

A para-marginal incision was performed and a full thickness flap raised from tooth number 6 up to tooth number 3 with two vertical relieving incisions (Figure 6B). Access to the lesion was created by means of the bur H255E.314.012 (Komet, Germany). A horizontal cut was made with the same bur both on the root and on the fixture apex and all the granulation tissue in the surrounding bone was scraped off (Figure 6C).

The retropreparation of tooth 5 was done with surgical retrotip (R1D, Piezomed, W&H, Bürmoos, Austria) and it was filled with Biodentine (Septodont, Saint-Maudefuse, France).

The flap was sutured tension-free and the patient was dismissed. After the healing period, the patient noted improvement of the symptoms. One year later, a periapical radiography was taken showing the healing of the periapical radiolucency, the fixture showed no signs and symptoms of peri-implantitis, and tooth number 15 showed no mobility and no symptoms. Probing depth was 2 mm around the tooth and 3 mm around the implant (Figure 6D).

The histological analysis of the surrounding tissue revealed the presence of a rich inflammatory tissue.

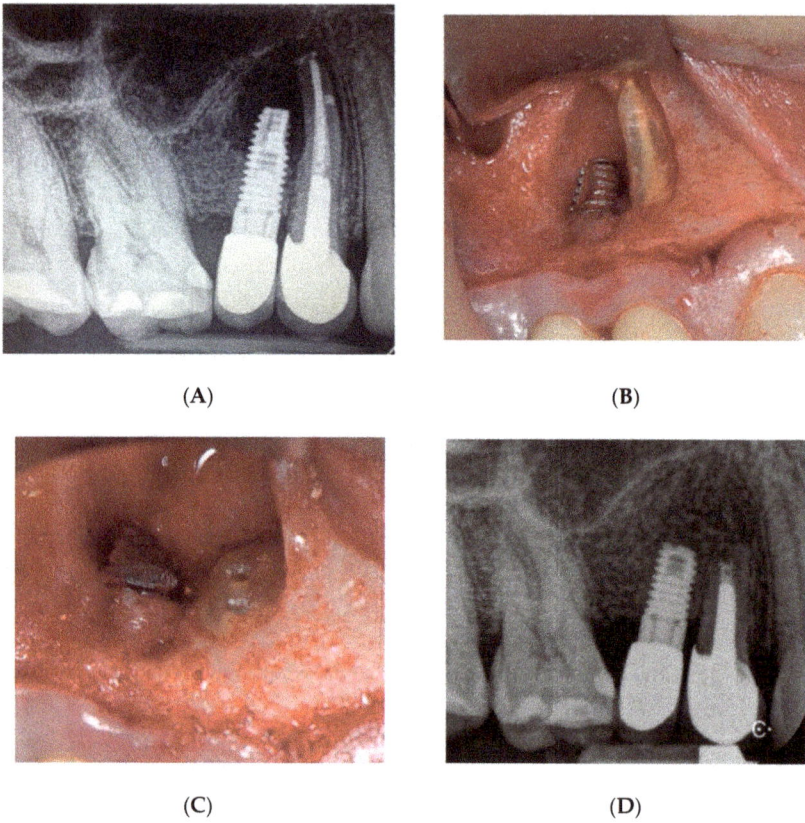

Figure 6. Case 2 (**A**) Preoperative image showing the presence of a radiolucency between the implant apex and the adjacent tooth. (**B**) Clinical view of the apex prior to the resection. (**C**) Implant apical resection and tooth apex resection with both root canals ready to receive the filling material. (**D**) 2 years follow-up.

4. Discussion

Among implant failures, a significant role seems to be played by apical peri-implantitis (IPL). Different researchers have described cases of IPL—as retrospective studies or case reports—with indications for treatment of this disease and suggestions for possible causes [8,9,11–29]. These include microfractures of the cortical bone, in the form of vestibular or lingual bony dehiscence and fenestration, osteitis or osteomyelitis secondary to bacterial contamination during the surgical procedure, overheating of the bony structure, or poor bone quality [7–9,11,19–23].

However, the best evidence-supported etiology of IPL suggested by the different researchers is bacterial in nature [8,11,12,19,22]. This etiology may be due either to transmission of endodontic periapical lesions, starting with dental structures adjacent to the implant, or to infected dental remnants present in the affected edentulous crest. If implants are inserted close to teeth with acute or chronic endodontic periapical lesions, or radicular fragments of extracted teeth remaining in the alveolus and not promptly eliminated, these can involve the surface implant and induce IPL [11,20,27–29].

From a statistical perspective, the region most affected by IPL is that of the maxillary premolars [8]. This may be due to the anatomy of these teeth, which often present with two roots. In many cases, incomplete flushing, shaping, and closure of the canal system can lead to failure of endodontic treatment and concomitant formation of apical inflammatory tissue, which in 26% of cases is not visible on radiography [24]. Extraction of the maxillary premolars and later revision of the alveolus with alveolar curettes can result in apical residues remaining permanently in the medullary bone if the procedures are not performed correctly. If not guided by precise radiographic examinations, substitution of the extracted structure with an implant in the infected zone can induce peri-implantitis in the apical area of the fixture. This occurrence can precipitate pain symptoms in the patient immediately after the intervention, as in our case, or even several weeks or years after the implantation [8,15,17,18,21,25,26].

IPL has been attributed in a histological study to the amide present on the latex of the gloves. In fact, the presence of amide from gloves has been detected inside neutrophilic granulocytes. However, this may not be the primary cause of IPL in the first case report, since the clinical symptomatology was manifested approximately one month after implant insertion and the adjacent dental structure presented an endodontic apical lesion [18].

Confirmation of the bacterial origin of apical IPL is supported by the finding of types of bacteria in the apical portion of the implant that are very similar to those in endodontic infections, such as Porphyromonas endodontalis, Porphyromonas gingivalis, and Prevotella intermedia, while contrariwise, bacteria typical of periodontal lesions are found in classic peri-implantitis [30–38].

Our study is one of the few available in the literature that reports an implant affected by apical IPL. The histological analysis revealed complete osteointegration of the coronal two-third of the fixture, whereas the apical portion remained free of contact to bone. This could be due to necrotic tooth remnants found upon CT scan examination.

The osteotomy use of surgical burs or the fixture placement itself may have reactivated a latent infection around these tooth fragments, causing an inflammatory reaction in the apical portion of the implant. Our failure in the histological examination to find inflammatory tissue may be due to detachment or to its seclusion within the mandibular bone during drilling of the implant [8,9].

Other research has also reported the presence of root fragments—not detected during the implantation—which induced inflammatory apical reactions to the fixture [8].

Radiopaque zones in edentulous crests are very frequent in areas where a dental extraction has previously been performed. These may be due to focal osteosclerosis, a non-expansible radiopaque alteration of trabecular bone of unknown origin, asymptomatic, with various shapes and sizes, affecting both the maxilla and the mandible, with higher prevalence in the mandibular molar and premolar region. Its radiopacity may resemble other pathologies of the jaws, such as condensing osteitis, root segments, hypercementosis, cementoblastoma, impacted teeth, focal cemento-osseous dysplasia, and odontomas [39–41].

Focal osteosclerosis can be present in proximity to the retained root tips or in the edentulous crest region [42]. In our case, previous extraction of a dental structure may have resulted in focal osteosclerosis, possibly reactivated on the occasion of implant insertion in the area of interest. This suggestion would explain the area of radiopacity visible on both CT and intraoral radiography at teeth 46–47. As far as we know, however, there are no other published studies of implants with IPL in proximity to areas of focal osteosclerosis.

Another possible approach that would explain the patient's painful symptomatology could be injury to the vascular-neural bundle of the alveolar canal occurring during preparation of the implant site. This may be seen also on radiography as an area of radiolucency involving the apex of the implant in close contact with the underlying alveolar canal. However, despite the fact that trunk anesthesia was not performed—to maintain neural sensitivity during the intervention—the patient did not experience any pain during placement of the implant or post-operative paresthesia.

Treatment of local IPL consists in the removal of the implant (case report n.1) or removal of its apical portion (case report n.2), with consequent elimination of the inflammatory tissue [26]. Removal of the apical portion of the implant requires the remaining integrated part to be capable of bearing the masticatory load [9]. In case report n.1, we decided to remove the implant in toto since excision of its apical portion alone could have caused permanent injury to the vascular-neural bundle of the inferior alveolar nerve, with consequent neuro-sensory changes in the patient's right lower lip. Instead, in case report n.2, the apical portion of the implant as well as the adjacent tooth apex were surgically removed and periapical lesion successfully healed with no signs and symptoms of IPL. In the first clinical case, the fixture was implanted in another surgical site; therefore, the healing times are crucial. However, it was a four-wall defect, which is a common post-extraction site. In the second case, the lesion had endodontic origin; thus, improvement was noticed 12 months after baseline.

Early surgical treatment is essential in order to limit progression of the lesion to the osseointegrated part of the fixture. Our histological study shows that this surgical therapy may be helpful in the treatment of IPL since the coronal two-thirds portion of the implant is fully osseointegrated. According to the present literature, some dental remnants may be intentionally left in post-extraction sites without causing infectious complications like the ones experienced by the authors in the first case report. This confirms that infections proceeding from neighboring teeth may cause IPL in fixtures' periapical tissue. As far as investigated by the authors, only one failure for infectious reasons has been described with the socket shield technique because the apex was left during the surgical procedure. Indeed, the tooth apex and endodontium need to be accurately removed when performing this technique in order to achieve clinical success; only a buccal sliver is meant to be left in situ [43,44].

5. Conclusions

Because of the ever-increasing number of people undergoing implant-based treatment in recent years, there has been an increased incidence of apical IPL. The presence of infected root remnants or endodontic periapical lesions seems to be the major cause of this type of implant failure. Treatment of apical IPL should be directed toward elimination of the bacterial noxae and limitation of progression of the lesion to the osseointegrated part of the implant. Removal of the apical portion of the implant appears to be a valid therapeutic option, since the remaining part of the fixture appears from our histological examination to be optimally osseointegrated and not affected by the inflammatory process. Good initial treatment planning seems fundamentally important. It should be targeted toward the identification of local etiological factors present either in the edentulous crest or the adjacent dental structures, and their preventive elimination before insertion of the fixture so as not to compromise implant predictability.

Author Contributions: C.B.: Conceptualization (lead); Investigation (equal); Methodology (equal); Supervision (lead); Writing–original draft (equal); Writing–review & editing (equal), F.F.: Investigation (equal); Data curation (equal); Formal analysis (equal); Methodology (equal); Validation (lead); Writing–review & editing (equal); R.L.: Conceptualization (equal); Data curation (equal); Investigation (equal); Visualization (lead); Writing–review & editing (equal), A.V.: Project administration (lead); Resources (equal); Writing–review & editing (equal), G.B.: Investigation (equal); Methodology (equal); Formal analysis (lead); Writing–review & editing (equal), E.P.: Data curation (equal); Investigation (lead); Software (equal); Validation (equal); Writing–review & editing (equal), A.S.: Data curation (equal); Methodology (equal); Writing–review & editing (equal), T.T.: Conceptualization (equal); Methodology (equal); Data curation (equal); Writing–original draft (lead). All authors have read and agreed to the published version of the manuscript.

Funding: This study received no external funding.

Institutional Review Board Statement: Not applicable.

Informed Consent Statement: Informed consent was obtained from all subjects involved in the study.

Data Availability Statement: The data supporting the findings of the present study are available from the corresponding author upon reasonable request.

Conflicts of Interest: The authors declare no conflict of interest.

References

1. Esposito, M.; Hirsch, J.; Lekholm, U.; Thomsen, P. Differential diagnosis and treatment strategies for biologic complications and failing oral implants: A review of the literature. *Int. J. Oral Maxillofac. Implants* **1999**, *14*, 473–490. [PubMed]
2. Esposito, M.; Hirsch, J.M.; Lekholm, U.; Thomsen, P. Biological factors contributing to failures of osseointegrated oral implants. I: Success criteria and epidemiology. *Eur. J. Oral Sci.* **1998**, *106*, 527–551. [CrossRef]
3. Esposito, M.; Hirsch, J.M.; Lekholm, U.; Thomsen, P. Biological factors contributing to failures of osseointegrated oral implants. II: Etiopathogenesis. *Eur. J. Oral Sci.* **1998**, *106*, 721–764. [CrossRef]
4. Esposito, M. On Biological Failures of Osseointegrated Oral Implants. Ph.D. Thesis, University of Gothenburg, Gothenburg, Sweden, 1999.
5. El Askary, A.S.; Meffert, R.M.; Griffin, T. Why do implants fail? Part I. *Implant Dent.* **1999**, *8*, 173–185. [CrossRef] [PubMed]
6. Meffert, R.M. Periodontitis and peri-implantitis: One and the same? *Pract. Periodontics Aesthet. Dent.* **1993**, *5*, 79–80, 82.
7. McAllister, B.S.; Masters, D.; Meffert, R.M. Treatment of implants demonstrating periapical radiolucencies. *Pract. Periodontics Aesthet. Dent.* **1992**, *4*, 37–41. [PubMed]
8. Park, S.H.; Sorensen, W.P.; Wang, H.L. Management and prevention of retrograde peri-implant infection from retained root tips: Two case reports. *Int. J. Periodontics Restor. Dent.* **2004**, *24*, 422–433. [CrossRef]
9. Reiser, G.M.; Nevins, M. The implant periapical lesion: Etiology, prevention, and treatment. *Compend. Contin. Educ. Dent.* **1995**, *16*, 768, 770, 772.
10. Quirynen, M.; Vogels, R.; Alsaa, G.; Naert, I.; Jacobs, R.; van Steenberghe, D. Predisposing conditions for retrograde peri-implantitis, and treatment suggestions. *Clin. Oral Implants Res.* **2005**, *16*, 599–608. [CrossRef]
11. Sussman, H.I. Periapical implant pathology. *J. Oral Implantol.* **1998**, *24*, 133–138. [CrossRef]
12. Sussman, H.I. Implant pathology associated with loss of periapical seal of adjacent tooth: Clinical report. *Implant Dent.* **1997**, *6*, 33–37. [CrossRef] [PubMed]
13. Piattelli, A.; Scarano, A.; Piattelli, M.; Podda, G. Implant periapical lesions: Clinical, histological, and histochemical aspects. A case report. *Int. J. Periodontics Restor. Dent.* **1998**, *18*, 181–187.
14. Piattelli, A.; Scarano, A.; Balleri, P.; Favero, G.A. Clinical and histological evaluation of an active "implant periapical lesion": A case report. *Int. J. Oral Maxillofac. Implants* **1998**, *13*, 713–716.
15. Piattelli, A.; Scarano, A.; Piattelli, M. Abscess formation around the apex of a maxillary root form implant: Clinical and microscopical aspects. A case report. *J. Periodontol.* **1995**, *66*, 899–903. [CrossRef]
16. Scarano, A.; Di Domizio, P.; Petrone, G.; Iezzi, G.; Piattelli, A. Implant periapical lesion: A clinical and histological case report. *J. Oral Implantol.* **2000**, *26*, 109–113. [CrossRef]
17. Chaffee, N.R.; Lowden, K.; Tiffee, J.C.; Cooper, L.F. Periapical abscess formation and resolution adjacent to dental implants: A clinical report. *J. Prosthet. Dent.* **2001**, *85*, 109–112. [CrossRef]
18. Nedir, R.; Bischof, M.; Pujol, O.; Houriet, R.; Samson, J.; Lombardi, T. Starch-induced implant periapical lesion: A case report. *Int. J. Oral Maxillofac. Implant.* **2007**, *22*, 1001–1006.
19. Flanagan, D. Apical (retrograde) peri-implantitis: A case report of an active lesion. *J. Oral Implantol.* **2002**, *28*, 92–96. [CrossRef]
20. Jalbout, Z.N.; Tarnow, D.P. The implant periapical lesion: Four case reports and review of the literature. *Pract. Periodontic Aesthet. Dent.* **2001**, *13*, 107–112.
21. Oh, T.J.; Yoon, J.; Wang, H.L. Management of the implant periapical lesion: A case report. *Implant Dent.* **2003**, *12*, 41–46. [CrossRef]
22. Ayangco, L.; Sheridan, P.J. Development and treatment of retrograde peri-implantitis involving a site with a history of failed endodontic and apicoectomy procedures: A series of reports. *Int. J. Oral Maxillofac. Implants* **2001**, *16*, 412–417. [PubMed]
23. Talacko, A.A.; Aldred, M.J.; Abbott, P.V.; Smith, A.C.; Nerwich, A.H. Periapical biopsy? *Oral Surg. Oral Med. Oral Pathol. Oral Radiol. Endod.* **2000**, *89*, 532–534. [CrossRef]
24. Abou-Rass, M.; Bogen, G. Microorganisms in closed periapical lesions. *Int. Endod. J.* **1998**, *31*, 39–47. [CrossRef] [PubMed]
25. Brisman, D.L.; Brisman, A.S.; Moses, M.S. Implant failures associated with asymptomatic endodontically treated teeth. *J. Am. Dent. Assoc.* **2001**, *132*, 191–195. [CrossRef]
26. Balshi, S.F.; Wolfinger, G.J.; Balshi, T.J. A retrospective evaluation of a treatment procedure for dental implant periapical lesions: Long-term results of 39 implant apicoectomies. *Int. J. Oral Maxillofac. Implants* **2007**, *22*, 267–272. [PubMed]
27. Tseng, C.C.; Chen, Y.H.; Pang, I.C.; Weber, H.P. Peri-implant pathology caused by periapical lesion of an adjacent natural tooth: A case report. *Int. J. Oral Maxillofac. Implants* **2005**, *20*, 632–635. [PubMed]
28. Shaffer, M.D.; Juruaz, D.A.; Haggerty, P.C. The effect of periradicular endodontic pathosis on the apical region of adjacent implants. *Oral Surg. Oral Med. Oral Pathol. Oral Radiol. Endod.* **1998**, *86*, 578–581. [CrossRef]
29. Sussman, H. Endodontic pathology leading to implant failure—A case report. *J. Oral Implantol.* **1997**, *23*, 112–115. [PubMed]
30. Haapasalo, M. *Bacteroides* spp. in dental root canal infections. *Endod. Dent. Traumatol.* **1989**, *5*, 1–10. [CrossRef]
31. Pinheiro, E.T.; Gomes, B.P.; Ferraz, C.C.; Teixeira, F.B.; Zaia, A.A.; Souza Filho, F.J. Evaluation of root canal microorganisms isolated from teeth with endodontic failure and their antimicrobial susceptibility. *Oral Microbiol. Immunol.* **2003**, *18*, 100–103. [CrossRef] [PubMed]
32. Sundqvist, G.; Johansson, E.; Sjögren, U. Prevalence of black-pigmented bacteroides species in root canal infections. *J. Endod.* **1989**, *15*, 13–19. [CrossRef]

33. van Winkelhoff, A.J.; van Steenbergen, T.J.; de Graaff, J. Porphyromonas (Bacteroides) endodontalis: Its role in endodontal infections. *J. Endod.* **1992**, *18*, 431–434. [CrossRef]
34. Bogen, G.; Slots, J. Black-pigmented anaerobic rods in closed periapical lesions. *Int. Endod. J.* **1999**, *32*, 204–210. [CrossRef] [PubMed]
35. Mombelli, A. Etiology, diagnosis, and treatment considerations in peri-implantitis. *Curr. Opin. Periodontol.* **1997**, *4*, 127–136. [PubMed]
36. Blaya-Tárraga, J.A.; Cervera-Ballester, J.; Peñarrocha-Oltra, D.; Peñarrocha-Diago, M. Periapical implant lesion: A systematic review. *Med. Oral Patol. Oral Cir. Bucal.* **2017**, *22*, e737. [CrossRef]
37. Qu, C.; Meng, H.; Han, J. Implant periapical lesion—A review and a case report with histological evaluation. *Clin. Oral Implant. Res.* **2014**, *25*, 1099–1104. [CrossRef] [PubMed]
38. Ramanauskaite, A.; Juodzbalys, G.; Tözüm, T.F. Apical/Retrograde Periimplantitis/Implant Periapical Lesion: Etiology, Risk Factors, and Treatment Options: A Systematic Review. *Implant Dent.* **2016**, *25*, 684–697. [CrossRef] [PubMed]
39. Bsoul, S.A.; Alborz, S.; Terezhalmy, G.T.; Moore, W.S. Idiopathic osteosclerosis (enostosis, dense bone islands, focal periapical osteopetrosis). *Quintessence Int.* **2004**, *35*, 590–591. [PubMed]
40. Sisman, Y.; Ertas, E.T.; Ertas, H.; Sekerci, A.E. The frequency and distribution of idiopathic osteosclerosis of the jaw. *Eur. J. Dent.* **2011**, *5*, 409–414. [CrossRef]
41. Araki, M.; Matsumoto, N.; Matsumoto, K.; Ohnishi, M.; Honda, K.; Komiyama, K. Asymptomatic radiopaque lesions of the jaws: A radio-graphic study using cone-beam computed tomography. *J. Oral Sci.* **2011**, *53*, 439–444. [CrossRef] [PubMed]
42. Yonetsu, K.; Yuasa, K.; Kanda, S. Idiopathic osteosclerosis of the jaws: Panoramic radiographic and computed tomographic findings. *Oral Surg. Oral Med. Oral Pathol. Oral Radiol. Endod.* **1997**, *83*, 517. [CrossRef]
43. Hurzeler, M.B.; Zuhr, O.; Schupbach, P.; Rebele, S.F.; Emmanouilidis, N.; Fickl, S. The socket-shield technique: A proof-of-principle report. *J. Clin. Periodontol.* **2010**, *37*, 855–862. [CrossRef] [PubMed]
44. Gandhi, Y.; Bhatavadekar, N. Inappropriate socket shield protocol as a probable cause of peri-implant bone resorption: A case report. *J. Maxillofac. Oral Surg.* **2020**, *19*, 359–363. [CrossRef]

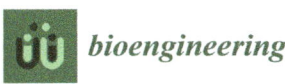

Review

Disinfection Procedures and Their Effect on the Microorganism Colonization of Dental Impression Materials: A Systematic Review and Meta-Analysis of In Vitro Studies

Louis Hardan [1,†], Rim Bourgi [1,†], Carlos Enrique Cuevas-Suárez [2,*], Monika Lukomska-Szymanska [3], Elizabeth Cornejo-Ríos [2], Vincenzo Tosco [4], Riccardo Monterubbianesi [4], Sara Mancino [5], Ammar Eid [6], Davide Mancino [7,8,9], Naji Kharouf [7,8,*,‡] and Youssef Haikel [7,8,9,‡]

1. Department of Restorative Dentistry, School of Dentistry, Saint-Joseph University, Beirut 1107 2180, Lebanon; louis.hardan@usj.edu.lb (L.H.); rim.bourgi@net.usj.edu.lb (R.B.)
2. Dental Materials Laboratory, Academic Area of Dentistry, Autonomous University of Hidalgo State, Circuito Ex Hacienda La Concepción S/N, San Agustín Tlaxiaca 42160, Mexico; elizabeth_cornejo@uaeh.edu.mx
3. Department of General Dentistry, Medical University of Lodz, 251 Pomorska St., 92-213 Lodz, Poland; monika.lukomska-szymanska@umed.lodz.pl
4. Department of Clinical Sciences and Stomatology, Polytechnic University of Marche, 60121 Ancona, Italy; v.tosco@pm.univpm.it (V.T.); r.monterubbianesi@univpm.it (R.M.)
5. Faculty of Pharmacy, Strasbourg University, 67400 Strasbourg, France; sara.mancino@etu.unistra.fr
6. Department of Endodontics, Faculty of Dental Medicine, Damascus University, Damascus 0100, Syria; ammarendo89@gmail.com
7. Department of Biomaterials and Bioengineering, INSERM UMR_S 1121, Biomaterials and Bioengineering, 67000 Strasbourg, France; endodontiefrancaise@outlook.com (D.M.); youssef.haikel@unistra.fr (Y.H.)
8. Department of Endodontics, Faculty of Dental Medicine, Strasbourg University, 67000 Strasbourg, France
9. Pôle de Médecine et Chirurgie Bucco-Dentaire, Hôpital Civil, Hôpitaux Universitaire de Strasbourg, 67000 Strasbourg, France
* Correspondence: cecuevas@uaeh.edu.mx (C.E.C.-S.); dentistenajikharouf@gmail.com (N.K.); Tel.: +52-(771)-7-2000 (C.E.C.-S.); +33-36-6752-2841 (N.K.)
† These authors contributed equally to this work.
‡ These authors contributed equally to this work.

Citation: Hardan, L.; Bourgi, R.; Cuevas-Suárez, C.E.; Lukomska-Szymanska, M.; Cornejo-Ríos, E.; Tosco, V.; Monterubbianesi, R.; Mancino, S.; Eid, A.; Mancino, D.; et al. Disinfection Procedures and Their Effect on the Microorganism Colonization of Dental Impression Materials: A Systematic Review and Meta-Analysis of In Vitro Studies. *Bioengineering* 2022, 9, 123. https://doi.org/10.3390/bioengineering9030123

Academic Editor: Chengfei Zhang

Received: 15 February 2022
Accepted: 11 March 2022
Published: 16 March 2022

Publisher's Note: MDPI stays neutral with regard to jurisdictional claims in published maps and institutional affiliations.

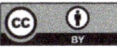

Copyright: © 2022 by the authors. Licensee MDPI, Basel, Switzerland. This article is an open access article distributed under the terms and conditions of the Creative Commons Attribution (CC BY) license (https://creativecommons.org/licenses/by/4.0/).

Abstract: Dental impressions are contaminated with potentially pathogenic microorganisms when they come into contact with patient blood, saliva, and plaque. Numerous disinfectants are used; however, no sole disinfectant can be designated as universal for all the impression materials. Thus, the aim of this study is to systemically review the literature to evaluate the effect of the existing disinfection procedures on the bacterial colonization of dental impression materials. This systematic review and meta-analysis was conducted according to the PRISMA statement. PubMed (MEDLINE), Web of Science, Scopus, EMBASE, and SciELO databases were screened up to April 2021. Eligibility criteria included in vitro studies reporting the antibacterial activity of disinfectant solutions in dental impression materials. The meta-analysis was performed using Review Manager (version 5.3.5). A global comparison was performed with the standardized mean difference based on random-effect models at a significance level of $\alpha = 0.05$. A total of seven studies were included in the meta-analysis. The included studies described the effect of disinfection processes with chlorhexidine gluconate, alcohol, sodium hypochlorite, glutaraldehyde, and hydrogen peroxide in alginate, polyvinyl siloxane, and polyether impression materials. The meta-analyses showed that the use of chlorhexidine, alcohol, glutaraldehyde, and sodium hypochlorite reduced the colony-forming units by a milliliter (CFU/mL) in alginate ($p < 0.001$). On the other hand, glutaraldehyde, sodium hypochlorite, and alcohol reduced the CFU/mL in polyvinyl siloxane ($p < 0.001$). Finally, alcohol and glutaraldehyde reduced the CFU/mL in polyether material ($p < 0.001$). High heterogeneity was observed for the alginate and polyvinyl siloxane materials ($I^2 = 74\%$; $I^2 = 90\%$). Based on these in vitro studies, the disinfection of impression materials with several disinfection agents reduces the CFU/mL count.

Keywords: antibacterial effect; dental impressions; disinfectant agents; disinfection; oral bacteria

1. Introduction

Dental impressions are certainly contaminated with possibly pathogenic microorganisms when they come into contact with patient blood, saliva, and plaque [1,2]. This could be the source of disease transmitters and cross-infections for dentists, dental assistants, and laboratory technicians [3,4]. Consequently, sanitizing the impressions efficiently before transportation to the laboratory technician ensembles is crucial [5]. Indeed, when the impressions are sterilized, this can avoid the transmission of disease, yet it is not the ideal way, since dimensional changes can occur [6].

Considering that, in some countries, tap water contains halogenated compounds, the Advisory British Dental Association Service recommends the rinsing of impression materials with tap water in daily dental practice; despite this, although some of the microorganisms adhered to the surface of a dental impression could be removed by this procedure, a high percentage still remains [7]. This has been exhibited to lessen the amounts of the bacteria on the surface of the impression presented by nearly 90% [8]. Nevertheless, a noteworthy number of bacteria would persist. More recent suggestions support the use of a disinfecting solution [9]. Knowledge evidently varies about the type, concentration, and immersion times of disinfection protocols, making it difficult to evaluate the most applicable method [10,11].

Numerous disinfectants are used regularly such as sodium hypochlorite, chlorhexidine, alcohol, glutaraldehyde, and hydrogen peroxide [12]. Since no sole disinfectant can be designated as a universal disinfectant for all impression materials, it is fundamental to select an ideal disinfectant agent with superior antimicrobial activity that does not disturb the recorded features, such as surface characteristics or dimensional stability of an impression materials [13,14].

Additionally, many combinations between impression materials and disinfectant could occur by knowing that a large range of branded impression materials (reversible and irreversible hydrocolloids, polyethers, polysulphides, and silicones) and gypsum-based casts existed in the marketplace. A disinfectant possesses a dual purpose: it needs to be an effective antimicrobial agent but produce no adverse effect on the dimensional accuracy of the impression material and resultant gypsum model. The latter is of significance in an attempt to deliver a functional and well-fitting finished appliance. Disagreement happens in the literature as to whether the disinfection procedure produces degradation or distortion of impressions [15–17].

The reaction of some specific brands of gypsum products and impression materials to disinfection process is diverse, advising a deficiency of compatibility between a given material and protocol. Hence, individual analysis of impression materials is needed to define the effectiveness of a specific disinfection method in different areas [18].

Accordingly, the aim of this study was to systemically review the literature of the existing disinfection procedures on the bacterial colonization of dental impression materials. The null hypothesis to be tested was that the use of disinfectant agents will not reduce the colony-forming units per milliliter (CFU/mL) adhered to the surface of impression materials used in dentistry.

2. Materials and Methods

This systematic review and meta-analysis was reported following the guidelines of the Preferred Reporting Items for Systematic Reviews and Meta-Analyses (PRISMA statement) [19]. The registration protocol was carried out in the Open Science Framework with the registration number 0000-0002-2759-8984. The following PICOS strategy was used: population, impression materials; intervention, use of disinfection materials; control, rinsing with tap water; outcome: antimicrobial activity; and type of study, in vitro studies. The research question was as follows: Does the use of disinfection procedures for impression materials in dental practice reduce the microbial count?

2.1. Search Strategy

The literature search was performed by two independent reviewers (E.C.R. and R.B.) up to April 22, 2021. The following databases were screened: PubMed (MEDLINE), Web of Science, Scopus, EMBASE, and SciELO. The search strategy was performed according to the keywords defined in Table 1. All studies were imported into Rayyan QCRI platform [20].

Table 1. Keywords used in search strategy.

Search Strategy	
#1	Dental models OR Dental impressions OR Irreversible hydrocolloid OR Alginate impressions OR Silicone impression OR Primary impression OR Polyvinyl siloxane
#2	Disinfection OR Sodium hypochlorite OR Disinfection techniques OR Sterilization OR Chemical disinfection OR Disinfection protocol OR Immersion disinfection OR Cross contamination OR Ultraviolet disinfection OR Microbial activity OR Disinfectant solutions OR Autoclave OR Disinfectant agents
#3	#1 and #2

2.2. Eligibility Criteria

The title and abstract of each identified article were reviewed by two independent reviewers (E.C.R. and R.B.) to determine if the article should be considered for full-text review according to the following eligibility criteria: (1) in vitro studies reporting the antibacterial activity of disinfectant solutions in dental impression materials; (2) included mean and standard deviation (SD) in CFU/mL; (3) included a control group where tap water was used; and (4) published in the English language. Case reports, case series, pilot studies, expert opinions, conference abstracts, and reviews were excluded. In the case of disagreements at the time of the selection of the studies for the full-text review, they were resolved by discussion and consensus by a third reviewer (C.E.C.-S).

2.3. Data Extraction

The Microsoft Office Excel 2019 program (Microsoft Corporation, Redmond, Washington, DC, USA) was used to extract the data of interest from the included manuscripts. These were placed on a standardized form. Two reviewers (L.H. and R.B.), who received training in this software, performed the analysis. The data recovered from each manuscript were author, year, impression material evaluated, disinfection agents used, type of microorganism evaluated, main outcome, and main results.

2.4. Quality Assessment

The risk of bias of the selected articles was assessed by two reviewers (R.B. and E.C.R.) according to the parameters of the previous systematic review [21]. The risk of bias of each article was evaluated according to the description of the following parameters: specimen randomization, single-operator protocol implementation, blinding of the operator, the presence of a control group, complete outcome data, and description of the sample size calculation. If the authors reported the parameter, the study received a "YES" for that specific parameter. In case of missing information, the parameter received a "NO". The risk of bias was classified according to the sum of "YES" answers received: 1 to 2 indicated a high bias, 3 to 4 indicated a medium risk of bias, and 5 to 6 indicated a low risk of bias.

2.5. Statistical Analysis

The meta-analyses were performed using Review Manager Software version 5.1 (The Nordic Cochrane Centre, The Cochrane Collaboration, Copenhagen, Denmark). The analyses were carried out using a random-effect model, and pooled-effect estimates were obtained by comparing the standardized mean difference between CFU/mL values obtained when a disinfection agent was used; against a control group when tap water was used. The standardized mean difference was performed since this statistic in meta-analysis is used when all the studies assess the same outcome but measure it in a variety of ways; for this to be appropriate, it must be assumed that between-study variation reflects only differences in measurement scales, such as the different scientific notation used among the studies included. Additionally, for comparison purposes, when a value of 0 was found in the data, this was replaced with "0.1" with a SD of "0.01" for the statistical analysis. The comparisons were made considering the type of impression material and the type of disinfection agent used. A p-value < 0.05 was considered statistically significant. Statistical heterogeneity of the treatment effect among studies was assessed using the Cochran Q test and the inconsistency I^2 test.

3. Results

The search resulted in the retrieval of 2598 records (Figure 1). After removal of duplicates, 2084 articles were screened, and 2027 were excluded based on the title or abstract. A total of 57 full-text articles were assessed for eligibility. Of these, nineteen were not considered for the qualitative analysis: seventeen did not evaluate the antibacterial activity and two were short communications, leaving thirty-eight studies for the qualitative analysis; from these, thirty-one were excluded from the quantitative analysis: in fourteen studies, the SD could not be retrieved, and in another thirteen studies, the results were not expressed in CFU/mL, two studies did not have any control group, and two studies did not have enough comparison groups. Finally, seven studies were considered for the meta-analysis. Table S1 describes the quantitative data extracted from studies included in the meta-analysis.

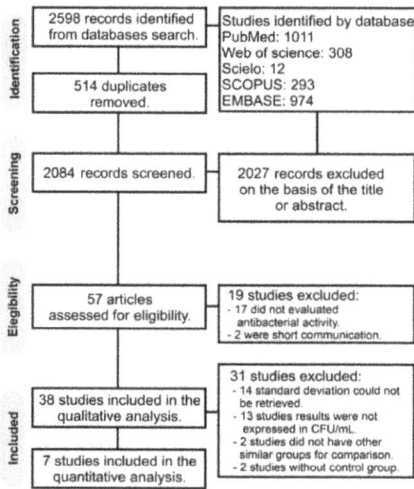

Figure 1. Search flowchart according to the PRISMA Statement.

The characteristics of the studies included in this systematic review are summarized in Table 2. Several disinfection agents were identified for the present review, including chlorhexidine, alcohol, sodium hypochlorite, glutaraldehyde, and hydrogen peroxide. Most of the studies included in this review evaluated the antibacterial activity to alginate and polyvinyl siloxane impressions, only two studies evaluated the effect of disinfection on polyether, while only one tested on condensation silicone. Utmost of the studies reported the effect of disinfection agents on CFU/mL, while a few reported inhibition halos.

Table 2. Characteristics of the included studies.

Study	Impression Material	Disinfection Agent	Type of Microorganism	Main Outcome	Main Results
Ahmed 2020 [22]	Alginate	Chlorhexidine Desident CaviCide Alcohol	Bacteria Fungi	Colony-forming units	Disinfectants killed the bacteria completely.
Al-Enazi 2016 [23]	Polyvinyl siloxane Alginate	Sodium hypochlorite Glutaraldehyde	Streptococcus diphtheroid Neisseria	Colony-forming units	Use of 1% sodium hypochlorite yielded better results than did 2% glutaraldehyde.
Al-Jabrah 2007 [24]	Alginate Polyether Polyvinyl siloxane	Dimenol Perform-ID® MD520® Haz-tabs®	Does not specify	Colony-forming units	All four disinfectant solutions tested produced effective disinfection of the impression materials investigated.
Alwahab 2012 [25]	Alginate	Chlorhexidine digluconate	Pseudomonas aeruginosa Staphylococcus aureus Candida albicans	Inhibition halos	The least antibacterial activity of chlorhexidine digluconate was observed against Pseudomonas aeruginosa.
Azevedo 2019 [26]	Polyvinyl siloxane	Hydrogen peroxide MD520® Sodium hypochlorite	Does not specify	Colony-forming units	All disinfectants tested showed high antimicrobial efficiency.
Bal 2007 [27]	Polyvinyl siloxane Polyether	Sodium hypochlorite Gludex spray Mikrozid spray	Staphylococcus aureus Enterococcus faecalis	Colony-forming units	The disinfectant spray was less effective than sodium hypochlorite or Gludex.
Benakatti 2017 [28]	Alginate	Chlorhexidine Gluconate solution	Staphylococcus aureus	Inhibition halos	This disinfection method was effective in the elimination of S. aureus.
Beyerle 1994 [29]	Alginate	Sodium Hypochlorite	Bacillus subtilis Mycobacterauii bovis	Colony-forming units	One-minute exposure resulted in very inconsistent killing in all instances.
Brauner 1990 [30]	Alginate	Blueprint asept®	Streptococcus mutans Streptococcus sanguis Streptococcus aureus Streptococcus pyogenes Staphylococcus aureus Actinomyces odontolyticus Escherichia coli Klebsiella pneumoniae Proteus mirabilis Enterobacter aerogenes Pseudomonas aeruginosa	Inhibition halos	Due to its bactericidal effect, Blueprint asept® can be recommended.
Bustos 2010 [31]	Alginate Condensation silicone Alginate	Sodium Hypochlorite Glutaraldehyde	Gram (+) and (−) cuccus and Gram (−) bacillus Candida	Colony-forming units	Alginate and silicone impressions can successfully be disinfected if they are immersed in either 0.5% NaOCl solution or 2% glutaraldehyde for 5 min.
Choudhury 2018 [32]	Alginate	Sodium Hypochlorite Epimax®	Staphylococcus aureus Candida albicans Pseudomonas aeruginosa	Colony-forming units	Both Epimax and 0.525% sodium hypochlorite can disinfect the alginate impression material against Candida albicans, Pseudomonas aeruginosa, and Staphylococcus aureus.

Table 2. Cont.

Study	Impression Material	Disinfection Agent	Type of Microorganism	Main Outcome	Main Results
Cserna 1994 [33]	Alginate	Chlorhexidine Quaternary ammonium salt	*Lactobacillus* *Streptococcus mutans*	Inhibition halos	Antimicrobial alginates are more effective than nonantimicrobial alginates in reducing the surface growth of the oral bacteria *Lactobacillus* and *Streptococcus mutans*.
Cubas 2014 [34]	Alginate	Chlorhexidine	*Streptococci* *Candida*	Colony-forming units	Chlorhexidine as a water substitute during impression taking offers decreased microbial contamination with no negative alterations of the resulting casts, thus providing an easy method for controlling cross-infection.
Demajo 2016 [35]	Alginate Polyvinyl siloxane	MD 520® Minuten®	Does not specify	Colony-forming units	Glutaraldehyde is more effective than alcohol-based chemical disinfectants.
Doddamani 2011 [36]	Alginate	Povidone Iodine Sodium Hypochlorite Glutaraldehyde Distilled Water	*Staphylococcus aureus* *Bacillus subtilis* *Streptococcus viridans*	Colony-forming units	Disinfectants work equally well on an irreversible hydrocolloid impression material.
Estafanous 2012 [37]	Polyvinyl siloxane Polyether	EcoTru [EnviroSystems] ProSpray [Certol] Sodium hypochlorite	*Pseudomonas aeruginosa* *Salmonella choleraesius* *Staphylococcus aureus*	Colony-forming units	Disinfectants investigated in this study will effectively disinfect Polyvinyl siloxane and polyether elastomeric impression materials.
Flanagan 1998 [38]	Alginate	Single quaternary ammonium compound Chlorhexidine Dual quaternary ammonium compound	Gram-positive cocci Gram-negative bacilli yeast	Colony-forming units	The alginate with chlorhexidine killed all the gram-negative bacilli and the majority (95–99%) of the gram-positive cocci and yeast.
Gerhardt 1991 [39]	Alginate	Sodium hypochlorite	*Staphylococcus aureus* *Pseudomonas aeruginosa* *Bacillus subtilis*	Inhibition halos	The results indicated that chlorine disinfecting solutions of sufficient concentration can be retained for periods up to 1 week and still maintain their effectiveness.
Ginjupalli 2016 [40]	Alginate	Silver nanoparticles	*E. coli* *S. aureus* *C. albicans*	Inhibition halos	The particles imparted significant antimicrobial activity to the alginate impression materials tested.
Goel, 2014 [41]	Alginate	Sodium hypochlorite Microwave irradiation	*Staphylococcus aureus* *Pseudomonas aeruginosa*	Colony-forming units	The results suggested that the microwave irradiated Kala stone casts proved to be a better disinfection method when compared with 0.07% sodium hypochlorite chemically disinfected incorporated cast.
Hiramine 2021 [42]	Alginate	Sodium dichloroisocyanurate NaClO	*Streptococcus mutans* *Escherichia coli* *Staphylococcus aureus* *Candida albicans* Dental plaque bacteria	Colony-forming units	The number of oral bacteria adhering to the surfaces of impressions markedly decreased following a 10 min immersion in the 1000 ppm sodium dichloroisocyanurate solution.

Table 2. Cont.

Study	Impression Material	Disinfection Agent	Type of Microorganism	Main Outcome	Main Results
Ishida 1991 [43]	Alginate Condensation silicone	UV light	Candida albicans C. glabrata C. tropicalis C. parapsilosis C. krusei C. guillermondi	Colony-forming units	UV light is effective in disinfecting impression materials that are contaminated with candida organisms.
Ismail 2016 [44]	Alginate	Povidone iodine powder	Streptococcus mutans and Staphylococcus aureus	Inhibition halos	Modified alginate impression material with 15 weight % povidone-iodine powered gives the material self-disinfected properties
Ivanovski 1995 [45]	Alginate	Sterile Water Chlorhexidine Glutaraldehyde Povidone-iodine Sodium hypochlorite with sodium chloride	Escherichia coli Staphylococcus aureus Enterobacter cloacae Pseudomonas aeruginosa Klebsiella pneumoniae Actinobacter alcoaceticus Bacillus subtilis Mycobacterium phlei Candida albicans.	Colony-forming units	When glutaraldehyde was used, all the microorganisms tested were killed after 1 h. Chlorhexidine was ineffective against most microorganisms.
Jennings 1991 [3]	Polysulfide rubber Alginate Polyvinyl siloxane	Chlorhexidine gluconate	C. alb cans P. aeruginosa	Colony-forming units	Chlorhexidine gluconate (0.2%) was found to be less effective than either glutaraldehyde (2%) or sodium hypochlorite (0.0125%).
Jeyapalan 2018 [46]	Polyvinyl siloxane	Electrolyzed oxidizing water Glutaraldehyde Sodium hypochlorite	Streptococci Staphylococci Pseudomonas Candida Proteus Klebsiella E. coli	Colony-forming units	All three chemical disinfectants employed in this study showed acceptable mean log reduction values and kill rate % for antimicrobial efficacy.
Mathew 2017 [47]	Polyvinyl siloxane	Radio frequency glow discharge	Gram-negative bacilli Gram-positive cocci Escherichia coli Staphylococcus aureus	Inhibition halos	Ratio glow discharge is a very rapid and handy device, which can disinfect saliva contaminated elastomeric impression material surfaces.
McNeill 1992 [48]	Alginate	Glutaraldehyde Hypochlorite solution chlorine Hygojet system	Streptococcus sanguis poliovirus	Colony-forming units	Washing the impression for 15 s followed by immersion in 2% glutaraldehyde for 20.0 min or a hypochlorite solution for 7.5 min effectively disinfected the impression.
Moura 2010 [49]	Alginate	Sodium hypochlorite	Does not specify	Colony-forming units	5.25% sodium hypochlorite can be used with antimicrobial efficacy, using the humidifier box and nebulizer box methods, and 2.5% sodium hypochlorite was not effective in the nebulizer box method.
Nascimento 2015 [50]	Alginate	Sodium hypochlorite Chlorhexidine	S. mutans S. sanguis E. faecalis	Colony-forming units	4% chlorhexidine was the most suitable disinfectant.

Table 2. Cont.

Study	Impression Material	Disinfection Agent	Type of Microorganism	Main Outcome	Main Results
Rweyendela 2009 [13]	Alginate	Chlorinated compounds: Aseptrol Presept	Candida albicans Staphylococcus aureus Pseudomonas aeruginosa Streptococcus mutans Bacillus subtilis spores	Colony-forming units	The compounds effectively disinfected the alginate in the presence of organic material, but Aseptrol did so after an immersion time of only 1.5 min.
Samra 2010 [51]	Alginate Polyvinyl siloxane	Glutaraldehyde Sodium hypochlorite Ultraviolet chamber	Streptococcus viridans Diphtheriids Streptococcus pneumoniae Candida albicans Pseudomonas aeruginosa Staphylococcus albus	Colony-forming units	All the disinfection systems were effective in reducing the microbial load with the ultraviolet chamber as the most effective.
Savabi 2018 [52]	Alginate	Ozonated water	Pseudomonas aeruginosa Staphylococcus aureus Candida albicans	Colony-forming units	Immersion of alginate impression material in ozonated water for 10 min will not lead to complete disinfection but decreases the microorganisms to a level that can prevent infection transmission.
Schwartz 1996 [53]	Alginate	Sodium hypochlorite	Staphylococcus aureus Salmonella choleraesuis Pseudomonas aeruginosa Mycobacterium bovis Bacillus subtilis	Colony-forming units	It was found that a 10 min immersion in solutions reduced to pH 7 to 11 consistently produced a 4-log (99.99%) or greater reduction in viable organisms.
Singla 2018 [54]	Polyether	Disinfectant spray Deconex	Escherichia coli Staphylococcus aureus Pseudomonas aeruginosa Candida albicans	Colony-forming units	The disinfectant used was effective.
Tanaka 1994 [55]	Alginate	Chlorhexidine	Streptococcus mitis Actinomyces naeslundii Staphylococcus aureus Veillonella parvula Porphyromonas gingivalis Candida albicans	Colony-forming units	The use of an impression material supplemented with 1% chlorhexidine, such as Coe Hydrophilic Gel, may protect clinical staff and dental technicians from at least some bacterial infections associated with impression procedures.
Trivedi 2019 [56]	Alginate	Aloe Vera	Staphylococcus aureus Pseudomonas aeruginosa Candida albicans	Colony-forming units	The effectiveness of aloe vera as a disinfectant was demonstrated.
Zhang 2017 [57]	Elastomer impression material	Glutaraldehyde Ultraviolet radiation	Human Immunodeficiency Virus Hepatitis 3 virus	Colony-forming units	Combined use of ultraviolet radiation and 2% glutaraldehyde immersion can eliminate both Human Immunodeficiency Virus and Hepatitis B virus.

Figures 2–4 show the result from the meta-analyses. With regards to alginate, the use of disinfection agents such as chlorhexidine, alcohol, glutaraldehyde, and sodium hypochlorite significantly reduced the CFU/mL count ($p < 0.001$). It is worth mentioning that a high heterogenicity was observed ($I^2 = 74\%$) (Figure 2).

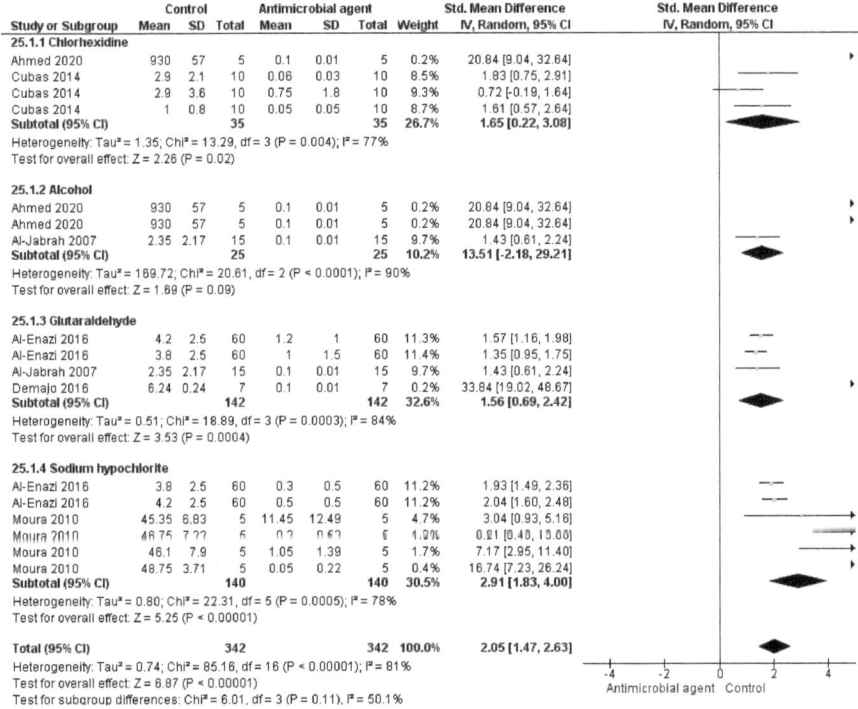

Figure 2. Forest plot of the analysis of CFU/mL count in alginate after disinfection.

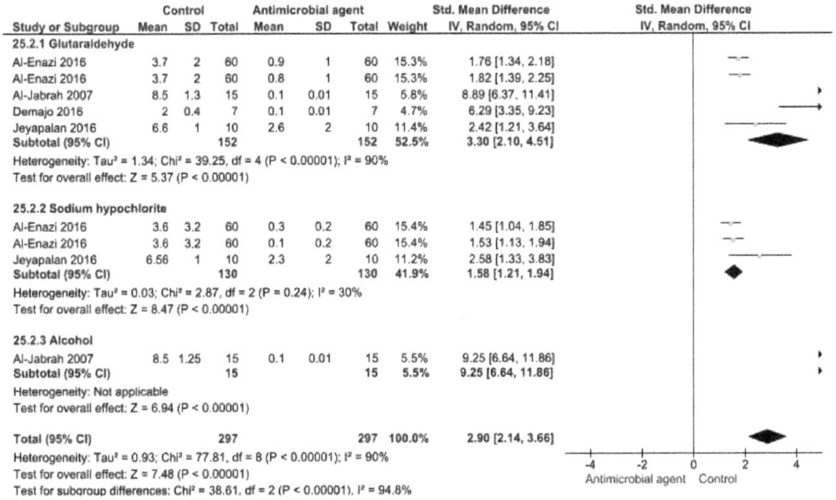

Figure 3. Forest plot of the analysis of CFU/mL count in polyvinyl siloxane after disinfection.

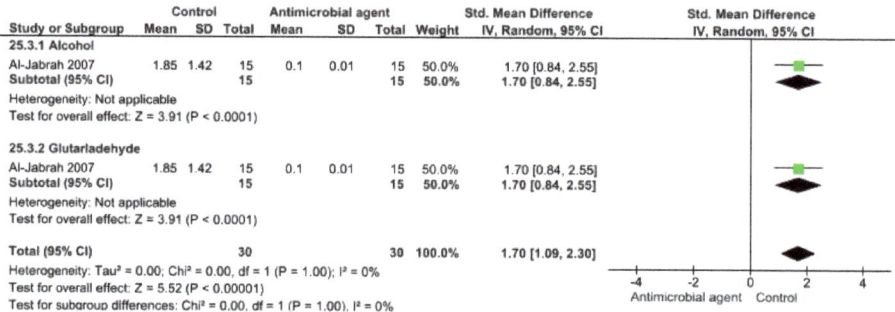

Figure 4. Forest plot of the analysis of CFU/mL count in polyether after disinfection.

Figure 3 shows the effect of different disinfection agents on polyvinyl siloxane material. According to the meta-analysis, all the disinfection agents tested significantly reduced the CFU/mL count ($p < 0.001$). Again, a high heterogenicity was observed in the comparisons (90%).

Finally, Figure 4 shows the effect of different disinfection agents on polyether impression material. According to the meta-analysis, both alcohol and glutaraldehyde significantly reduced the CFU/mL count ($p < 0.001$). As only one study was included in this analysis, a 0% heterogenicity was found.

The risk of bias analysis was shown that most of the studies were categorized with high and medium risk of bias (Table 3). Utmost of the manuscripts examined failed to report the single operator, operator blinded, and sample size calculation factors.

Table 3. The results of the risk of bias assessment.

Study	Specimen Randomization	Single Operator	Operator Blinded	Control Group	Complete Outcome Data	Sample Size Calculation	Risk of Bias
Ahmed 2020 [22]	NO	NO	NO	YES	NO	NO	High
Al-Enazi 2016 [23]	YES	NO	NO	YES	YES	NO	Medium
Al-Jabrah 2007 [24]	YES	NO	NO	YES	YES	NO	Medium
Alwahab 2012 [25]	NO	NO	NO	YES	YES	NO	High
Azevedo 2019 [26]	YES	NO	NO	YES	NO	NO	High
Bal 2007 [27]	NO	NO	NO	YES	NO	NO	High
Benakatti 2017 [28]	NO	YES	NO	YES	YES	NO	Medium
Beyerle 1994 [29]	NO	NO	NO	YES	NO	NO	High
Brauner 1990 [30]	YES	NO	NO	YES	NO	NO	High
Bustos 2010 [31]	YES	NO	NO	YES	YES	NO	Medium
Choudhury 2018 [32]	NO	NO	NO	YES	NO	NO	High
Cserna 1994 [33]	NO	NO	NO	YES	YES	NO	High
Cubas 2014 [34]	YES	NO	YES	YES	YES	YES	Low
Demajo 2016 [35]	NO	NO	NO	YES	YES	NO	High
Doddamani 2011 [36]	NO	NO	NO	YES	NO	NO	High
Estafanous 2012 [37]	NO	NO	NO	YES	NO	NO	High
Flanagan 1998 [38]	NO	NO	NO	YES	YES	NO	High
Gerhardt 1991 [39]	NO	NO	NO	YES	NO	NO	High
Ginjupalli 2016 [40]	NO	YES	NO	YES	YES	NO	Medium
Goel 2014 [41]	NO	NO	NO	YES	YES	NO	High
Hiramine 2021 [42]	NO	NO	NO	YES	YES	NO	High
Ishida 1991 [43]	NO	NO	NO	YES	YES	NO	High
Ismail 2016 [44]	NO	NO	NO	YES	NO	NO	High
Ivanovski 1995 [45]	NO	NO	NO	YES	YES	NO	High
Jennings 1991 [3]	YES	NO	NO	YES	YES	NO	Medium
Jeyapalan 2018 [46]	YES	NO	NO	YES	YES	NO	Medium
Mathew 2017 [47]	NO	NO	NO	YES	NO	YES	High
McNeill 1992 [48]	NO	NO	NO	YES	NO	NO	High
Moura 2010 [49]	YES	NO	NO	YES	YES	NO	Medium
Nascimento 2015 [50]	NO	NO	NO	YES	YES	NO	High
Rweyendela 2009 [13]	NO	NO	NO	YES	YES	NO	High
Samra 2010 [51]	NO	NO	NO	YES	NO	NO	High
Savabi 2018 [52]	NO	NO	NO	YES	YES	NO	High
Schwartz 1996 [53]	NO	NO	NO	YES	YES	NO	High
Singla 2018 [54]	NO	NO	NO	YES	NO	NO	High
Tanaka 1994 [55]	NO	NO	NO	YES	NO	NO	High
Trivedi 2019 [56]	NO	NO	NO	YES	YES	YES	Medium
Zhang 2017 [57]	YES	NO	NO	YES	NO	NO	High

4. Discussion

This systematic review and meta-analysis was directed towards testing the effect of disinfection agents on the bacterial colonization of different impression materials. This review focused on the study of the CFU/mL measure, since this is the most common measure used to determine the antibacterial activity. To the best of the authors knowledge, this is the first approach to prove that the application of disinfectant agents is effective to reduce the count of some oral pathogens on the surface of alginate, polyvinyl siloxane, and polyether impression materials and that this procedure can certainly reduce the possibility of cross-contamination. Accordingly, the hypothesis tested in this study was rejected.

Normally, chemical disinfectant agents were generally used in dental exercise because of their easy application. For the alginate materials, the use of disinfection agents such as chlorhexidine, alcohol, glutaraldehyde, and sodium hypochlorite significantly reduced the CFU/mL count ($p < 0.001$). Irreversible hydrocolloids, the frequent material used in dentistry, tend to absorb both blood and saliva [23]. Thus, research was focused on a solution to inhibit the colonization of microbe on the surface of these materials [11].

Collected data were established on the CFU in a media culture. These were recorded by using a colony counter, and the counts were expressed by a standard technique of estimating microbial colony count known as the CFU count. The bacteriological examination evidently exhibited that the CFU recorded after disinfection were fewer than before disinfection [23], thus making the disinfection process an important issue to solve after taking an impression in the dental world.

It is highlighted in a previous study [58] that the use of tap water on the surface of alginate impression failed to kill *Streptococcus Mutans* and *Lactobacilli*; however, by using chlorhexidine, a positive antimicrobial activity has been shown [59]. This could be possible by the binding between the positive site of chlorhexidine and negative sites of the bacterial cell, which resulted in interference with osmosis and escapes the constituents that lead to cell death [22]. In addition, alcohol was able to kill all the detected bacteria in this study by inactivating the growth of the bacteria on the alginate impression, and this was deemed probable by alkylating the amino and sulf hydral groups of bacterial proteins [60–62]. Further, for the other disinfectants, it was demonstrated that by using 2% glutaraldehyde solution or 1% sodium hypochlorite, gram-positive organisms will be modified by reducing their growth [11]. Indeed, this effect was most noticeable for 1% sodium hypochlorite, as described in this research.

A previous study denoted that after immersion in sterile water for 10 min, for some of impression materials, including alginate impression, the number of microorganisms counted was diminished, though alginate material still retained some of these microorganisms in comparison to other materials [24]. The physical nature of alginate impression could affect the capacity of disinfectants for doing their biocidal activity. In the oral environment, microorganisms might become integrated into the gelling impression material since the presence of oral fluids or saliva [29]. The set-up of these microorganisms in the alginate material restricted the efficacy of the water rinse, and the alginate gel assembly could hinder the penetration of the disinfectant [29,63]. Thus, this idea explained the results of this study as tap water did not reduce the microorganism counts in comparison to the other disinfectant solution. Overall, for alginate impressions, the use of disinfectant agents would be of great interest, and the efficacy of the disinfection ranged between 92% and 99.97% in all the situations [23].

According to the meta-analysis, all the disinfection agents significantly reduced the CFU/mL count ($p < 0.001$) on polyvinyl siloxane material. Among the numerous available impression materials in prosthodontics, this material was considered the material of choice, due to their fine detail reproduction, excellent physical properties, remarkable dimensional stability, good acceptance by the patient, and elastic recovery feature [64–66]. In addition, these materials were tasteless and odorless [46]. As stated above in alginate impression, using 2% glutaraldehyde solution or 1% sodium hypochlorite could be recommended also for disinfecting the polyvinyl siloxane impression [67,68]. In this manner, it is advisable to immerse these kinds of impressions in these solutions rather than spraying, as successful finding was observed in many previous studies, without harming the physical properties [15,18,31,69]. Seemingly, by putting the polyvinyl siloxane material in an alcohol-based disinfectant solution for a contact time of 15 min, a media free of microorganisms could be observed [24]. Accordingly, this can support the finding obtained in this study, as any kind of disinfectant solution tested showed promising results with polyvinyl siloxane impression material.

The present analysis noted that both alcohol and glutaraldehyde significantly reduced the CFU/mL count ($p < 0.001$) of polyether impression material. This could be explained by the fact that the contaminating bacteria could be reduced by 85% when soaking this kind of impression material in sterile water for 15 min; in addition, as found with polyvinyl siloxane impression, the use of alcohol-based solution produced effective disinfection of the polyether impression [24]. With regards to glutaraldehyde, the antimicrobial activity of this compound depends on the duration of dilution and its concentration. This could be elucidated by the fact that the biocidal activity of glutaraldehyde results from alkylation of sulfhydryl, hydroxyl, carboxyl, and amino groups of microorganisms, which alters RNA, DNA, and protein synthesis [70]. This conclusion seems to support the results in this meta-analysis.

From this review, various disinfectant agents were used to show the importance of reducing microorganisms on the surface of the impression materials used in dentistry. The results should be considered with caution since other brands of impression materials were available in the dental market and not included. In addition, there is the opportunity for slight changes in chemistry of these materials, causing significantly different reactions. Additionally, most of the studies included were classified as having high or medium risk of bias, and, therefore, better experimental designs should be conducted in order to obtain a higher degree of evidence. One of the limitations of this review relies on the fact that it is only focusing on the antibacterial efficacy of the application of a disinfectant on the surface of a dental impression; however, other variables should be taken into account, such as the effect of this procedure on the accuracy, precision, and surface quality of the resulting working models, especially when dental impressions are disinfected both in the dental office and in the dental laboratory. This led to controversy as to whether the disinfection process causes degradation or distortion of dental impressions and to what extent. Therefore, studying the effect of these disinfectants on the dimensional stability of the impression materials should be considered in further research. Additionally, viruses could be considered in future investigation by having the required equipment since their manipulation was considered dangerous for some researchers. Moreover, clinical studies were needed since testing of the efficacy of disinfectants from different patients derived impressions was scarce, knowing the differences in oral flora composition of individual person.

5. Conclusions

Based on in vitro studies, disinfection of alginate with chlorhexidine, alcohol, glutaraldehyde, and sodium hypochlorite reduced the CFU/mL count on the surface of alginate impressions. This trend was observed when polyvinyl siloxane impressions were disinfected with glutaraldehyde, sodium hypochlorite, and alcohol and when polyether was immersed in alcohol or glutaraldehyde. Therefore, these substances could be employed to reduce cross-contamination in the dental office.

Supplementary Materials: The following supporting information can be downloaded at: https://www.mdpi.com/article/10.3390/bioengineering9030123/s1, Table S1: Quantitative data extracted from studies included in the meta-analysis.

Author Contributions: Conceptualization, L.H., R.B. and C.E.C.-S.; methodology, L.H., R.B., N.K. and C.E.C.-S.; software, L.H., R.B. and C.E.C.-S.; validation, D.M., A.E., N.K., V.T. and Y.H.; formal analysis, L.H., R.B. and C.E.C.-S.; investigation, L.H., R.B., N.K., M.L.-S., E.C.-R., R.M., D.M. and

S.M.; resources, E.C.-R., Y.H., N.K., M.L.-S. and D.M.; data curation, L.H., R.B. and C.E.C.-S.; writing—original draft preparation, L.H., R.B. and C.E.C.-S.; writing—review and editing, M.L.-S., L.H., N.K. and Y.H.; visualization, N.K., E.C.-R., S.M., A.E., V.T., L.H., R.B. and R.M.; supervision, L.H.; project administration, L.H. All authors have read and agreed to the published version of the manuscript.

Funding: This research received no external funding.

Institutional Review Board Statement: Not applicable.

Informed Consent Statement: Not applicable.

Data Availability Statement: The data presented in this study are available in the article.

Acknowledgments: Authors Louis Hardan and Rim Bourgi would like to acknowledge the Saint-Joseph University of Beirut, Lebanon. Furthermore, the referees would also recognize the University of Hidalgo State, Mexico, the Medical University of Lodz, and the University of Strasbourg for accompanying this research.

Conflicts of Interest: The authors declare no conflict of interest.

References

1. Chidambaranathan, A.S.; Balasubramanium, M. Comprehensive Review and Comparison of the Disinfection Techniques Currently Available in the Literature. *J. Prosthodont.* **2019**, *28*, e849–e856. [CrossRef] [PubMed]
2. Ganavadiya, R.; Shekar, B.R.C.; Saxena, V.; Tomar, P.; Gupta, R.; Khandelwal, G. Disinfecting Efficacy of Three Chemical Disinfectants on Contaminated Diagnostic Instruments: A Randomized Trial. *J. Basic. Clin. Pharm.* **2014**, *5*, 98. [CrossRef] [PubMed]
3. Jennings, K.J.; Samaranayake, L.P. The Persistence of Microorganisms on Impression Materials Following Disinfection. *Int. J. Prosthodont.* **1991**, *4*, 382–387. [PubMed]
4. Samaranayake, L.P.; Hunjan, M.; Jennings, K.J. Carriage of Oral Flora on Irreversible Hydrocolloid and Elastomeric Impression Materials. *J. Prosthet. Dent.* **1991**, *65*, 244–249. [CrossRef]
5. Al Mortadi, N.; Al-Khatib, A.; Alzoubi, K.H.; Khabour, O.F. Disinfection of dental impressions: Knowledge and practice among dental technicians. *Clin. Cosmet. Investig. Dent.* **2019**, *11*, 103–108. [CrossRef]
6. Cottone, J.A.; Young, J.M.; Dinyarian, P. Disinfection/Sterilization Protocols Recommended by Manufacturers of Impression Materials. *Int. J. Prosthodont.* **1990**, *3*, 379–383.
7. British Dental Association. *The Control of Cross-Infection in Dentistry*; British Dental Association: London, UK, 1991; Volume 30.
8. Ghasemi, E.; Badrian, H.; Hosseini, N.; Khalighinejad, N. The effect of three different disinfectant materials on polyether impressions by spray method. *WJD* **2012**, *3*, 229–233. [CrossRef]
9. Blair, F.M.; Wassell, R.W. A Survey of the Methods of Disinfection of Dental Impressions Used in Dental Hospitals in the United Kingdom. *Br. Dent. J.* **1996**, *180*, 369–375. [CrossRef]
10. Amjadi, M.; Shakibamehr, A.H.; Sharifi, K.; Aalaei, S. General Dentists' Knowledge about Disinfecting Dental Impressions. *Teikyo Med.* **2021**, *44*, 837–842. [CrossRef]
11. Somasundram, J.; Geetha, R. Disinfection Of Impression Material-A Review. *Eur. J. Mol. Clin. Med.* **2020**, *7*, 2451–2460.
12. Stoeva, V.; Bozhkova, T.; Atanasowski, A.; Kondeva, V. Study of Knowledge of Hand Disinfection and Dental Impressions in Everyday Practice among Dental Students during a Pandemic by Coronavirus Disease 2019. *Open Access Maced. J. Med. Sci.* **2021**, *9*, 138–142. [CrossRef]
13. Rweyendela, I.H.; Patel, M.; Owen, C.P. Disinfection of Irreversible Hydrocolloid Impression Material with Chlorinated Compounds: Scientific. *S. Afr. Dent. J.* **2009**, *64*, 208–212.
14. Infection Control Recommendations for the Dental Office and the Dental Laboratory. *J. Am. Dent. Assoc.* **1996**, *127*, 672–680. [CrossRef] [PubMed]
15. Matyas, J.; Dao, N.; Caputo, A.A.; Lucatorto, F.M. Effects of Disinfectants on Dimensional Accuracy of Impression Materials. *J. Prosthet. Dent.* **1990**, *64*, 25–31. [CrossRef]
16. Tullner, J.B.; Commette, J.A.; Moon, P.C. Linear Dimensional Changes in Dental Impressions after Immersion in Disinfectant Solutions. *J. Prosthet. Dent.* **1988**, *60*, 725–728. [CrossRef]
17. Rueggeberg, F.A.; Beall, F.E.; Kelly, M.T.; Schuster, G.S. Sodium Hypochlorite Disinfection of Irreversible Hydrocolloid Impression Material. *J. Prosthet. Dent.* **1992**, *67*, 628–631. [CrossRef]
18. Adabo, G.L.; Zanarotti, E.; Fonseca, R.G.; dos Santos Cruz, C.A. Effect of Disinfectant Agents on Dimensional Stability of Elastomeric Impression Materials. *J. Prosthet. Dent.* **1999**, *81*, 621–624. [CrossRef]
19. Page, M.; McKenzie, J.; Bossuyt, P.; Boutron, I.; Hoffman, T.; Mulrow, C.; Shamseer, L.; Tetzlaff, J.; Akl, E.; Brennan, S.; et al. The PRISMA 2020 Statement: An Updated Guideline for Reporting Systematic Reviews. *MetaArXiv Preprint* **2020**. [CrossRef]
20. Ouzzani, M.; Hammady, H.; Fedorowicz, Z.; Elmagarmid, A. Rayyan—A Web and Mobile App for Systematic Reviews. *Syst. Rev.* **2016**, *5*, 210. [CrossRef]

21. Hardan, L.; Devoto, W.; Bourgi, R.; Cuevas-Suárez, C.E.; Lukomska-Szymanska, M.; Fernández-Barrera, M.Á.; CornejoRíos, E.; Monteiro, P.; Zarow, M.; Jakubowicz, N.; et al. Immediate Dentin Sealing for Adhesive Cementation of Indirect Restorations: A Systematic Review and Meta-Analysis. *Gels* **2022**, *8*, 175. [CrossRef]
22. Ahmed, H.M.A.; Jawad, R.R.; Nahidh, M. Effect of the Different Disinfectants on the Microbial Contamination of Alginate Impression Materials. *Indian J. Forensic Med. Toxicol.* **2020**, *14*, 793.
23. Al-Enazi, T.A.; Naik, A. Disinfection of Alginate and Addition Silicon Rubber-Based Impression Materials. *Int. J. Stomatol. Occlusion Med.* **2016**, *8*, 44–48. [CrossRef]
24. Al-Jabrah, O.; Al-Shumailan, Y.; Al-Rashdan, M. Antimicrobial Effect of 4 Disinfectants on Alginate, Polyether, and Polyvinyl Siloxane Impression Materials. *Int. J. Prosthodont.* **2007**, *20*, 299–307. [PubMed]
25. Alwahab, Z. Comparison of Antimicrobial Activities and Compressive Strength of Alginate Impression Materials Following Disinfection Procedure. *J. Contemp. Dent. Pract.* **2012**, *13*, 431–435. [CrossRef]
26. Azevedo, M.J.; Correia, I.; Portela, A.; Sampaio-Maia, B. A Simple and Effective Method for Addition Silicone Impression Disinfection. *J. Adv. Prosthodont.* **2019**, *11*, 155–161. [CrossRef] [PubMed]
27. Bal, B.T.; Yılmaz, H.; Aydin, C.; Al, F.D.; Sultan, N. Efficacy of Various Disinfecting Agents on the Reduction of Bacteria from the Surface of Silicone and Polyether Impression Materials. *Eur. J. Prosthodont.* **2007**, *15*, 177–182.
28. Benakatti, V.B.; Patil, A.P.; Sajjanar, J.; Shetye, S.S.; Amasi, U.N.; Patil, R. Evaluation of Antibacterial Effect and Dimensional Stability of Self-Disinfecting Irreversible Hydrocolloid: An in Vitro Study. *J. Contemp. Dent. Pract.* **2017**, *18*, 887–892. [CrossRef]
29. Beyerle, M.P.; Hensley, D.M.; Bradley, D.V., Jr.; Schwartz, R.S.; Hilton, T.J. Immersion Disinfection of Irreversible Hydrocolloid Impressions with Sodium Hypochlorite. Part I: Microbiology. *Int. J. Prosthodont.* **1994**, *7*, 234–238.
30. Brauner, A.W. In Vitro and Clinical Examination of the Effect of.an Antimicrobial Impression Material on the Oral microflora. *Dent. Mater.* **1990**, *6*, 201–203. [CrossRef]
31. Bustos, J.; Herrera, R.; González, U.; Martínez, A.; Catalán, A.; González, U. Effect of Inmersion Desinfection with 0.5% Sodium Hypochlorite and 2% Glutaraldehyde on Alginate and Silicone: Microbiology and SEM Study. *Int. J. Odontostomat.* **2010**, *4*, 169–177. [CrossRef]
32. Choudhury, G.K.; Chitumalla, R.; Manual, L.; Rajalbandi, S.K.; Chauhan, M.S.; Talukdar, P. Disinfectant Efficacy of 0.525% Sodium Hypochlorite and Epimax on Alginate Impression Material. *J. Contemp. Dent. Pract.* **2018**, *19*, 113–116. [CrossRef]
33. Cserna, A.; Crist, R.L.; Birk Adams, A.; Dunning, D.G. Irreversible Hydrocolloids: A Comparison of Antimicrobial Efficacy. *J. Prosthet. Dent.* **1994**, *71*, 387–389. [CrossRef]
34. De Azevedo Cubas, G.B.; Valentini, F.; Camacho, G.B.; Leite, F.R.M.; Cenci, M.S.; Pereira-Cenci, T. Antibacterial Efficacy and Effect of Chlorhexidine Mixed with Irreversible Hydrocolloid for Dental Impressions: A Randomized Controlled Trial. *Int. J. Prosthodont.* **2014**, *27*, 363–365. [CrossRef] [PubMed]
35. Demajo, J.K.; Cassar, V.; Farrugia, C.; Millan-Sango, D.; Sammut, C.; Valdramidis, V.; Camilleri, J. Effectiveness of Disinfectants on Antimicrobial and Physical Properties of Dental Impression Materials. *Int. J. Prosthodont.* **2016**, *29*, 63–67. [CrossRef]
36. Doddamani, S.; Patil, R.A.; Gangadhar, S.A. Efficacy of Various Spray Disinfectants on Irreversible Hydrocolloid Impression Materials: An in Vitro Study. *Indian J. Dent. Res.* **2011**, *22*, 764–769. [CrossRef] [PubMed]
37. Estafanous, E.W.; Palenik, C.J.; Platt, J.A. Disinfection of Bacterially Contaminated Hydrophilic PVS Impression Materials. *J. Prosthodont.* **2012**, *21*, 16–21. [CrossRef] [PubMed]
38. Flanagan, D.A.; Palenik, C.J.; Setcos, J.C.; Miller, C.H. Antimicrobial Activities of Dental Impression Materials. *Dent. Mater.* **1998**, *14*, 399–404. [CrossRef]
39. Gerhardt, D.E.; Williams, H.N. Factors Affecting the Stability of Sodium Hypochlorite Solutions Used to Disinfect Dental Impressions. *Quintessence Int.* **1991**, *22*, 587–591.
40. Ginjupalli, K.; Alla, R.K.; Tellapragada, C.; Gupta, L.; Perampalli, N.U. Antimicrobial Activity and Properties of Irreversible Hydrocolloid Impression Materials Incorporated with Silver Nanoparticles. *J. Prosthet. Dent.* **2016**, *115*, 722–728. [CrossRef]
41. Goel, K.; Gupta, R.; Solanki, J.; Nayak, M. A Comparative Study between Microwave Irradiation and Sodium Hypochlorite Chemical Disinfection: A Prosthodontic View. *J. Clin. Diagn. Res.* **2014**, *8*. [CrossRef]
42. Hiramine, H.; Watanabe, K.; Inaba, K.; Sasaki, H.; Hamda, N. Evaluation of Antimicrobial Effects on Dental Impression and Biofilm Removal by Sodium Dichloroisocyanurate. *Biocontrol. Sci.* **2021**, *26*, 17–25. [CrossRef]
43. Ishida, H.; Nahara, Y.; Tamamoto, M.; Hamada, T. The Fungicidal Effect of Ultraviolet Light on Materials Impression. *J. Prosthet. Dent.* **1991**, *65*, 532–535. [CrossRef]
44. Ismail, H.A.; Asfour, H.; Shikho, S.A. A Self-Disinfecting Irreversible Hydrocolloid Impression Material Mixed with Povidone Iodine Powder. *Eur. J. Dent.* **2016**, *10*, 507–511. [CrossRef] [PubMed]
45. Ivanovski, S.; Savage, N.W.; Brockhurst, P.J.; Bird, P.S. Disinfection of Dental Stone Casts: Antimicrobial Effects and Physical Property Alterations. *Dent. Mater.* **1995**, *11*, 19–23. [CrossRef]
46. Jeyapalan, V.; Krishnan, C.S.; Ramasubramanian, H.; Sampathkumar, J.; Azhagarasan, N.S.; Krishnan, M. Comparative Evaluation of the Antimicrobial Efficacy of Three Immersion Chemical Disinfectants on Clinically Derived Poly (Vinyl Siloxane) Impressions. *J. Prosthodont.* **2018**, *27*, 469–475. [CrossRef] [PubMed]
47. Mathew, S.; Alani, M.M.; Velayudhan Nair, K.N.; Haridas, S.; Reba, P.B.; Thomas, S.A. Radiofrequency Glow Discharge as a Mode of Disinfection for Elastomeric Impression Materials. *J. Contemp. Dent. Pract.* **2017**, *18*, 131–136. [CrossRef]

48. McNeill, M.; Coulter BDS, W.; Hussey BOS, D. Disinfection of Irreversible Hydrocolloid Impressions: A Comparative Study. *Int. J. Prosthodont.* **1992**, *5*, 563–567.
49. Moura, C.D.v; Moura, W.L.d.; França, F.M.G.; Martins, G.A.S.; Feltrim, P.P.; Zanetti, R.V. Disinfection of Irreversible Hydrocolloid Impressions with Sodium Hypochlorite Steam: Assessment of Antimicrobial Efficacy. *Rev. Odonto. Ciênc.* **2010**, *25*, 182–187.
50. Nascimento, P.L.A.d.; Ribeiro, R.B.; Gadê-Neto, C.R.; Dias, A.H.d.M. Incorporation of Disinfectants for Obtaining Dental Stone: Microbiological and Dimensional Evaluation. *Rev. Odontol. UNESP* **2015**, *44*, 24–30. [CrossRef]
51. Samra, R.K.; Bhide, S.V. Efficacy of Different Disinfectant Systems on Alginate and Addition Silicone Impression Materials of Indian and International Origin: A Comparative Evaluation. *J. Indian Prosthodont. Soc.* **2010**, *10*, 182–189. [CrossRef]
52. Savabi, O.; Nejatidanesh, F.; Bagheri, K.P.; Karimi, L.; Savabi, G. Prevention of Cross-Contamination Risk by Disinfection of Irreversible Hydrocolloid Impression Materials with Ozonated Water. *Int. J. Prev. Med.* **2018**, *9*, 14. [CrossRef] [PubMed]
53. Schwartz, R.; Hensley, D.H.; Bradley, D. Immersion Disinfection of Irreversible Hydrocolloid Impressions in PH-Adjusted Sodium Hypochlorite. Part 1: Microbiology. *Int. J. Prosthodont.* **1996**, *7*, 217–222.
54. Singla, Y.; Pachar, R.B.; Poriya, S.; Mishra, A.; Sharma, R.; Garg, A. Evaluation of the Efficacy of Different Mixing Techniques and Disinfection on Microbial Colonization of Polyether Impression Materials: A Comparative Study. *J. Contemp. Dent. Pract.* **2018**, *19*, 296–300. [CrossRef] [PubMed]
55. Tanaka, H.; Ebara, S.; Sugawara, A.; Nishiyama, M.; Hayashi, K. Basic Properties of an Alginate Impression Material Supplemented with Chlorhexidine I. Disinfectant Effects on Oral Microbes. *J. Nihon. Univ. Sch. Dent.* **1994**, *36*, 135–138. [CrossRef]
56. Trivedi, R.; Sangur, R.; Bathala, L.R.; Srivastava, S.; Madhav, S.; Chaubey, P. Evaluation of Efficacy of Aloe Vera as a Disinfectant by Immersion and Spray Methods on Irreversible Hydrocolloid Impression Material and Its Effect on the Dimensional Stability of Resultant Gypsum Cast—An in Vitro Study. *J. Med. Life Sci.* **2019**, *12*, 395–402. [CrossRef]
57. Zhang, W.; Mao, H.; Zhou, G. Effect of Ultraviolet Radiation Combined with Immersion Disinfection of Silicone Impressions Infected with Hepatitis B Virus and HIV. *Biomed. Res.* **2017**, *28*, 6377–6380.
58. Kollu, S.; Hedge, V.; Chakravarthy, K. Efficacy of Chlorhexidine in Reduction of Microbial Contamination in Commercially Available Alginate Materials—In-Vitro Study. *Glob. J. Med. Res.* **2013**, *13*, 1–7.
59. Nakagawa, T.; Hosaka, Y.; Ishihara, K.; Hiraishi, T.; Sato, S.; Ogawa, T.; Kamoi, K. The Efficacy of Povidone-Iodine Products against Periodontopathic Bacteria. *Dermatology* **2006**, *212*, 109–111. [CrossRef]
60. Hamzah, R.A.M.; Saloom, H.F. Efficacy of Various Disinfectants on Bacterial and Fungal Contamination of Clamping Tweezers. *Int. J. Med. Sci. Public Health* **2018**, *7*, 41–45.
61. Huang, P.Y.; Masri, R.; Romberg, E.; Driscoll, C.F. The Effect of Various Disinfectants on Dental Shade Guides. *J. Prosthet. Dent.* **2014**, *112*, 613–617. [CrossRef]
62. Severa, J.; Klaban, V. Desident CaviCide a New Disinfectant. *Cas. Lek.* **2009**, *148*, 269–270.
63. Gryshkov, O.; Mutsenko, V.; Tarusin, D.; Khayyat, D.; Naujok, O.; Riabchenko, E.; Nemirovska, Y.; Danilov, A.; Petrenko, A.Y.; Glasmacher, B. Coaxial Alginate Hydrogels: From Self-Assembled 3D Cellular Constructs to Long-Term Storage. *Int. J. Mol. Sci.* **2021**, *22*, 3096. [CrossRef] [PubMed]
64. Chee, W.W.L.; Donovan, T.E. Polyvinyl Siloxane Impression Materials: A Review of Properties and Techniques. *J. Prosthet. Dent.* **1992**, *68*, 728–732. [CrossRef]
65. Donovan, T.E.; Chee, W.W.L. A Review of Contemporary Impression Materials and Techniques. *Dent. Clin. N. Am.* **2004**, *48*, 445–470. [CrossRef] [PubMed]
66. Mandikos, M.N. Polyvinyl Siloxane Impression Materials: An Update on Clinical Use. *Aust. Dent. J.* **1998**, *43*, 428–434. [CrossRef]
67. Estrela, C.; Estrela, C.R.A.; Barbin, E.L.; Spanó, J.C.E.; Marchesan, M.A.; Pécora, J.D. Mechanism of Action of Sodium Hypochlorite. *Braz. Dent. J.* **2002**, *13*, 113–117. [CrossRef]
68. Taylor, R.L.; Wright, P.S.; Maryan, C. Disinfection Procedures: Their Effect on the Dimensional Accuracy and Surface Quality of Irreversible Hydrocolloid Impression Materials and Gypsum Casts. *Dent. Mater.* **2002**, *18*, 103–110. [CrossRef]
69. Atabek, D.; Alaçam, A.; Tüzüner, E.; Polat, S.; Sipahi, A.B. In-Vivo Evaluation of Impression Material Disinfection with Different Disinfectant Agents. *J. Hacettepe Fac. Dent.* **2009**, *33*, 52–59.
70. Stonehill, A.A.; Krop, S.; Borick, P.M. Buffered Glutaraldehyde—A New Chemical Sterilizing Solution. *Am. J. Hosp. Pharm.* **1963**, *20*, 458–465. [CrossRef]

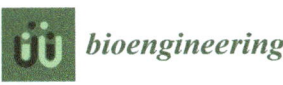

Article

In Vitro Qualitative Evaluation of Root-End Preparation Performed by Piezoelectric Instruments

Calogero Bugea [1,*], Federico Berton [2], Antonio Rapani [2], Roberto Di Lenarda [2], Giuseppe Perinetti [2], Eugenio Pedullà [3], Antonio Scarano [4] and Claudio Stacchi [2]

1. Independent Researcher, 73100 Lecce, Italy
2. Department of Medical, Surgical and Health Sciences, University of Trieste, 34100 Trieste, Italy; fberton@units.it (F.B.); rapani.antonio@gmail.com (A.R.); rdilenarda@units.it (R.D.L.); gperinetti@units.it (G.P.); claudio@stacchi.it (C.S.)
3. Department of General Surgery and Surgical-Medical Specialties, University of Catania, 95100 Catania, Italy; eugenio.pedulla@unict.it
4. Department of Medical, Oral and Biotechnological Sciences, University of Chieti-Pescara, 66100 Chieti, Italy; ascarano@unich.it
* Correspondence: calogerobugea@yahoo.it

Abstract: Although the application of ultrasounds in endodontic surgery allows for effective debridement of the root canal, incorrect device setting or inefficient tips seem to generate cracks during root-end retropreparation. The primary aim of this in vitro study was to establish the presence, or absence, of a correlation between ultrasonic root-end preparation and the formation of cracks. The present study was conducted on human teeth, extracted for periodontal reasons. After root canal treatment, roots were resected 3 mm from the anatomical apex by using a high-speed handpiece and carbide burs. The resected teeth were retroprepared by using an ultrasonic tip (R1D, Piezomed, W&H, Bürmoos, Austria), setting the piezoelectric device at maximum power available for the tip. Time required for the retropreparation was recorded. Before and after retropreparation, all roots were photographed under a stereomicroscope and analyzed by two different operators to evaluate: (a) the presence and extension of dentinal cracks and (b) the morphology of root-end preparation. Finally, piezoelectric tips were analyzed by scanning electron microscopy (SEM) to evaluate morphologic changes after use. A total of 43 single roots (33 with one root canal, 10 with two root canals) were treated. Average preparation time was 1 minute and 54 seconds. None of the roots without initial cracks developed new cracks after retropreparation. Quality of the preparation margins was fairly equal among the prepared specimens. None of the piezoelectric tips broke during instrumentation, and SEM analysis showed minimal surface wear of the tips after performing 11 retropreparations. Within the limits of the present study, the tested piezoelectric system does not seem to represent a major cause for root crack formation. Pre-existing cracks may expand after ultrasound root-end preparation.

Keywords: piezoelectric surgery; endodonticsurgery; crack formation; ultrasonic tip; retropreparation

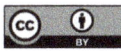

1. Introduction

Ultrasounds were first introduced in endodontic surgery by Richman [1], with the aim of improving the effectiveness of root canal debridement and of performing both resection and retropreparation of the apical part of the dental root. Today, clinicians often choose ultrasonic root-end preparation, mainly because of the unmatched visibility this technology allows. This advantage is due to the angled shape of the tips, and to the cavitation effect, and allows to reduce the angle of the resection bevel [2–8]. Despite the excellent results obtained with the ultrasonic tips, some drawbacks have been associated with the use of this technique [9], including the presence of dentinal cracks on the resected root-end [10] and risk of perforation.

The contact between the instrument and root canal walls during preparation creates stress concentration in dentin and microcrack formation [11]. These microcracks are important because they may further develop into vertical root fractures. A recent study demonstrated that root fracture is not an instant event but rather a gradual propagation of tiny, less pronounced craze lines in the tooth structure [12].

In recent years, the occurrence of root fracture in either sound or endodontically treated/restored teeth has become a major concern in endodontics [13–15]. Some authors demonstrated that the endodontic procedures may increase the incidence of dentinal defects, such as Shemesh et al. [16] and Bier et al. [17]. Great interest was placed on the dentinal microcrack phenomenon by clinicians, academics and researchers over the following years. In a recent narrative review conducted on crack formation, Versiani et al. analyzed how the root dentinal microcracks observed in cross-sectional images of extracted teeth are not caused by canal-shaping procedures, and dehydration often causes cracking of the dentinal tissue, regardless of canal instrumentation [18].

In endodontic surgery, Layton et al. [19] suggested that ultrasonic root-end preparation might increase the risk of crack formation and found different types of cracks which they classified as follows:

- Intra-canal cracks start at the inner part of the canal and run through the dentine. They can be complete, if reaching the root surface, or incomplete, if ending inside the dentin.
- Intra-dentin cracks only affect the dentin, are usually distal or mesial to the canal and develop from buccal to lingual, and vice versa.
- Cement cracks start inside the cement and expand to the cement–dentin junction in a radial pattern.

The primary aim of this work was to investigate in vitro the influence of ultrasonic root-end preparation on the formation of different types of cracks. The ultrasonic tips used were evaluated by assessing the overall quality of the retrograde cavities and the effect of multiple uses on the tip itself.

2. Materials and Methods

This in vitro study investigated the integrity of human single roots after retrograde cavity preparation performed with a piezoelectric device. Quality and operative time of the preparations were evaluated, as well as the presence of cracks before and after ultrasonic instrumentation. Cracks were also recorded based on location and extension. Piezoelectric tips were examined after using scanning electron microscopy (SEM) to evaluate surface and shape alterations.

2.1. Specimen Selection

A total of 56 human teeth extracted for periodontal reasons from patients of 57 to 84 years old were cleaned from calculus and decay and stored in HBSS Solution (Hanks' Balanced Salt Solution) at room temperature for a period of two to four weeks. A preliminary evaluation of the existence of fractures or dentinal cracks due to the extraction procedure was performed, using a microscope at $16\times$ magnification (Leica 320, Leica Microsystems, Wetzlar, Germany). Teeth exhibiting radicular alterations or with incomplete or reabsorbed apices were discarded. A total of 33 single-rooted premolars and 10 mesial roots of mandibular molars were selected for treatment.

2.2. Specimen Preparation and Analysis

The crowns were resected to simplify the endodontic procedure and iconographic acquisition. All the teeth were endodontically treated following a crown-down approach. Canals were shaped to the working length with a rotary sequence (Protaper Universal, Dentsply Maillefer, Ballaigues, Switzerland) up to the F3 instrument. Canals were then obturated using warm vertical condensation [20] and sealer (Pulp Canal Sealer EWT™, Kerr Dental, Orange, CA, USA). Backpacking was performed by condensation of thermolasticized gutta-percha (Obtura III, Obtura Spartan, Algonquin, IL, USA).

All roots were resected 3 mm from the anatomical apex by using a high-speed handpiece with multiblade carbide bur (H847KRG314.016/018, Komet, Besigheim, Germany) under water spray. Each carbide bur was replaced after resecting ten roots. The resected roots were soaked in blue ink (Pelikan, Schindellegi, Switzerland) balanced with salt for 48 h, then rinsed, photographed and examined under an optical microscope (Leica MZ16, Leica Microsystems, Wetzlar, Germany) at 16× magnification to evaluate the presence of cracks prior to the retropreparation.

2.3. Root-End Preparation

Both root resection and root-end preparation were performed by the same expert endodontist (C.B.) under microscope magnification (Leica M320, Leica Microsystems, Wetzlar, Germany). All the root-ends were prepared using a piezoelectric device (Piezomed, W&H, Bürmoos, Austria), set to power (40/100) as suggested by the manufacturer for the use of the dedicated tip (R1D, Piezomed, W&H, Bürmoos, Austria), under continuous saline irrigation. Each specimen was prepared following a standard protocol, with an up and down motion until creating a 3 mm deep preparation, measured by means of a periodontal probe. The tip was only activated when in contact with the tooth. Each tip was used to perform 11 retropreparations and then replaced. Cavities were then rinsed with 5 mL of saline solution to eliminate debris and remnants.

2.4. Image Recording and Analysis

All specimens were photographed under 16 × magnification (Leica MZ16, Leica Microsystems, Wetzlar, Germany) after root-end resection and after retropreparation. The photographs were paired and coded by an independent assessor (C.S.) and then evaluated by two blinded assessors (F.B. and A.R.). Comparison of paired photographs determined presence, characteristics and time of occurrence of each crack.

2.5. Crack Evaluation

Crack evaluation was conducted and scored according to Abedi's method [21], as follows:

- Roots with no cracks after root resection (before root-end preparation) and no cracks after root-end preparation;
- Roots with no cracks after root resection (before root-end preparation) that developed cracks after root-end preparation;
- Roots with cracks after root resection (before root-end preparation), which became longer or wider after root-end preparation, or that developed new cracks during root-end preparation.

Cracks were also classified as follows:

- Intracanal: cracks originating within the canal and extending into dentin;
- Intradentinal: cracks enclosed within the dentin and separate from the root surface and the canal;
- Extracanal: cracks originating at the root surface and extending into dentin;
- Communicating: cracks extending from root surface to the canal.

2.6. Retrograde Cavity Evaluation

The quality of the root-end cavity margins was scored according to the degree of defects [22] as follows: (0) ideal preparation, no detectable defects; (1) imprint, a single visible defect, likely produced by the contact between the angulated portion of the tip and the cavity margin; (2) microchipped, ragged margin; (3) chipped, ragged margin together with defects likely caused by the tip bouncing off the root surface.

2.7. Tip Analysis

A qualitative analysis of the effects of usage on tip shape and surface topography was performed by using scanning electron microscopy (FEG ESEM XL 30; FEI, Hillsboro, OR, USA). The entire sample was divided into four groups (3 groups of 11 teeth and 1 group of 10 teeth): images of the ultrasonic tip used in each group were captured at 35×, 100× and 200× magnification and compared by 2 different investigators (F.B. and A.R.) with the images of a brand-new tip.

2.8. Working Time

The entire retropreparation procedure was timed with a professional stopwatch from the first contact of the tip to the root-end to the last passage of the retropreparation (HS-80TW-1EF, Casio, Shibuya, Japan).

These data were then elaborated separately for roots with one single canal and roots with two canals.

2.9. Statistical Analysis

Average mean crack between the assessors (as ordinal data) was calculated for both the PRE and POST time points and used to assess the significance of the difference between the time points by means of the Mann–Whitney U-test. Inter-rater repeatability was evaluated using the percentage of agreement and by both unweighted and linear-weighted kappa coefficients presented as mean (95% CI). The kappa coefficient ranges from 0 for no agreement to 1 for perfect agreement. The following standards for strength of agreement for the coefficient have been proposed: 0.01–0.20, slight; 0.21–0.40, fair; 0.41–0.60, moderate; 0.61–0.80, substantial; and >0.80 almost perfect [2]. Crack type was scored as follows: intracanal (1); intradentinal (2); extracanal (3) and communicating (4). Wilcoxon paired signed-rank test assessed the significance of the difference in the crack type between the 'pre' and 'post' root-end preparation. A p value less than 0.05 was used for the rejection of the null hypothesis.

3. Results

3.1. Examiners' Agreement

Overall median (25th; 75th percentile) of the crack modality was 1.0 (0–3.0) and 2.3 (0–4.0) at the PRE and POST time points, respectively. The difference between the time points was not significant ($p = 0.258$ Mann–Whitney; $p = 0.136$ Wilcoxon).

The overall percentage of agreement between the raters was 72.7% (32 cases out of 44) for both the PRE and POST time point assessments, respectively (Table 1). For the PRE time point, unweighted and weighted kappa coefficients were 0.639 (0.466–0.811) and 0.700 (0.533–0.868), respectively. For the POST time point, unweighted and weighted kappa coefficients were 0.610 (0.437–0.783) and 0.741 (0.599–0.884), respectively.

Table 1. Crosstabulation of the different crack modalities between the assessors according to the time points.

Time Point	Assessor FB	Assessor AR				
		None	Intracanal	Intradentinal	Extracanal	Communicating
Pre	None	12	1	0	0	0
	Intracanal	2	8	0	0	2
	Intradentinal	0	0	2	1	1
	Extracanal	0	0	0	3	1
	Communicating	0	3	0	1	7
Post	None	13	2	0	0	0
	Intracanal	1	4	0	2	2
	Intradentinal	0	0	0	0	2
	Extracanal	0	2	0	1	2
	Communicating	0	1	0	0	14

3.2. Crack Presence and Evaluation

Of the 43 prepared roots, 34 were not affected by resection of the apex, while 9 roots showed the presence of cracks, namely 4 intracanal cracks, 2 intradentin cracks, 2 extracanal cracks and 1 communicating crack. After retropreparation, none of the sound roots showed newly formed cracks, while one intracanal crack was eliminated during retropreparation. The only communicating crack was unvaried after retropreparation. All the other cracks (i.e., 3 intracanal, 2 extracanal, 2 intradentin) turned into communicating cracks. Analysis of pre- and post-treatment crack type variation was reported in Table 2.

Table 2. Pre- and post-treatment crack type variation analyzed by Wilcoxon paired signed rank test.

Crack Type	Mean ± SD	Diff. *
Pre	0.42 ± 0.96	<0.05; S *
Post	0.74 ± 1.57	

* Diff.—significance of the difference; S—statistically significant.

3.3. Quality of the Retrograde Cavity

There was a total of 31 roots showing ideal preparation (0); 3 roots showing microchipping, ragged margin (2); 5 roots showing chipping (3); and 4 roots showing imprint (1) (Figures 1 and 2).

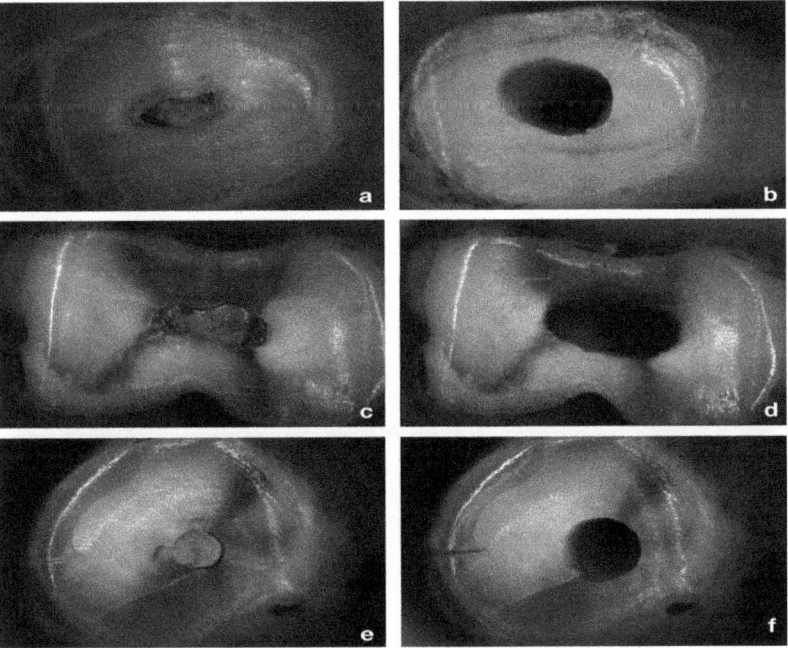

Figure 1. (**a**) Preoperative view of a single canal root; (**b**) Postoperative view of canal (**a**), absence of cracks; (**c**) Preoperative view of a mesial root; (**d**) Postoperative view of (**c**), note the precision of the preparation; (**e**) Preoperative view of a single canal root with the presence of cracks; (**f**) Postoperative view of (**e**), note the development of the crack.

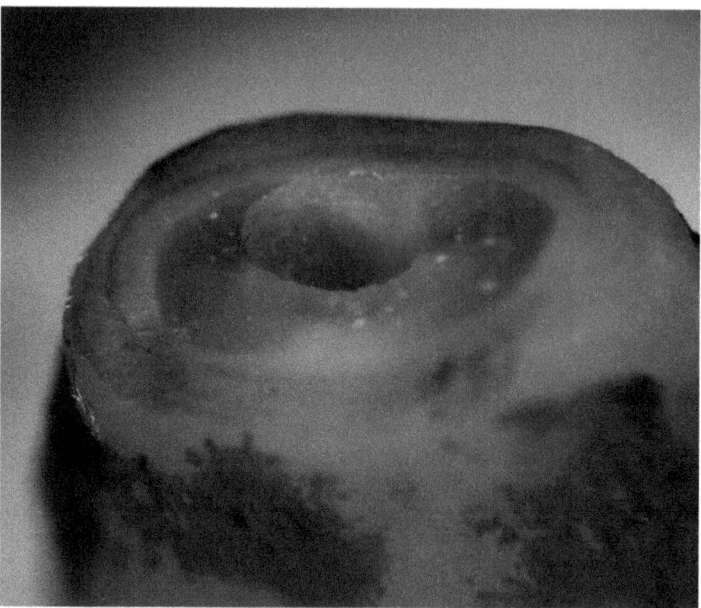

Figure 2. Details of the preparation.

3.4. Working Time

The working time was registered for the entire time for preparation of all specimens (total time 01:21:31). Mean root-end preparation time was 114.00 ± 69.32 seconds. In Table 3 are reported the data for single canals and double canals.

Table 3. Time evaluation.

	Minutes	Seconds
mean	01:54	113.74
SD	01:09	69.32
mode	01:32	92.00
median	01:33	93.00
sd single canal	01:08	67.61
mode single canal	01:32	92.00
median single canal	01:32	93.00
mean double canal	02:23	142.6
sd single double canal	01:09	69.28
mode double canal	N/A *	N/A *
median double canal	02:44	164.00

* N/A—not applicable.

3.5. SEM Evaluation of the Tips

Surface modifications of the R1D tips after 11 root-end preparations were minimal. Slight rounding of the diamond crystal edges was found, and very few crystals were lost during instrumentation (Figure 3). No relevant difference was found based on the working time of each tip. Tip 1 was used for 27 min 23 s, tip 2 for 18 min 58 s, tip 3 for 15 min 8 s, and tip 4 for 20 min 2 s.

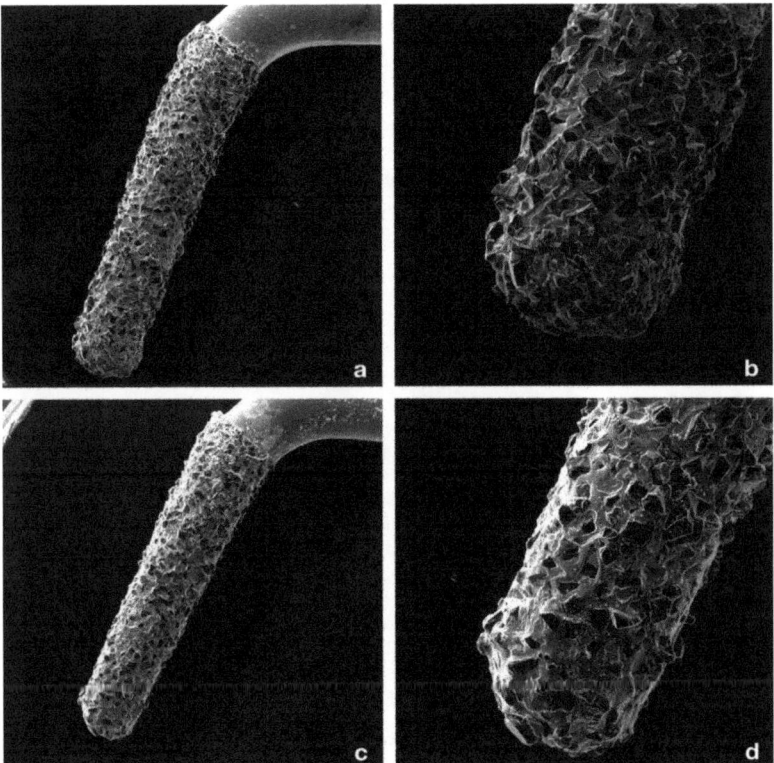

Figure 3. (a) SEM magnification of tip R1D (Piezomed, W&H, Bürmoos, Austria); (b) Details of the tip; note the regular position of the diamonds; (c) SEM magnification of tip R1D (Piezomed, W&H, Bürmoos, Austria) after utilization (20 min and 2 s); (d) Details of the tip; note the reduction of the number of diamonds compared to (a).

4. Discussion

The clinical outcomes of endodontic surgery have greatly improved in recent years, thanks to the adoption of microsurgical instruments, which have made management of the apical third [2,3,23] more efficient. To date, it is unknown if root-end alterations induced by retro-tips could affect the short and long-term clinical outcome, but any approach aimed at minimizing adverse effects (e.g., cracks) should be considered [22].

The present in vitro study was performed on human teeth extracted for periodontal reasons. Some teeth presented cracks prior to the root-end preparation, which could have been present prior to extraction or may have occurred during the extraction maneuvers or during the shaping procedures [18,24]. In fact, in vitro preparation may cause cracks more often than in vivo because of the shock-absorbing capacity of the periodontal ligament and because of the dehydration occurring during the shaping procedure [7,25]. In the present study, cracks were visible after root resection, while no cracks developed during ultrasonic root-end preparation. This result is in contrast to the supposed augmented risk of developing cracks upon ultrasonic root-end instrumentation. On the other hand, 77.8% (seven out of nine) of the present cracks were found to have worsened after preparation of the retrograde cavity. These results suggest that intact roots are at low risk of developing a crack. Existing cracks may extend or change in morphology.

Few studies have investigated the different types of cracks produced after root-end preparation with ultrasonic retro-tips [24–26]. Rainwater et al. [24] found no significant difference in prevalence and type of crack when comparing a stainless-steel and a diamond retro-tip, the ultrasonic device set at low power. Beling et al. [26] found intradentinal and incomplete cracks after root-end preparation using a stainless-steel retro-tip, the ultrasonic device set at low power.

Margin quality of the retrograde cavities does not seem to be affected by the power setting and the oscillations of the piezoelectric device, in agreement with other studies [10,27–29]. Moreover, tips were changed every 11 preparations to standardize the approach, but the operator did not notice a decrease in cutting efficacy, as verified upon SEM examination of the used tips which did not show significant signs of surface wear [30–33].

5. Conclusions

The present study showed encouraging results in retro-preparation performed with W&H Piezomed (W&H, Bürmoos, Austria). Although ultrasound root-end preparation did not cause any cracks, it seems that existing cracks might expand upon ultrasonic instrumentation [34].

Author Contributions: C.B.: Conceptualization (lead); Investigation (equal); Methodology (equal); Supervision (lead); Writing–original draft (equal); Writing–review & editing (equal), F.B.: Investigation (equal); Data curation (equal); Formal analysis (equal); Methodology (equal); Validation (lead); Writing–review & editing (equal), A.R.: Conceptualization (equal); Data curation (equal); Investigation (equal); Visualization (lead); Writing–review & editing (equal), R.D.L.: Project administration (lead); Resources (equal); Writing–review & editing (equal), G.P.: Investigation (equal); Methodology (equal); Formal analysis (lead); Writing–review & editing (equal), E.P.: Data curation (equal); Investigation (lead); Software (equal); Validation (equal); Writing–review & editing (equal), A.S.: Data curation (equal); Methodology (equal); Writing–review & editing (equal), C.S.: Conceptualization (equal); Methodology (equal); Data curation (equal); Writing–original draft (lead). All authors have read and agreed to the published version of the manuscript.

Funding: This study received no external funding.

Institutional Review Board Statement: Not applicable.

Informed Consent Statement: Not applicable.

Data Availability Statement: The data supporting the findings of the present study are available from the corresponding author upon reasonable request.

Conflicts of Interest: The authors declare no conflict of interest.

References

1. Richman, R.J. The use of ultrasonics in root canal therapy and root resection. *Med. Dent. J.* **1957**, *12*, 12–18.
2. Wang, Z.H.; Zhang, M.M.; Wang, J.; Jiang, L.; Liang, Y.H. Outcomes of Endodontic Microsurgery Using a Microscope and Mineral Trioxide Aggregate: A Prospective Cohort Study. *J. Endod.* **2017**, *43*, 694–698. [CrossRef] [PubMed]
3. Nagendrababu, V.; Jayaraman, J.; Suresh, A.; Kalyanasundaram, S.; Neelakantan, P. Effectiveness of ultrasonically activated irrigation on root canal disinfection: A systematic review of in vitro studies. *Clin. Oral Investig.* **2018**, *22*, 655–670. [CrossRef]
4. Floratos, S.; Kim, S. Modern Endodontic Microsurgery Concepts: A Clinical Update. *Dent. Clin. N. Am.* **2017**, *61*, 81–91. [CrossRef] [PubMed]
5. Kang, M.; In Jung, H.; Song, M.; Kim, S.Y.; Kim, H.C.; Kim, E. Outcome of nonsurgical retreatment and endodontic microsurgery: A meta-analysis. *Clin. Oral. Investig.* **2015**, *19*, 569–582. [CrossRef] [PubMed]
6. Carr, G. Advanced techniques and visual enhancement for endodontic surgery. *Endod. Rep.* **1992**, *7*, 6–9.
7. Tidmarsh, B.G.; Arrowsmith, M.G. Dentinal tubules at the root ends of apicected teeth: A scanning electron microscopic study. *Int. Endod. J.* **1989**, *22*, 184–189. [CrossRef]
8. Plotino, G.; Pameijer, C.H.; Grande, N.M.; Somma, F. Ultrasonics in endodontics: A review of the literature. *J. Endod.* **2007**, *33*, 81–95. [CrossRef] [PubMed]
9. Khabbaz, M.G.; Kerezoudis, N.P.; Aroni, E.; Tsatsas, V. Evaluation of different methods for the root-end cavity preparation. *Oral Surg. Oral Med. Oral Pathol. Oral Radiol. Endodontol.* **2004**, *98*, 237–242. [CrossRef]
10. Del Fabbro, M.; Tsesis, I.; Rosano, G.; Bortolin, M.; Taschieri, S. Scanning electron microscopic analysis of the integrity of the root-end surface after root-end management using a piezoelectric device: A cadaveric study. *J. Endod.* **2010**, *36*, 1693–1697. [CrossRef]

11. Abou El Nasr, H.M.; Abd El Kader, K.G. Dentinal damage and fracture resistance of oval roots prepared with single-file systems using different kinematics. *J. Endod.* **2014**, *40*, 849–851. [CrossRef] [PubMed]
12. Milani, A.S.; Froughreyhani, M.; Rahimi, S.; Jafarabadi, M.A.; Paksefat, S. The effect of root canal preparation on the development of dentin cracks. *Iran. Endod. J.* **2012**, *7*, 177–182. [PubMed]
13. Llena-Puy, M.C.; Forner-Navarro, L.; Barbero-Navarro, I. Vertical root fracture in endodontically treated teeth: A review of 25 cases. *Oral Surg. Oral Med. Oral Pathol. Oral Radiol. Endodontol.* **2001**, *92*, 553–555. [CrossRef] [PubMed]
14. Toure, B.; Faye, B.; Kane, A.W.; Lo, C.M.; Niang, B.; Boucher, Y. Analysis of reasons for extraction of endodontically treated teeth: A prospective study. *J. Endod.* **2011**, *37*, 1512–1515. [CrossRef]
15. Yoshino, K.; Ito, K.; Kuroda, M.; Sugihara, N. Prevalence of vertical root fracture as the reason for tooth extraction in dental clinics. *Clin. Oral Investig.* **2015**, *19*, 1405–1409. [CrossRef]
16. Shemesh, H.; Bier, C.A.; Wu, M.K.; Tanomaru-Filho, M.; Wesselink, P.R. The effects of canal preparation and filling on the incidence of dentinal defects. *Int. Endod. J.* **2009**, *42*, 208–213. [CrossRef]
17. Bier, C.A.S.; Shemesh, H.; Tanomaru-Filho, M.; Wesselink, P.R.; Wu, M.K. The ability of different nickel-titanium rotary instruments to induce dentinal damage during canal preparation. *J. Endod.* **2009**, *35*, 236–238. [CrossRef]
18. Versiani, M.A.; Cavalcante, D.M.; Belladonna, F.G.; Silva, E.J.N.L.; Souza, E.M.; De-Deus, G. A critical analysis of research methods and experimental models to study dentinal microcracks. *Int. Endod. J.* **2021**, 1–49. [CrossRef]
19. Layton, C.A.; Marshall, J.G.; Morgan, L.A.; Baumgartner, J.C. Evaluation of cracks associated with ultrasonic root-end preparation. *J. Endod.* **1996**, *22*, 157–160. [CrossRef]
20. Schilder, H. Filling root canals in three dimensions. *J. Endod.* **2006**, *32*, 281–290. [CrossRef]
21. Abedi, H.R.; Van Mierlo, B.L.; Wilder-Smith, P.; Torabinejad, M. Effects of ultrasonic root-end cavity preparation on root apex. *Oral Surg. Oral Med. Oral Pathol. Oral Radiol. Endodontol.* **1995**, *80*, 207–213. [CrossRef]
22. De Bruyne, M.A.; De Moor, R.J. SEM analysis of the integrity of resected root apices of cadaver and extracted teeth after ultrasonic root-end preparation at different intensities. *Int. Endod. J.* **2005**, *38*, 310–319. [CrossRef] [PubMed]
23. Tsesis, I.; Rosen, E.; Taschieri, S.; Telishevsky Strauss, Y.; Ceresoli, V.; Del Fabbro, M. Outcomes of surgical endodontic treatment performed by a modern technique: An updated meta-analysis of the literature. *J. Endod.* **2013**, *39*, 332–339. [CrossRef] [PubMed]
24. Rainwater, A.; Jeansonne, B.G.; Sarkar, N. Effects of ultrasonic root-end preparation on microcrack formation and leakage. *J. Endod.* **2000**, *26*, 72–75. [CrossRef] [PubMed]
25. Engel, T.K.; Steiman, H.R. Preliminary investigation of ultrasonic root end preparation. *J. Endod.* **1995**, *21*, 443–445. [CrossRef]
26. Beling, K.L.; Marshall, J.G.; Morgan, L.A.; Baumgartner, J.C. Evaluation for cracks associated with ultrasonic root-end preparation of gutta-percha filled canals. *J. Endod.* **1997**, *23*, 323–326. [CrossRef]
27. Waplington, M.; Lumley, P.J.; Walmsley, A.D. Incidence of root face alteration after ultra-sonic retrograde cavity preparation. *Oral Surg. Oral Med. Oral Pathol. Oral Radiol. Endodontol.* **1997**, *83*, 387–392. [CrossRef]
28. Gutmann, J.L.; Saunders, W.P.; Nguyen, L.; Guo, I.Y.; Saunders, E.M. Ultrasonic root-end preparation Part 1. SEM. analysis. *Int. Endod. J.* **1994**, *27*, 318–324. [CrossRef]
29. Mehlhaff, D.S.; Marshall, J.G.; Baumgartner, J.C. Comparison of ultrasonic and high-speed bur root-end preparations using bilaterally matched teeth. *J. Endod.* **1997**, *23*, 448–452. [CrossRef]
30. Lin, Y.H.; Mickel, A.K.; Jones, J.J.; Montagnese, T.A.; González, A.F. Evaluation of cutting efficiency of ultrasonic tips used in orthograde endodontic treatment. *J. Endod.* **2006**, *32*, 359–361. [CrossRef]
31. Navarre, S.W.; Steiman, R. Root-End fracture during retropreparation: A comparison between zirconium nitride-coated and stainless steel microsurgical ultrasonic instruments. *J. Endod.* **2002**, *28*, 330–332. [CrossRef] [PubMed]
32. Godfrey, M.P.; Kulild, J.C.; Walker, M.P. A comparison of the dentin cutting efficiency of 4 pointed ultrasonic tips. *J. Endod.* **2013**, *39*, 897–900. [CrossRef] [PubMed]
33. Brent, P.; Morgan, L.; Marshall, J.; Baumgartner, J.C. Evaluation of diamond-coated ultrasonic instruments for root-end preparation. *J. Endod.* **1999**, *25*, 672–675. [CrossRef]
34. Tawil, P.Z. Periapical Microsurgery: Can Ultrasonic Root-end Preparations Clinically Create or Propagate Dentinal Defects? *J. Endod.* **2016**, *42*, 1472–1475. [CrossRef] [PubMed]

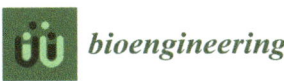

Systematic Review

What Is the Most Effective Technique for Bonding Brackets on Ceramic—A Systematic Review and Meta-Analysis

Inês Francisco [1,*], Raquel Travassos [1], Catarina Nunes [1], Madalena Ribeiro [1], Filipa Marques [1], Flávia Pereira [1], Carlos Miguel Marto [2,3,4,5,6], Eunice Carrilho [2,3,4,5], Bárbara Oliveiros [3,7], Anabela Baptista Paula [1,2,3,4,5] and Francisco Vale [1]

1. Institute of Orthodontics, Faculty of Medicine, University of Coimbra, 3004-531 Coimbra, Portugal; raqueltravassos.91@gmail.com (R.T.); mcal9497@hotmail.com (C.N.); anabelabppaula@sapo.pt (M.R.); filipa.p.s.marques@gmail.com (F.M.); fppereira_@hotmail.com (F.P.); madalenaprata@hotmail.com (A.B.P.); fvale@fmed.uc.pt (F.V.)
2. Institute of Integrated Clinical Practice, Faculty of Medicine, University of Coimbra, 3004-531 Coimbra, Portugal; cmiguel.marto@uc.pt (C.M.M.); eunicecarrilho@gmail.com (E.C.)
3. Coimbra Institute for Clinical and Biomedical Research (iCBR), Area of Environment Genetics and Oncobiology (CIMAGO), Faculty of Medicine, University of Coimbra, 3004-531 Coimbra, Portugal; boliveiros@fmed.uc.pt
4. Centre for Innovative Biomedicine and Biotechnology (CIBB), University of Coimbra, 3004-531 Coimbra, Portugal
5. Clinical Academic Center of Coimbra (CACC), 3004-531 Coimbra, Portugal
6. Institute of Experimental Pathology, Faculty of Medicine, University of Coimbra, 3004-531 Coimbra, Portugal
7. Laboratory of Biostatistics and Medical Informatics (LBIM), Faculty of Medicine, University of Coimbra, 3004-531 Coimbra, Portugal
* Correspondence: ines70.francisco@gmail.com

Abstract: *Background*: There has been an increase in demand for orthodontic treatment within the adult population, who likely receive restorative treatments using ceramic structures. The current state of the art regarding the most effective method to achieve an appropriate bond strength of brackets on ceramic surfaces isn't consensual. This systematic review aims to compare the available surface treatments to ceramics and determine the one that allows to obtain the best bond strength. *Methods*: This systematic review followed the PRISMA guidelines and the PICO methodology was used, with the question "What is the most effective technique for bonding brackets on ceramic crowns or veneers?". The research was carried out in PubMed, Web of Science, Embase and Cochrane Library databases. In vitro and ex vivo studies were included. The methodological quality was evaluated using the guidelines for reporting of preclinical studies on dental materials by Faggion Jr. *Results*: A total of 655 articles searched in various databases were initially scrutinized. Seventy one articles were chosen for quality analysis. The risk of bias was considered medium to high in most studies. The use of hydrofluoric acid (HF), silane and laser afforded the overall best results. HF and HF plus laser achieved significantly highest bond strength scores in felsdphatic porcelain, while laser was the best treatment in lithium disilicate ceramics. *Conclusions*: The most effective technique for bonding brackets on ceramic is dependent on the type of ceramic.

Keywords: adhesion; bonding; dental porcelain; glass ceramics; orthodontic bracket; shear strength

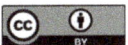

1. Introduction

In recent years there has been an increase in demand for orthodontic treatment within the adult population. As of 2015, according to the American Association of Orthodontics, the demand within this age group has doubled over a four year period and this number is set to increase further in the future [1]. This can be attributed not only to evergrowing aesthetic concerns [2] but also to the expeditious evolution of orthodontic techniques [1]. In this age group, there is a high likelihood that an orthodontist will encounter complex restorative treatments using ceramic structures [1–3] due to their numerous advantages, namely biocompatibility, excellent aesthetics, reduced bacterial plaque accumulation, low thermal expansion, resistance to abrasion or fracture along with colour stability [4–7]. The most used ceramic used in dental practices are feldsphatic, lithium and zirconia [4,8].

Nonetheless, these types of restorations can reveal themselves quite complex for orthodontists, since achieving a reasonable bond strength on ceramic surfaces is challenging due to the presence of a glaze layer that hinders the adhesion process [7–10]. This is evident in the clinical practice as well with some studies having reported bracket adhesion failure rates on ceramic surfaces of around 9.8% after two years [7]. Consequently, orthodontists may encounter difficulties in achieving an optimal adhesion force on ceramic surfaces that is not only effective but also harmless [3,7], that is, an adhesion force that is resistant to orthodontic and masticatory forces while also retaining the function and aesthetics that are provided by this type of restoration after bracket debonding [3,7,10,11]. Recurrent bracket debonding reduces the success of orthodontic treatment, as it creates adverse consequences in terms of appliance efficiency, cost, treatment duration and patient's comfort which can all be avoided by achieving adequate adhesion [4,10,12].

As a response to the referred difficulties, different conditioning methods of ceramic surfaces have emerged, whether they are mechanical, chemical or a combination of both, these are applied to change the ceramics' properties and increase bonding strength [9,13]. Mechanical methods like sandblasting with aluminium oxide, the use of diamond burs and laser irradiation help produce micromechanical retentions. As for chemical methods, which are used to establish a porous surface on the ceramic, the most commonly used products include phosphoric acid (PhA), hydrofluoric acid (HF), silane and, as of recently, universal adhesives [1,4,8–10,13–15].

However, it is not only the ceramic surface treatment method that influences the bond strength, factors such as ceramic type, bracket material and design, light curing source, adhesive system properties and clinician's experience are as equally important when trying to achieve the best results [4,7,8,13,15].

According to the current available literature, the most commonly used protocol for ceramic surface treatment starts with an oxide aluminium sandblasting, followed by conditioning with hydrofluoric acid, application of silane, and lastly the placement of bonding resin [10,16]. Despite being a highly successful technique in terms of adhesion strength, this protocol also presents itself with a few handicaps. This sequence is not only long and complex, but the use of hydrofluoric acid requires a very careful application due to its high corrosiveness, meaning that in the sequence of a direct contact it can lead to soft tissue necrosis [2,9,16,17].

The current state of the art isn't consensual regarding the most effective and safest method to achieve a reasonable bond strength of brackets on ceramic surfaces. Several studies were performed with different ceramic types and used different surface treatment protocols. As such, it becomes necessary to gather and evaluate all the scientific information presently available to determine the best protocol.

2. Materials and Methods

This systematic review was drawn up in accordance with the Preferring Items for Systematic and Meta-Analyses and Meta-Analyses (PRISMA) guidelines and was registered in PROSPERO with the ID 282131 number. The Population, Intervention, Comparison and Outcome (PICO) question is outlined in Table 1.

Table 1. The PICO question.

Population	Ceramic subtracts (crowns, veneers) . . .
Intervention	Adhesion Techniques . . .
Comparison	Diverse techniques (fluoride acid, sand blasting, adhesive, silane) . . . .
Outcome	Which is the most effective . . . .

PICO question: What is the most effective technique for bonding brackets on ceramic crowns or veneers?

The literature search was carried out in several databases, namely PubMed (www.ncbi.nlm.nih.gov/pubmed), Web of Science Core Collection (webofknowledge.com/WOS), Cochrane Library (www.cochranelibrary.com), and EMBASE (www.embase.com).

The last search was performed on 1 September 2021. The search formula for was the following: (bracket * OR 'brace'/exp OR brace OR 'orthodontic bracket'/exp OR 'orthodontic bracket' OR 'orthodontic device'/exp OR 'orthodontic device') AND ('dental porcelain'/exp OR 'dental porcelain' OR porcelain * OR 'glass ceramics'/exp OR 'glass ceramics') AND ('shear strength'/exp OR 'shear strength' OR 'dental bonding'/exp OR 'dental bonding' OR 'adhesion'/exp OR adhesion OR bond *). The same formula was applied was applied to the other databases. Articles published from 2011 to 2021 in English, Portuguese, and Spanish were searched.

Four independent reviewers scrutinized the studies, in accordance with defined inclusion criteria: in vitro or ex vivo studies evaluating the shear bond strength of brackets to ceramic substrate. There were included metallic, polycarbonate, sapphire, zirconia and ceramic brackets. Excluded criteria were all subtracts that differ from ceramic such as gold, amalgam, other metallic alloy, resins and polycarbonate/polycarboxylate; ex-vivo studies with enamel surfaces, polymerization techniques studies and surface characteristics studies.

Three external elements were consulted in case of doubt or in the absence of consensus. For each study the following information was extracted: author and date, study design, adhesion technique type (type, time, clinical application), porcelain type, sample size, test group and control group, bracket type, intervention test, results, and main conclusions.

Two reviewers independently assessed the methodological quality of included studies. In the case of discrepancies, a third reviewer was consulted. The methodological quality was checked using the guidelines for reporting of preclinical studies on dental materials by Faggion Jr. [18].

Statistical Analysis

Studies were polled by surface treatment and porcelain type (either feldspathic or lithium disilicate). For each porcelain, treatments were compared using an ANOVA with post-hoc comparisons through the Mann-Whitney test with Bonferroni correction. To perform the comparisons, the sample variability was computed for each study considering the pool of studies which have analyzed the same treatment, and study weights were computed as a percentage of the total sample variance.

The IBM SPSS Statistics for Windows, Version 27.0 (IBM Corp.: Armonk, NY, USA) was used to perform the statistical analysis.

The synthetic measure based on weighted means for each treatment, as well as its variance, were used to plot the confidence intervals on a descriptive forest plot, using Excel (Microsoft Corporation, Redmond, WA, USA) and a bubble plot.

3. Results

The search results and the initial number of abstracts selected according to the selection criteria from the various databases are provided in Figure 1. From the 655 studies collected from all the databases based on their title and abstract, 90 studies were screened by title and abstract. 71 articles satisfied the final selection criteria and were included in the present systematic review and meta-analysis. Figure 1 presents the PRISMA flow of the article selection process.

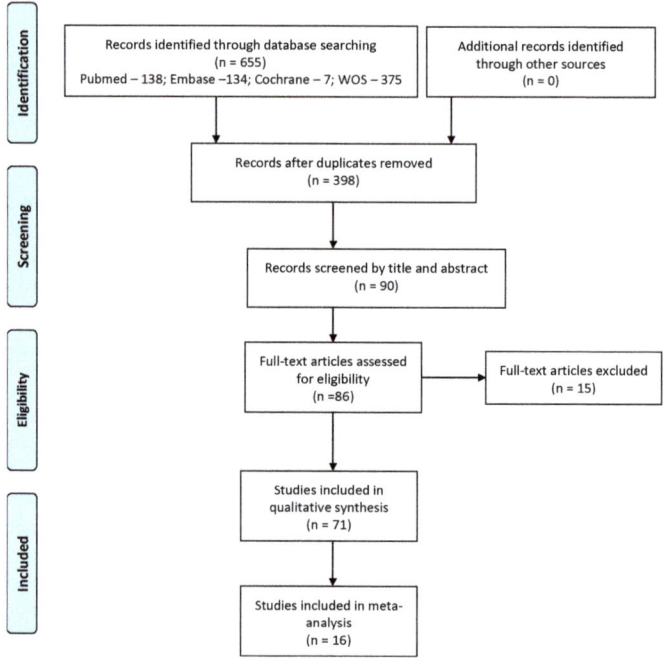

Figure 1. PRISMA flow diagram of studies selection.

The results are described in detail in Table 2. The sample size (n) ranged from 8 to 960, obtaining a total sample of n = 7246. The final selection of studies was 64 in vitro, 5 ex vivo e 2 in vitro/ex vivo, from 2011 to 2021.

All the articles evaluated various methods of conditioning the ceramic surface to obtain an adequate bond strength when bonding brackets. The types of adhesion technique mostly present in the included articles are application of orthophosphoric acid or hydrofluoric acid in various concentrations, silane application, sandblasting/air abrasion with aluminum oxide or silicon dioxide, diamond bur roughening, single bond universal adhesive and the application of different types of lasers such as Er:YAG laser, CO_2 laser, Er:CrYSGG laser, Nd:YAG laser, Cr:YSGG laser, FS laser.

All types of porcelain (feldsphatic, lithium dissilicate glass ceramic, leucite reinforced glass ceramic, monolithic zirconia, hybrid porcelain, silica-based ceramic, lithium dissilicate-reinforced ceramic, fluoroapatite-leucite glass-ceramic, fluoroapatite, and leucite-reinforced ceramic, glazed ceramic porcelain fused to metal) were studied.

Regarding the type of brackets, metallic, ceramic, polycarbonate, sapphire, and zirconia brackets were included.

All articles used shear bond test for the application of force, except for one study that used tensile strength test [19] and another one that used the adhesion strength test [20].

3.1. Risk of Bias

The results of the quality assessment of the in vitro studies included are reported in Figure 2.

Table 2. Summary of parameters and results from in vitro and ex vivo included studies.

Authors, Year	Study Design	Type of Adhesion Technique (Type, Time, Clinical Application)	Type of Porcelain	Sample Size (n)	Test Group	Control Group	Bracket Type	Intervention Test	Results	Conclusions
Mohammed et al., 2019 [21]	Ex vivo	Five different surface conditioning methods: G1: 37% H_3PO_4 acid gel (30 s) + washed + air dried + primer & bonding agent; G2: 9% HF acid (90s) G3: sandblasting for 2–3 s + 9% HF acid; G4: Sandblasting (2–3 s) + Silane, G5: Fine diamond bur roughening + silane	Porcelain	60	50 ceramic crowns fabricated onto the premolar teeth following crown preparation	Natural teeth were acid etched in conventional manner using 37% H_3PO_4 acid (n = 10)	Metallic	SBST	G4 produced maximum bond strength of 12.34 ± 0.95 MPa comparable or even better than the control group 11.03 ± 1.63 MPa; G2 and G3 9% HF acid 11.48 ± 0.98 MPa; G5 F 9.28 ± 1.11 MPa. Ceramic surfaces conditioned with 37% H_3PO_4 acid produced least SBST of 5.51 ± 0.88 MPa and hence not suitable for bonding Orthodontic brackets in a clinical scenario.	G4 produced maximum bond strength comparable or even better than the control group followed by G3 and G5. G2 produced least SBST and hence not suitable for bonding Orthodontic brackets in a clinical scenario.
Dilber et al., 2016 [22]	In vitro	Three surface conditioning methods: G1: fine diamond burr; G2: fine diamond burr + air abrasion with 30 μm SiO_2 + silane G3: fine diamond burr +9.5% HF acid + silane	Feldspathic ceramic; Lithium disilicate glass ceramic; Nanocomposite; Polymer infiltrated ceramic network	204	CAD/CAM blocks (n = 204, n = 17 per group) of (a) VITA Mark II (VM), (b) IPS e.max CAD (IP), (c) Lava Ultimate (LU), (d)VITA ENAMIC (VE); C-Control: (fine diamond bur); CJ: (fine diamond bur + air abrasion with 30 μm SiO_2 + silane) HF: (fine diamond bur +9.5% HF acid + silane)	Specimens were mechanically roughened with fine diamond burrs placed with their shafts parallel to the specimen axes. Then, they were washed and rinsed thoroughly to remove the debris, and air-dried	Metallic	SBST	Mean bond strength (MPa) values were significantly affected by the surface conditioning method ($p < 0.001$) but not the CAD/CAM material type ($p = 0.052$); Bond strengths for all CJ and HF-conditioned specimens were two-fold higher (11.83 ± 1.95 – 9.44 ± 1.63) than those for control specimens with all materials (4.73 ± 0.93 – 6.02 ± 0.69). Significantly lower mean values were obtained in LU-CJ (9.78 ± 1.61) and LU-HF (9.44 ± 1.63) than those for other groups (11.83 ± 1.95 – 10.93 ± 1.33) groups ($p < 0.05$).	All CAD/CAM materials tested benefitted from additional surface conditioning either with HF acid or silica coating and silanization; Weibull parameters indicated more reliable adhesion of metal brackets to feldspathic ceramic when their graze was removed with fine diamond bur and then conditioned with either hydrofluoric acid or silica coating followed by silanization compared to those of other material combinations;

Table 2. Cont.

Authors, Year	Study Design	Type of Adhesion Technique (Type, Time, Clinical Application)	Type of Porcelain	Sample Size (n)	Test Group	Control Group	Bracket Type	Intervention Test	Results	Conclusions
Miersch et al., 2019 [23]	In vitro	(1) Roughening, etching with 9% buffered HF acid; (2) Sandblasting and silane; (3) Roughening, and an experimental single component ceramic primer containing ammonium polyfluoride and trimethoxysilylpropyl methacrylate; (4) Applying the experimental single-component ceramic primer without prior roughening; (5) Only roughening;	Leucite reinforced glass ceramic	60	60 identical molar crowns with the morphology of tooth 36 were computer-aided designed and computer-aided manufactured (CAD/CAM) from a leucite-reinforced glass ceramic. G1: roughening, hydrofluoric acid, silane; G2: roughening, silane; G3: roughening, experimental coupling agent; G4: experimental coupling agent; G5: roughening;	In group 6 (control), the buccal tube was positioned directly on the untreated ceramic surface only using the luting composite, which was polymerized by light curing (n = 10)	Metallic	SBST	The highest mean value of SBST was examined in group 1 (61.56 MPa), followed by group iii (45.53 MPa), group 2 (41.65 MPa), and group 4 (23.14 MPa). The comparison between groups 1–4 (with coupling agent) and group 5 (without coupling agent) revealed statistically significant differences ($p \leq 0.002$), with the exception of the comparison between groups 4 and 5. Within groups 1–4, statistically significant results were determined between groups 1 and 4 as well as between groups 3 and 4 ($p < 0.001$). The SBST of group 6 was not calculated as the buccal tubes debonded after the incubation period.	A suitable coupling agent system produced clinically acceptable shear bond strengths capable of withstanding orthodontic forces.
Kurt et al., 2019 [24]	In vitro	G1: HF acid 9.6% for 2 min + silane; G2: Sandblasting with Al$_2$O$_3$ applied from a distance of 10 mm for 10 s in circling motions at 2.5 bar pressure + silane; G3: Silica coating with cojet under 2.5 bar pressure, at a 10-mm distance for 10 s + silane; G4: Roughening with diamond burr at 40,000 rpm for 10 s+ silane	Feldspathic porcelain monolithic zirconia hybrid porcelain	168	56 feldspathic porcelain, 56 monolithic zirconia, and 56 hybrid porcelain samples were divided into 4 surface treatment subgroups.	NR	Metallic	SBST	Of the materials conditioned with HF acid, the feldspathic porcelain group had the significantly highest bonding resistance (8.84). The surface-conditioning method did affect the SBST on different surfaces.	Variations of surface types of the materials affected the bonding resistance of orthodontic attachments. Comparisons of the materials with each other showed the highest bonding resistance to be for the feldspathic porcelain in HF acid group.

Table 2. Cont.

Authors, Year	Study Design	Type of Adhesion Technique (Type, Time, Clinical Application)	Type of Porcelain	Sample Size (n)	Test Group	Control Group	Bracket Type	Intervention Test	Results	Conclusions
Zhang et al., 2016 [25]	In vitro	G1: 9.6% HF acid for 2 min (HF); G2: HF acid for 2 min and silane (HFS); G3: Sandblasting from a distance of 10 mm at a pressure of 3 bar for 10 s, then washed and dried for 1 min and silane (sas); G4: Silica-coating by using the intraoral sandblaster filled with 30 mL silica-modified aluminum trioxide at 3 bar pressure, from a distance of 10 mm for 10 s and silane was applied afterward (sis).	Silica based ceramic	80	G1 (HF); G2 (HFS); G3 (sas); G4 (sis).	NR	Metallic	SBST	The HF-acid-treated group revealed the lowest bond strength value (3.1 MPa), which was significantly lower than those of the other three groups (p = 5.82 9 10−13). Silica-coating with silane (12.3 MPa) and sandblasting with silane (11.6 MPa) groups yielded similar bond strengths (p = 0.14), and both showed significantly higher shear bond strength than that of the HF acid with silane group.	Shear bond strengths exceeded the optimal range of ideal bond strength for clinical practice, except for the isolated HF group. HF acid etching followed by silane was the best suited method for bonding on IPS Classic.
Recen et al., 2021 [26]	In vitro	Four surface conditioning methods: G1: cojet sand from a 10 mm distance at a pressure of 0.25 MPa for 15 s; G2: MEP was applied and agitated into the FC surface for 20 s; G3: 9% HF acid etching for 90 s. Followed by silane coupling agent for 60 s; G4: Diamond burr for 3 s followed by silane coupling agent for 60 s.	Feldspathic porcelain	40	G1: Sandblasting; G2: Monobond® Etch & Prime (MEP); G3: 9% HF and Silane coupling agent G4: Roughening and silane.	NR	Metallic	SBST	No statistically significant difference ($p > 0.05$) was found in SBST between the groups	Considering the mean SBST values, all treatment methods except use of a diamond bur followed by a silane coupling agent can all be used for the bonding of metal brackets to the FC restorations with sufficient SBST for clinical performance. The clinical application of MEP has been found promising since it presented with comparably high SBST values to cojet and HF with safe ARI scores. Also, it eliminates the need for extra steps, minimizing the probability of contamination or the necessity to purchase additional instruments but also excludes potential detrimental effects of HF or sandblasting.

Table 2. *Cont.*

Authors, Year	Study Design	Type of Adhesion Technique (Type, Time, Clinical Application)	Type of Porcelain	Sample Size (n)	Test Group	Control Group	Bracket Type	Intervention Test	Results	Conclusions
Mehta et al., 2016 [27]	In vitro	Hydrofluoric acid 4% (HF), porcelain conditioner silane primer, reliance assure primer, reliance assures plus primer, and z prime plus zirconia primer	Feldspathic porcelain and zirconia	72	36 zirconia specimens divided into 2 groups: G1-sandblasting + HF + silane + ra primer; G2-sandblasting + silane + ra plus primer. 36 glazed feldspathic porcelain specimens divided into two groups: G1-sandblasting + z prime plus primer. G2-sandblasting + ra plus primer.	One control group for zirconia porcelain group (sandblasting + porcelain conditioner (silane)) and one control group for feldspathic porcelain group (sandblasting + porcelain conditioner (silane))	Metallic	TBST	No statistically significant mean differences were found in tbs among the different bonding protocols for feldspathic and zirconia, p values = 0.369 and 0.944, respectively.	Silanization following sandblasting resulted in tensile bond strengths comparable to other bonding protocols for feldspathic and zirconia surface.
Xu et al., 2018 [28]	In vitro	G1 9% HF acid for 2 min; G2 and G3 Er:YAG laser with two energy parameters: 250 mJ, 20 Hz and 300 mJ, 20 Hz; G4 and G5 Er:YAG laser with two energy parameters: 250 mJ, 20 Hz and 300 mJ, 20 Hz + 9% HF acid for 2 min	NR	90	90 ceramic chips were divided into five groups (n = 18 each):	NR	NR	SBST	The SBST in G2 and G3 (treated by laser only) were low, only 2.97 and 3.11 MPa respectively; it was 5.28 MPa in G1 (HF). The SBST of G4 and G5, treated by both laser and HF, were 6.73 and 7.09 MPa respectively, much more than G1, G2, and G3. Based on the comparison between G1 and G2, there is a statistical difference in SBST ($p < 0.05$). By comparing G1 and G3, the SBST has statistical difference ($p < 0.05$). The comparison between G2 and G4 indicates the statistical difference in SBST ($p < 0.05$). Moreover, the statistical difference in SBST exists between G2 and G5 ($p < 0.05$), G3 and G5 ($p < 0.05$).	The exclusive use of HF acid, or Er:YAG laser could not achieve sufficient bracketing bonding strength. The bonding strength of combination strategy of 250 mJ, 20 Hz Er:YAG laser and HF acid on porcelain restoration surface can be satisfied for orthodontic bracket bonding.

Table 2. Cont.

Authors, Year	Study Design	Type of Adhesion Technique (Type, Time, Clinical Application)	Type of Porcelain	Sample Size (n)	Test Group	Control Group	Bracket Type	Intervention Test	Results	Conclusions
Ahrari et al., 2013 [29]	In vitro	G1, G2, G3: CO_2 laser for 10 s a silane coupling agent was applied before bracket bonding; G4: 9.6% hydrofluoric HF acid gel was used for 2 min.	Feldspathic porcelain	80	Four groups of 20: the specimens in G1 to G3 were treated with a fractional CO_2 laser for 10 s using 10 mJ of energy, frequency of 200 Hz, and powers of 10 W (G1), 15 W (G2) and 20 W (G3). In G4: a 9.6% hydrofluoric HF acid gel was used for 2 min.	NR	NR	SBST	Deglazing caused significant increase in SBST of laser treated porcelain surfaces ($p < 0.05$) but had no significant effect on SBST when HF acid was used for etching ($p < 0.137$). ANOVA revealed no significant difference in SBST values of the study groups when glazed surfaces were compared ($p < 0.269$). However, a significant between group difference was found among the deglazed specimens ($p < 0.001$). Tukey test revealed that the bond strengths of 10 W and 15 W laser groups were significantly higher than that of the HF acid group ($p < 0.05$).	Application of 9.6% hydrofluoric acid produced bond strength values that surpassed the minimum strength required in clinical conditions, either used on glazed or deglazed porcelain; due to the significantly higher bond strength, porcelain treatment with a fractional CO_2 laser could be recommended as a suitable alternative technique to HF acid for bonding orthodontic brackets to deglazed feldspathic porcelain.
Mirhashemi et al., 2018 [30]	In vitro	G1: 9% HF for 2 min; G2: etching with the 9% HF for 2 min followed by irradiation with the Er:CrYSGG laser for 10 s; G3: etching with the 9% HF for 2 min followed by irradiation with the Er:YAG laser for 10 s; G4: irradiation with the Er:CrYSGG laser for 10 s without acid etching; G5: irradiation with the Er:YAG laser	Feldspathic porcelain	60	60 specimens of maxillary incisor crown were prepared and randomly assigned to five groups: G.1: etching with the 9% HF + Er:CrYSGG laser; G2: etching with the 9% HF + Er:YAG laser; G3: etching with the 3% HF + Er:YAG laser. G4: Er:CrYSGG laser G5: Er:YAG laser	NR	Metallic	SBST	The average SBST [mean ± SD] values in the five groups were as follows: HF (32.58 ± 9.21 MPa), Er:CrYSGG + HF (27.81 ± 7.66 MPa), Er:YAG + HF (23.08 ± 9.55 MPa), Er:CrYSGG (14.11 ± 9.35 MPa), and Er:YAG (6.30 ± 3.09 MPa). A statistically significant difference in SBST existed between the first three groups and the two laser groups (df = 4, F = 18.555, $p < 0.001$).	The Er:YAG laser with the stated specifications is not a suitable alternative to HF etching. In the case of Er:CrYSGG laser, although the conditioning outcome met the bond strength requirement for orthodontic brackets (that is, 6–8 MPa). Therefore, the bond strength must be further improved by fine-tuning the irradiation details.

183

Table 2. Cont.

Authors, Year	Study Design	Type of Adhesion Technique (Type, Time, Clinical Application)	Type of Porcelain	Sample Size (n)	Test Group	Control Group	Bracket Type	Intervention Test	Results	Conclusions
Alavi et al., 2021 [16]	In vitro	G1: 9.6% hydrofluoric acid HF; G2: neodymium-doped yttrium aluminium garnet (Nd:YAG) laser; G3: carbon dioxide (CO_2) laser; The glass ceramic surfaces were primed with a silane, and the brackets were bonded using a light-cured composite resin.	lithium disilicate–reinforced ceramic	36	36 lithium disilicate ceramic blocks were assigned to three groups (n = 12): G1: 9.6% HF; G2: neodymium-doped yttrium aluminium garnet (Nd:YAG) laser; G3: carbon dioxide (CO_2) laser	NR	Metallic	SBST	The median and interquartile range of SBST values in three groups were 6.48 (1.56–15.18), 1.26 (0.83–1.67), and 0.99 MPa (0.70–2.10), respectively.	Neither CO_2 nor Nd:YAG lasers resulted in adequate surface changes for bonding of brackets on ceramics compared with the samples conditioned with HF.
Girish et al., 2012 [31]		G2: Bur for 10 s; G3: hydrofluoric acid HF; G4: sandblasting for 10 s; G5: bur for 10 s + silane; G6: Hydrofluoric acid + silane; G7: sandblasting+ silane	NR	70	G2: bur; G3: hydrofluoric acid HF; G4: sandblasting; G5: burt+silane; G6: hydrofluoric acid HF + silane; G7: sandblasting+ silane.	G1-untreated surface (n = 10)	Metallic	SBST	Sandblasting with silane produced the highest SBST among all the groups and showed a mean value of 15.18 MPa. The weakest SBST was seen in the control group with a mean of 1.57 MPa. The statistical results showed that there was a significant difference between all the groups.	Sandblasting with silane combination produced the highest SBST, so it is a clinically suitable method for bonding orthodontic metal brackets onto ceramic surface.
Ji-Yeon Lee et al., 2015 [32]	In vitro	G0: No-primer (np); G1:porcelain conditioner (pc); G2: z prime plus (zp); G3: monobond plus (mp); G4: zirconia liner premium (zl)	Zirconia	100	Four primer groups (n = 20 per group), and each primer was divided into two subgroups (n = 10 each) to examine by thermocycling protocols.	1 control group (np) (n = 20)	Metallic	SBST	The SBST of all experimental groups decreased after thermocycling. Before thermocycling, the SBST was G4, G2 ≥ G3 ≥ G1 > G0 but after thermocycling, the SBST was G4 ≥ G3 ≥ G2 > G1 = G0 ($p > 0.05$).	Surface treatment with a zirconia primer increases the SBST relative to no-primer or silane primer application between orthodontic brackets and zirconia prostheses.
Ihsan et al., 2019 [33]	In vitro	G1: transbondtm XT primer; G2: single bond universal adhesive for 20 s, and also air dried for 5 s, and then light cured for 10 s; G3: theracem, was done in the same way as described with the previous groups except that no priming or bonding agent to the zirconia surfaces was needed according to manufacturer instructions.	Zirconia	30	Single bond universal adhesive group (n = 10); Theracem group (n = 10).	G1: control group (n = 10)	Metallic	SBST	The highest value of the mean shear bond strength was in G2 (16.299 ± 2.201 MPa), followed by that of G3 (15.373 ± 1.575 MPa), while the G1 had the lowest value (5.337 ± 1.274 MPa). ANOVA showed that there was a statistically highly significant difference ($p \leq 0.01$) among the mean values of the shear bond strength of all groups.	The two types of 10-mdp-containing adhesive systems provide good value of shear bond strength for buccal tubes bonded to zirconia surface, however, single bond universal adhesive/composite resin is the best.

Table 2. Cont.

Authors, Year	Study Design	Type of Adhesion Technique (Type, Time, Clinical Application)	Type of Porcelain	Sample Size (n)	Test Group	Control Group	Bracket Type	Intervention Test	Results	Conclusions
Mehmeti et al., 2019 [8]	In vitro	Two different etching materials were used for conditioning of the surface of ceramic crowns: 5% HF and 37% H_3PO_4 for 120 s, and subsequently silane.	Zirconia and lithium-disilicate ceramics	96 (all-ceramic crowns, of which 48 full contour zirconia and 48 lithium disilicate)	Eight groups: G1: Metallic bracket bonded to zirconia surface etched with H_3PO_4; G2: Metallic bracket bonded to zirconia surface etched with HF; G3: Ceramic bracket bonded to zirconia surface etched with H_3PO_4; G4: Ceramic bracket bonded to zirconia surface etched with HF; G5: Metallic bracket bonded to lithium disilicate surface etched with H_3PO_4; G6: Metallic bracket bonded to lithium disilicate surface etched with HF; G7: Ceramic bracket bonded to lithium disilicate surface etched with H_3PO_4; G8: Ceramic bracket bonded to lithium disilicate surface etched with HF.	NR	Ceramic and metallic orthodontic brackets	SBST	Lithium-disilicate showed better bond strength in almost all groups. However, no significant difference between the groups was noticed and none of the factors had a significant influence on the mean values of SBST ($p > 0.05$).	The use of HF for surface etching of zirconia and lithium-disilicate, does not cause a significant increase in the SBST values as compared to etching with H_3PO_4 and silane application.
Costa et al., 2012 [34]	In vitro	G1 and C2: 10% hydrofluoric acid gel for 20s with or without silane; G3 and G4: 10% hydrofluoric acid gel for 60s with or without silane.	Feldspathic porcelain	8	G1 and G2: cylinders were etched using 10% hydrofluoric acid gel for 20 s only (n = 2) and 10% hydrofluoric acid gel for 20 s and silane (n = 2); G3 and G4: cylinders were etched using 10% hydrofluoric acid gel for 60s only (n = 2) and 10% hydrofluoric acid gel for 60s and silane (r = 2).	NR	Metallic	SBST	Silane application increased bond strength significantly ($p < 0.05$) compared with no silane application; the bonding material transbond XT promoted a significantly higher ($p < 0.05$) shear bond strength than fuji ortho lc, with or without silane application and for both etching times. The specimens etched for 20 s showed significantly lower ($p < 0.05$) shear bond strengths than those etched for 60s, for both bonding materials.	Etching time of 60 s, application of silane and transbond XT resin significantly improved the shear bond strength of brackets to feldspathic ceramics.

Table 2. *Cont.*

Authors, Year	Study Design	Type of Adhesion Technique (Type, Time, Clinical Application)	Type of Porcelain	Sample Size (n)	Test Group	Control Group	Bracket Type	Intervention Test	Results	Conclusions
Dalaie et al., 2016 [35]	In vitro	9% hydrofluoric acid for 2 min and silane	Feldspathic porcelain	40	40 porcelain-fused-to-metal restorations and four different bracket base designs were bonded to these specimens	NR	Metallic and ceramic	SBST	One-way ANOVA showed that the SBST values were significantly different among the four groups ($p < 0.001$). Groups 1, 2, and 4 were not significantly different, but group 3 had significantly lower SBST ($p < 0.001$).	The bracket base design significantly affects the SBST of brackets to feldspathic porcelain.
Juntavee et al., 2020 [15]	In vitro	9.6% HF for 15 s	Feldspathic based ceramic; lithium disilicate glass-ceramic; fluoroapatite-leucite glass-ceramic; BIS-GMA, BIS-EMA, TEGDMA 73–77% silanated quartz and silica; UDMA, TEGDMA, sodium fluoride, 85% fused silica; uncured methacrylate monomer, inert material fillers, fused silica.	60	Machined ceramic specimens (10 × 10 × 2 mm) were prepared from vitablocs mark II (vita) and IPS e.max® CAD (ivoclar). Layered porcelain fused to metal was used to fabricate PFM specimens. Half of specimens (n = 30) were etched. Three resin bonding systems were used for attaching metal brackets to each group (n = 10): transbond™ XT (3 m), light bond™ (reliance), or bluglo™ (Ormco), all cured with LED curing unit.	Control group (n = 30) specimens nonetched	Metallic	SBST	There were significant effects on SBST of metal bracket to the ceramic veneering materials due to the factor of different types of ceramic materials, surface treatment, resin cement ($p < 0.05$). The mean SBST of metal bracket bonded to vitablocs™ mark II was higher than bonded to IPS e.max® CAD and bonded to IPS d.SIGN® porcelain ($p < 0.05$). The mean SBST of metal bracket bonded to vitablocs™ mark II ceramic materials was significant lower than the mean SBST of metal bracket bonded to vitablocs™ mark II ceramic materials ($p < 0.05$). Also, the mean SBST of metal bracket bonded to IPS e.max® CAD ceramic reveals significantly lower than the mean SBST of metal bracket bonded to vitablocs™ mark II ceramic materials ($p < 0.05$).	Etching ceramic surface enhanced ceramic-bracket bond strength. However, bond strengths in nontreated ceramic surface groups were still higher than bond strength required for bonding in orthodontic treatment.

Table 2. *Cont.*

Authors, Year	Study Design	Type of Adhesion Technique (Type, Time, Clinical Application)	Type of Porcelain	Sample Size (n)	Test Group	Control Group	Bracket Type	Intervention Test	Results	Conclusions
Kaygisiz et al., 2015 [36]	In vitro	G1: Sandblasting with Al_2O_3 for 4 s; G2: Er:CrYSGG laser; G3: sandblasting + etching with HF + silane; G4: etching with HF + silane	Three groups: metal, sapphire and zirconia (n = 28/group).	84	The mounted specimens were randomly divided into four groups: G1: sandblasting with Al_2O_3; G2: Er:CrYSGG laser; G3: sandblasting, etching with HF and silane; G4: etching with HF and silane application) (n = 7/group)	NR	Metallic, saphire and zirconia	SBST	Statistical analysis indicated significant differences among surface treatment procedures ($p < 0.0001$). In addition, the effect of the first and second bonding factors on SBST behaviors was shown to be significant for the brackets ($p < 0.001$).	The use of sandblasting, HF treatment and silanization procedure could be used for improving the rebond shear bond strength of zirconia brackets to porcelain surface.
Topcuoglu et al., 2013 [37]	Ex vivo	Sandblasted + 9.6% HF gel for 2 min; Er:YAG laser short pulse (sp); Er:YAG laser super short pulse (ssp); sandblasted+ sp, or sandblasted + ssp	Porcelain-fused-to-metal	150	Nine groups differing in adhesive system and surface treatment. In five groups, the adhesive system was Relyx u 200 and in the other four, Transbond XT was used. For each adhesive system, the porcelain surfaces were treated in one of five different ways: sandblasted + HF, Er:YAG laser sp, Er:YAG ssp, sandblasted + sp, or sandblasted – ssp.	Sandblasted group with transbond XT (n = 15)	Metallic	SBST	There were statistically significant differences among groups ($p = 0.002$). The highest SBST were observed in G2 (8.83–3.3 MPa), followed by groups 1, 8, 10, and 9 (in that order) with values of 8.25–3.2, 3.48–1.7, 3.11–0.93, and 1.56–0.86 MPa, respectively. The results of the independent samples t-test indicated that there were no statistically significant differences between G1 and the control group ($p = 0.635$). There were no statistically significant differences between G8 and G10 ($p = 0.502$).	Er:YAG laser application did not allow for elimination of the hydrofluoric acid step.
Gonçalves et al., 2011 [38]	In vitro	G1: 10% hydrofluoric acid for 20 s + silane; G2: 10% hydrofluoric acid for 60 s + silane (after application of silane on the ceramic surface, metallic brackets were bonded to the cylinders using Transbond XT).	Feldspathic ceramic	60	The specimens for each etching time were assigned to four groups (n = 15), according to the light source: xl2500 halogen light, Ultralume 5 LED, Accure 3000 argon laser, and Apollo 95e plasma arc. Light-activation was carried out with total exposure times of 40, 40, 20 and 12 s, respectively.	NR	Metallic	SBST	Specimens etched for 20 s presented significantly lower bond strength ($p < 0.05$) compared with those etched for 60 s.	Only the etching time had significant influence on the bond strength of brackets to ceramic.

Table 2. Cont.

Authors, Year	Study Design	Type of Adhesion Technique (Type, Time, Clinical Application)	Type of Porcelain	Sample Size (n)	Test Group	Control Group	Bracket Type	Intervention Test	Results	Conclusions
Akpinar et al., 2015 [39]	In vitro	G1: SB for 3 s with Al_2O_3; G2: 9.6% HF gel for 4 min (hf); G3: Nd:YAG laser irradiation (ny) for 20 s; G4: performance of femtosecond laser pulses; after surface conditioning, all specimens were cleaned for 380 sec in an ultrasonic cleaner and were air dried in air stream before bonding.	Feldspathic porcelain	80	G1: Group sandblasting; G2: group HF; G3: group any LASER; G4: performance of femtosecond laser pulses (each group, n = 20)	NR	Metallic	SBST	The bond strength in G3 (5.11–1.53) was significantly lower than the other groups ($p < 0.05$). There were no statistically significant differences among G1 (9.07–3.76), G2 (9.09–3.51), and G4 (11.58–4.16) ($p = 0.28$).	G4 treatment produced high SBST of the processes assessed; therefore, it appears to be an effective method for bonding orthodontic metal brackets to prepared porcelain surfaces.
Asiry, et al., 2018 [40]	In vitro	G1: HF; G2:deglazing using diamond burr (DB); G3: sand blasting (SB) with 25 μm aluminum trioxide (Al_2O_3); G4: tribochemical silica coating (TS) with 30 μm silica coated aluminum trioxide (Al_2O_3)	NR	120	Four groups of 30 specimens: G1: group HF; G2: group DB; G3: group SB; G4 group TS; 15 specimens from each group were subjected to thermocycling and the remaining 15 specimens served as the baseline (n = 15).	60	NR	SBST	Group 4 exhibited highest SBST at baseline (14.68 ± 0.28) and after thermo-cycling (12.67 ± 0.22) while G1 specimens exhibited lowest SBST at baseline (6.32 ± 0.15) and after thermo-cycling (4.32 ± 0.26). G1 specimens demonstrated lowest SBST; and G4 specimens showed the highest SBST.	Increased surface roughness enhanced SBST of the specimens.
Erdur et al., 2015 [41]	In vitro	G1: Sandblasting for 20 s; G2: etching with 5% HF acid for 20 s;G3: Nd:YAG laser for 20 s; G4: Er:YAG laser for 20 s; G5: Ti:sapphire laser; After conditioning all ceramic surfaces, silane was applied to the ceramic surfaces.	Feldspathic and IPS Empress e-Max	150	150 ceramic discs were prepared and divided into two groups. In each group, the following five subgroups (n = 15) were set up: G5 Ti:sapphire laser, G3: Nd:YAG laser, C4: Er:YAG laser, G1: sandblasting, and G2: HF acid.	NR	NR	SBST	Feldspathic and IPS Empress e-Max ceramics had similar SBST values. The Ti:sapphire femtosecond laser (16.76–1.37 MPa) produced the highest mean bond strength, followed by sandblasting (12.79–1.42 MPa) and HF acid (11.28–1.26 MPa). The Er:YAG (5.43–1.21 MPa) and Nd:YAG laser (5.36–1.04 MPa) groups were similar and had the lowest SBST values.	Ti:sapphire laser- treated surfaces had the highest SBST values. Therefore, this technique may be useful for the pretreatment of ceramic surfaces as an alternative to conventional techniques.

Table 2. Cont.

Authors, Year	Study Design	Type of Adhesion Technique (Type, Time, Clinical Application)	Type of Porcelain	Sample Size (n)	Test Group	Control Group	Bracket Type	Intervention Test	Results	Conclusions
Asiry et al., 2018 [42]	In vitro	G1: IPS ceramic etching gel™ and Monobond plus™; G2: Monobond etch and prime™.	Lithium disilicate	40	The specimens were randomly assigned to two experimental groups (n = 20). G1 specimens were treated with two-step surface conditioning system (IPS ceramic etching gel™ and Monobond plus™) and G2 specimens were treated with one-step conditioning system (Monobond etch and prime™). Ten randomly selected specimens from each group were subjected to thermo-cycling and the remaining ten served as baseline.	N = 20	NR	SBST	The specimens treated with two-step conditioning system had higher bond strength than one-step conditioning system.	Traditional two-step conditioning provides better bond strength. The clinical importance of the study is that, the silane promoted adhesion significantly reduces on exposure to thermo-cycling.
Franz et al., 2019 [43]	In vitro	The bonding agent G1: Monobond S (Ivoclar Vivadent) or G2: Monobond Etch & Prime	Zirconia	20	The ceramic blocks (r = 20) were randomized and divided into two groups and fixation of brackets was done either by using the bonding agent Monobond S (Ivoclar Vivadent) or Monobond Etch & Prime	NR	Metallic	SBST	SBST resulted in significantly higher shear bond values when Monobond Etch & Prime was used compared to the use of Monobond S.	The use of Monobond Etch & Prime has great potential for the bonding of brackets on dental zirconia ceramics.
Yu et al., 2021 [44]	In vitro	All specimens were etched with 9.5% hydrofluoric acid for 20 s. The etched specimens were randomly assigned to one of four groups according to the adhesive used and the use (or not) of additional silane pretreatment for 20 s.	Lithium disilicate glass ceramic	80	Four groups (n = 20) defined by the pretreatment and adhesive used: G1 Adper Single Bond 2 (SB2); G2 silane + Adper Single Bond 2 (S@SB2); G3 Single bond Universal (SBU); and G4 silane + Single Bond Universal (S@SBU).	NR	Metallic	SBST	In all groups, the mean SBST values were statistically significantly lower ($p < 0.001$) after thermocycling than before. Furthermore, specimens in groups S@SB2 and S@SBU, both of which had silane pretreatment, showed statistically significantly higher mean SBST values than did the corresponding groups without silane pretreatment ($p < 0.05$).	The application of a silane-containing universal adhesive without silane pretreatment achieves adequate durability of the bond of metal brackets to dental glass ceramics

Table 2. *Cont.*

Authors, Year	Study Design	Type of Adhesion Technique (Type, Time, Clinical Application)	Type of Porcelain	Sample Size (n)	Test Group	Control Group	Bracket Type	Intervention Test	Results	Conclusions
Abdelnaby, 2011 [45]	In vitro	G1: 9.6% HF for 2 min; G2: 9.6% HF for 2 min + silane; G3: sandblasting for 10 s+ 9.6% HF for 2 min; G4: sandblasting for 10 s+ 9.6% HF for 2 min+ silane.	Feldspathic porcelain	100	The specimens were divided into four equal groups (n = 25). Porcelain surfaces were conditioned with different protocols. In G1, hydrofluoric acid and Embrace First-Coat primer were utilized. G2, hydrofluoric acid and silane were utilized. G3 and G4, sandblasting with aluminum oxide powder was done instead of etching.	NR	Metallic	SBST	Embrace First-Coat and silane exhibited a comparable SBST. The sandblasting process significantly increased SBST. No significant difference was found in bond SBST utilizing either hydrofluoric acid and Embrace First-Coat or sandblasting and silane. With regard to CSBS, the use of sandblasting and Embrace First-Coat revealed the highest significant CSBS value, followed by sandblasting and silane. Etching with hydrofluoric acid prior to application of either primer exhibited the least CSBS values; however, no significant difference was found between them. The SBST was significantly higher than CSBS.	Embrace First-Coat primer could be used successfully as an alternative to silane. Sandblasting provides higher bond strength than did hydrofluoric acid. Cyclic loading significantly decreased bond strength.
Cevik et al., 2017 [46]	In vitro	G1: 37.5% orthophosphoric acid for 4 min; G2: 9.6% hydrofluoric acid for 3 min; G3: Nd:YAG laser irradiation for 30 s; G4: sandblasting with 50 μm Al_2O_3 particles for 10 s; G5: grinding with a diamond bur for 30 s. All samples were primed with silane before the bracket bonding, including the control group.	Feldspathic and lithium disilicate	120	Five subgroups depending on surface treatment (n = 10) G1: 37.5% orthophosphoric acid; G2: 9.6% hydrofluoric acid; G3: Nd:YAG laser irradiation; G4: sandblasting with 50 μm Al_2O_3 particles; G5: grinding with a diamond bur.	Control group (n = 10)	Metallic	SBST	G4 demonstrated significantly higher shear bond strengths than other groups	Surface conditioning methods, except for sandblasting and grinding, were associated with lower shear bond strengths; however, thermocycling may have had negative effects on bond strengths of specimens. Furthermore, in each ceramic system, there was a significant difference between surface-conditioning methods and surface roughness with regard to shear bond strength.

Table 2. Cont.

Authors, Year	Study Design	Type of Adhesion Technique (Type, Time, Clinical Application)	Type of Porcelain	Sample Size (n)	Test Group	Control Group	Bracket Type	Intervention Test	Results	Conclusions
Saraç et al., 2011 [47]	In vitro	G1: Air-particle abrasion (APA) with 25 mm for 4 s Al_2O_3; G2: silica coating with 30 mm Al_2O_3 particles modified by silica for 4 s. Then silane application.	Feldspathic, fluoro-apatite, and leucite-reinforced ceramic.	60	20 feldspathic, 20 fluoro-apatite, and 20 leucite-reinforced ceramic specimens were examined following two surface-conditioning methods: G1: APA with 25 mm Al_2O_3 and G2: silica coating with 30 mm Al_2O_3 particles modified by silica.	NR	Metallic	SBST	The lowest SBST was with APA for the fluoro-apatite ceramic (11.82 MPa), which was not significantly different from APA for the feldspathic ceramic (13.58 MPa). The SBST for the fluoro-apatite ceramic was significantly lower than that of leucite-reinforced ceramic with APA (14.82 MPa). The highest SBST value was obtained with silica coating of the leucite-reinforced ceramic (24.17 MPa), but this was not significantly different from the SBST for feldspathic and fluoroapatite ceramic (23.51 and 22.18 MPa, respectively). The SBST values with silica coating showed significant differences from those of APA.	Chairside tribochemical silica coating significantly increased mean bond strength values; With all surface-conditioning methods, leucite-reinforced ceramic, in general, showed a higher SBST than feldspathic and fluoro-apatite ceramics.
Hsu et al., 2015 [48]	In vitro	G1: 37% phosphoric acid solution for 60 s, and porcelain primer (H_3PO_4) was applied to the etched porcelain crown surface for another 60 s; G2: 9% HF acid solution for 60 s and silane for 60 s; G3: 9% HF solution for 60 s and generic/pentron silane for 60 s; G4: 37% phosphoric acid etching solution for 60 s and ultradent silane for 60 s; G5: 37% phosphoric acid etching solution for 60 s and generic/pentron silane for 60 s.	Glazed ceramic porcelain fused to metal (PFM)	50	Five groups for bonding, each group n = 10; G1 (H_3PO_4-Porcelain Primer group) G2 (HF-Ultradent Silane); G3 (HF-Jeneric/Pentron Silane); G4 (H_3PO_4-Ultradent Silane)Ultradent; G5 (H_3PO_4-Jeneric/Pentron Silane).	NR	Metallic	SBST	The Porcelain Primer group had the lowest bond strengths and the H_3PO_4-Jeneric/Pentron silane group had the highest bond strengths ($p < 0.0005$). Cross-matching of acid and silane showed that acid had a statistically significant effect on bond strength. The H_3PO_4-Jeneric/Pentron silane group had the highest bond strength among all acid silane groups.	The Porcelain Primer group had the lowest bond strength, showing statistically significant differences to those of the Jeneric/Pentron groups (either phosphoric acid or HF acid etching) ($p < 0.0005$). Although acid might be more important than silane ($p = 0.005$) for bond strength, there were no statistically significant differences in bond strength among the other four etching-silane groups (phosphoric acid vs. HF acid; Ultradent vs. Jeneric/Pentron).

Table 2. Cont.

Authors, Year	Study Design	Type of Adhesion Technique (Type, Time, Clinical Application)	Type of Porcelain	Sample Size (n)	Test Group	Control Group	Bracket Type	Intervention Test	Results	Conclusions
Durgesh et al., 2016 [49]	In vitro	A silane-based primer consisting of 1.0 vol-% of 3 acryloxypropyltrimethoxysilane (ACPS) in ethanol/water, with a ph of 4.5; experimental primer, a novel silane system consisting of 0.5 vol-% of a cross-linker silane monomer bis-1,2-(triethoxysilyl) ethane (BTSE) which was added to 1.0 vol-% of acps, corresponding to a final 1.5 vol-% of silanes.	Glazed ceramic porcelain fused to metal (PFM)	180	Two groups of 90 specimens, according to the primer used. Each group was further divided into three subgroups according to the surface treatment to be received, thus there were 6 study groups; three with 3-acryloxypropyltrimethoxysilane (ACPS) silane primer, namely 1a (pretreatment with hydrofluoric acid, HF), 1b (pretreatment with grit-blasting) and 1c (pretreatment with tribochemical silica-coating) and 3 with a novel silane system (ACPS + bis-1,2(triethoxysilyl) ethane (BTSE)) assigned as 2a (HF), 2b (grit-blast), and 2c (tribochemical silica coating).	NR	NR	SBST	The highest SBST at baseline (26.8 + 1.7 MPa) and after thermocycling (24.6 + 1.7 MPa) was observed in group 2c, and the lowest (9.6 + 1.5 MPa and 4.5 + 1.1 MPa) was found in G1a.	The application of experimental silane primer system on specimens pretreated with tribochemical silica-coating demonstrated increased adhesion of orthodontic brackets making it an excellent choice in orthodontic bonding for a relatively long term use.
Bavbek et al., 2014 [50]	In vitro	Air abrasion with 30-µm silica coated aluminum oxide (Al_2O_3) particles (cojet) for 20 s; air abrasion with 50-µm Al_2O_3 particles.	Monolithic zirconium oxide ceramic (mz).	120	Two types of MZ (BruxZir Solid Zirconia, n = 60; Prettau-Zirkon, n = 60) with two types of surface finish (glazed, n = 30 per group; polished, n = 30 per group) were tested after two surface conditioning methods: 1. air abrasion with 30-µm silica coated aluminum oxide (Al_2O_3) particles (CoJet), or 2. air abrasion with 50-µm Al_2O_3 particles.	The non-conditioned group acted as the control.	NR	SBST	Mean µSBST values (MPa) did not show a significant difference between the two brands of MZ ($p > 0.05$). In both glazed (44 ± 6.4) and polished (45.9 ± 4.8) groups, CoJet application showed the highest µSBST values ($p < 0.001$). The control group (34.4 ± 6) presented significantly better results compared to that of Al_2O_3 (30 ± 3.8) ($p < 0.05$) on glazed surfaces, but it was the opposite in the polished groups (control: 20.3 ± 4.7; Al_2O_3: 33.8 ± 4.7; $p < 0.001$).	Air abrasion with CoJet followed by the application of universal primer improved the µSBST (microshear bond strength) of orthodontics resin to both the polished and glazed monolithic zirconium oxide materials tested

Table 2. Cont.

Authors, Year	Study Design	Type of Adhesion Technique (Type, Time, Clinical Application)	Type of Porcelain	Sample Size (n)	Test Group	Control Group	Bracket Type	Intervention Test	Results	Conclusions
Sandoval et al., 2020 [51]	In vitro	Hydrofluoric acid 10% + silane; sandblasting with aluminum oxide + silane; hydrofluoric acid 10% + Single Bond Universa; blasting with aluminum oxide + Single Bond Universal.	NR	60	G1: hydrofluoric acid – 10% silane; G2: blasting with aluminum oxide + silane; G3: hydrofluoric acid 10% + Single Bond Universa and G4: blasting with aluminum oxide + Single Bond Universal.	NR	Metallic	SBST	The average shear strengths were: G1 = 24.2 MPa; G2 = 21.3 MPa; G3 = G4 = 19.1 MPa to 14.2 MPa. There were differences between all groups ($p < 0.05$) except for G3 ($p > 0.05$).	Single Bond Universal treated with blasting aluminum oxide had the best performance, and promoted good shear strength, it caused less cohesive damage to the ceramic.
Najafi et al., 2014 [52]	In vitro	Roughened with a diamond bur and etched with hydrofluoric acid (HF) gel for 4 min; roughened with a bur and irradiated by a CO_2 laser with a 2W power setting for 20 s; CO_2 laser; sandblasted with 50 μm aluminum oxide for 20 s. Before bonding, the bracket silane was applied on the porcelain surfaces.	Feldspathic porcelain fused to metal.	48	Four groups: G1: Deglazed + HF group; G2: Deglazed + CO_2 group; G3: CO_2 group; G4: Sandblasted group. In the four groups, a silane coupling agent) was applied.	NR	Metallic	SBST	ANOVA revealed significant differences in SBS among the four groups ($p < 0.001$). G1 demonstrated significantly higher bond strength (13.13–2.47) when compared with the other groups. G2 showed higher bond strength (9.60–1.91) when compared with G4 (6.40–1.67) ($p = 0.016$).	Deglazing combined with HF etching produced the highest bond strength, but CO_2 laser irradiation provided adequate bond strength and allowed for elimination of the HF step. Deglazing is not recommended as a preliminary step before CO_2 laser conditioning.
Durgesh, 2020 [20]	In vitro	Grit-blasted with various distance (5 mm, 10 mm and 15 mm) with 1.0 vol. % 3 methacryloyloxypropyltrimethoxy-silane (ep1) or their blends with 0.5% (ep2), and 1.0 vol. % (ep3) 1, 2-bis-(triethoxysilyl) ethane (all in ethanol/water).	Zirconia	180	A total of 180 zirconia specimens were used for three test groups (n = 60), and then grit-blasted with various distance (5 mm, 10 mm and 15 mm). The grit-blasted specimen were allocated to three silanizations (n = 30): with 1.0 vol. % 3 methacryloyloxypropyltrimethoxysilane (EP1) or their blends with 0.5% (EP2), and 1.0 vol. % (EP3) 1, 2-bis-(triethoxysilyl) ethane (all in ethanol/water)	NR	NR	AST	ANOVA showed a significant influence of the grit-blasting distance, silane blend and artificial aging on the shear bond strength values ($p < 0.05$). The highest adhesion strengths were obtained for baseline specimens irrespective of the grit-blasting distance or the silane primer blend system used.	Grit-blasting at 10 mm and silane primer blend of 1.0 vol. % 3-MPS and 0.5 vol. % BTSE provided acceptable orthodontic bonding with least surface damage to zirconia surface. Adhesion strength values significantly decreased following thermo-cycling, irrespective of the grit-blasting distance and the silane primer blend system used.

193

Table 2. Cont.

Authors, Year	Study Design	Type of Adhesion Technique (Type, Time, Clinical Application)	Type of Porcelain	Sample Size (n)	Test Group	Control Group	Bracket Type	Intervention Test	Results	Conclusions
Garcia-Sanz et al., 2019 [53]	In vitro	Air particle abrasion (APA) with alumina particles (Al_2O_3) for 20 s; femtosecond Ti:sapphire laser for 12 min.	Zirconia	180	Five groups (n = 30) according to surface treatment: G1: air-particle abrasion (APA); G2: FS laser irradiation (300 mW output power, 60 μm inter-groove distance); G3: FS laser irradiation (200 mW, 100 μm); G4: FS laser irradiation (40 mW, 60 μm); G5: FS laser irradiation (200 mW, 60 μm).	G1- control group: No treatment applied (n = 30).	NR	SBST	SBST in groups 3 and 6 was significantly higher than the other groups (5.92 ± 1.12 MPa and 5.68 ± 0.94 MPa). No significant differences were found between groups 1, 2, 4, and 5 (3.87 ± 0.77 MPa, 4.25 ± 0.51 MPa, 3.74 ± 0.10 MPa, and 3.91 ± 0.53 MPa).	FS laser at 200 mW, 60 μm can be recommended as the ideal settings for treating zirconia surfaces, producing good SBST and more economical energy use.
Stella et al. 2015 [54]	In vitro	G1: 37% gel phosphoric acid etching for one minute + Silane application for one minute; G2: 37% liquid phosphoric acid etching for one minute+ Silane application for one minute; G3: 10% hydrofluoric acid etching for one minute; G4: 10% hydrofluoric acid etching for one minute + Silane application for one minute.	NR	52	Four experimental groups (n = 13) were set up according to the ceramic conditioning method: G1: 37% phosphoric acid etching followed by silane application; G2: 37% liquid phosphoric acid etching, no rinsing, followed by silane application; G3: 10% hydrofluoric acid etching alone. G4: 10% hydrofluoric acid etching followed by silane application.	NR	Metallic	SBST	The highest shear bond strength values were found in groups G3 and G4 (22.01 ± 2.15 MPa and 22.83 ± 3.32 Mpa, respectively), followed by G1 (16.42 ± 3.61 MPa) and G2 (9.29 ± 1.95 MPa).	Acceptable levels of bond strength for clinical use were reached by all methods tested; however, liquid phosphoric acid etching followed by silane application (G2) resulted in the least damage to the ceramic surface.
Epperson et al, 2021 [55]	Ex vivo	9.6% HF was for 4 min; 35% phosphoric acid (PA) with subsequent silanation; 50 μ aluminum oxide microetching (MIC)	Hybrid ceramics	60	G1: Lava (HF); G2: Lava (PA); G3 Lava (MIC); G1 Enamic (HF); G2 Enamic (PA); G3 Enamic (MIC).	Enamel control group (n = 10) (35% phosphoric acid for 30s and rinsed for 10 s. An adhesive primer, Transbond™ XT Primer was applied for 5 s and lightly air-thinned for 1 s.	Metallic	SBST	The SBST of all groups, except the HF Enamic® group, were significantly lower than the mean SBS of the enamel control group (8.8 MPa). The mean shear bond strength values of Enamic® were significantly higher than those of Lava™ Ultimate (p-values < 0.05).	Statistically, only Enamic® treated with HF exhibited sufficient SBST when compared with the enamel control.

Table 2. Cont.

Authors, Year	Study Design	Type of Adhesion Technique (Type, Time, Clinical Application)	Type of Porcelain	Sample Size (n)	Test Group	Control Group	Bracket Type	Intervention Test	Results	Conclusions
Al-Hity et al., 2012 [19]	In vitro	The influence of using different combinations of bracket, adhesive, and light-curing source on the tensile bond strength to porcelain Tensile tests were performed using: one ceramic bracket versus one metal bracket, two orthodontic composites; type bisphenol A-glycidyldimethacrylate and urethane dimethacrylate (UDMA), and four light-curing units with the same range of emission spectrum but various light intensities: three light-emitting diode (LED) units and one halogen-based unit.	Fluorapatite glass-ceramic.	160	160 porcelain samples were randomly divided into 16 equal groups. The porcelain surface was conditioned with 9% hydrofluoric acid before silane application. The composite was photo-polymerized for 40 s.	NR	Metallic and ceramic	TBST	The bond strength in all groups was sufficient to withstand orthodontic treatment (>6 MPa). There was no statistical difference between the adhesives, but comparing bracket × light interaction, it was significantly higher with the ceramic bracket. No significant differences were seen between the metal bracket groups, but for the ceramic bracket, the results were significantly higher with the LED light	No significant difference between adhesives' composition related to the bonding strength on porcelain. Bonding strength of ceramic brackets on porcelain is significantly higher than metal bracket. Bonding strength of ceramic bracket is significantly higher when an LED LCU of high light intensity is used compared to halogen-based or LED LCU with low intensity.
Ghozy et al., 2020 [13]	In vitro	9.5% HF for 1 min; 37% PA gel for 1 min.	VITABLOCS Mark II, VITAENAMIC, and IPS e.max CAD.	120	120 CAD/CAM ceramic blocks in 12 groups were fabricated from three different CAD/CAM ceramic materials: VITABLOCS Mark II, VITAENAMIC, and IPS e.max CAD. Each ceramic material group was divided into two etching groups: 60 metal (BM) and ceramic brackets (CB) of the upper right central incisor were bonded to the HF-treated blocks. Another 60 metal and CBs were bonded to the PA treated blocks.	NR	Metallic and ceramic	SBST	There were no significant differences in SBS values between the three CAD/CAM ceramic materials. The HF-treated specimens exhibited significantly higher SBS values than the PA-treated specimens. Also, the SBS values of CBs were significantly higher than the BM.	The CAD/CAM ceramic type did not influence SBST; however, HF exhibited significantly higher SBST compared to PA.

Table 2. Cont.

Authors, Year	Study Design	Type of Adhesion Technique (Type, Time, Clinical Application)	Type of Porcelain	Sample Size (n)	Test Group	Control Group	Bracket Type	Intervention Test	Results	Conclusions
Ramos et al., 2012 [56]	Ex vivo	G2: Diamond bur and processed with phosphoric acid 37% for 30 s; G3: Etching with HF 10% for 1 min; G4: etching with HF 10% for 1 min and application of 2 layers of silanization agent.	NR	40	n = 10 for each group. G2: fine diamond bur – orthophosphoric acid gel 37%; G3: HF 10%; G4: HF 10% + silane.	G1-control group: No surface treatment (n = 10).	Ceramic	SBST	There was a significant difference ($p < 0.05$) between the control group and all other groups. There was no significant difference ($p < 0.05$) between treated porcelain surface with diamond bur + orthophosphoric acid gel 37% (4.8 MPa) and HF 10% (6.1 MPa), but the group treated with HF 10% had clinically acceptable bond strength values. The group treated with HF 10% + silane (17.5 MPa) resulted in a statistically significant higher tensile bond strength ($p < 0.05$). In G4, 20% of the porcelain facets displayed damage.	Etching of the surface with HF 10% increased the bond strength values. Silane application was recommended to bond a ceramic bracket to the porcelain surface to achieve bond strengths that are clinically acceptable.
Mehmeti et al., 2018 [57]	In vitro	G1: 5% HF for 2 min; G2: 37% phosphoric acid for 2 min, and subsequently, silane.	Feldspar-based porcelain PFM.	48	Four groups (n = 12): G1: Metal bracket bonded after surface conditioning with 37 per cent phosphoric acid and silane; G2: Metal bracket bonded after surface conditioning with 5% HF and silane; G3: Ceramic bracket bonded after surface conditioning with 37% phosphoric acid and silane; G4: Ceramic bracket bonded after surface conditioning with 5% HF and silane.	NR	Metallic and ceramic	SBST	SBST values of the groups etched with HF and silane, compared to the groups etched with phosphoric acid and silane, are not significantly increased. However, ceramic brackets show significantly higher SBST values than metallic brackets.	Both types of ceramic surface conditioning procedures have similar features and provide strong enough SBST values to realize the orthodontic treatment. Also, the assumption that only the type of bracket significantly affects the SBST value can be accepted.

Table 2. Cont.

Authors, Year	Study Design	Type of Adhesion Technique (Type, Time, Clinical Application)	Type of Porcelain	Sample Size (n)	Test Group	Control Group	Bracket Type	Intervention Test	Results	Conclusions
Baeshen, 2021 [58]	In vitro	G1: Er-YAG laser for about 30 s + S coupling agent for 30 s; G2: Photodynamic therapy (PDT) using methylene blue (MB) photosensitizer at a concentration of 100 mg/L; G3: 9.5% of HF acid for 60 s +S coupling agent was applied and air dried for 60 s; G4: 9.5% HF acid for 60 s + ultrasonic bath with UB along with distilled water and air dried for 120 s + S; G5: Sandblasting with Al_2O_3 particles for 15 s; G6: SECP (Monobond etch and prime) for 60s followed by rinse for 20 s; G7: Er,Cr:YSGG for 60 s + S.	Lithium di silicate (LDC)	70	Seven groups according to ceramic surface conditioning. G1: surface treated with Er-YAG laser and saline (S); G2: PDT using MBP + S; G3: HF (Hydrofluoric acid) +saline. G4: HF (Hydrofluoric acid) +ultrasonic bath (UB + S; G5: sand blasting the glass ceramic surface with 120 um Al_2O_3. G6: LDC surface conditioned with SECP (Etch and Prime); G7: Er,Cr:YSGG + S on was irradiated on LDC.	G3 HF + S (control).	Metallic	SBST	SBST values of G2 HF acid + S displayed highest bond durability (22.28 ± 1.09 MPa) Whereas, specimens in G4 surface treated with 120 μm Al_2O_3 displayed lowest SBST scores (11.81 ± 0.55 MPa) and these bond scores were comparable to PDT using MBP + S (12.54 ± 1.09 MPa) ($p > 0.05$). LDC surface treated by Er,Cr:YSGG + S (21.11 ± 3.85 MPa), HF + UB + S (19.28 ± 0.52 MPa) exhibited results comparable to HF acid + S ($p > 0.05$).	LDC conditioned with HF-S still remains as gold standard. Use of PDT for surface treatment of LDC and bonded to metallic bracket is not recommended as it results in decreased bond durability. Use of Er,Cr:YSGG-S and HF + UB + S has a potential to be used alternatively to HF-S for LDC conditioning.
Tahmasbi et al., 2020 [9]	In vitro	G1: universal adhesive (Scotchbond™ Universal adhesive) 20 s, air spray 5 s, light cured 10 s 650 mW/cm³; G2: universal adhesive/silane 1min, air spray 30 s, Scotchbond Universal adhesive 20 s, air spray 5 s, light curinf 10 s; G3: conventional adhesive—two layers of Single Bond 2 conventional adhesive 20 s, air sprayed 5 s, light cured 10 s; G4: conventional adhesive/silane–silane 1 min, air spray 30 s, two layers of Single Bond 2 conventional adhesive 20 s, air spray 5 s, light cured 10 s.	Feldspathic porcelain	56	n = 14–universal adhesive; n = 14–universal adhesive/silane; n = 14–conventional adhesive; n = 14–conventional adhesive/silane.	NR	NR	SBST	The highest SBST was noted in the universal adhesive/silane group (12.7 MPa) followed by conventional adhesive/silane (11.9 MPa), conventional adhesive without silane (7.6 MPa), and universal adhesive without silane (4.4 MPa).	SBST of bracket to porcelain mainly depends on the use of silane rather than the type of adhesive. Both universal and conventional adhesives yield significantly higher SBST in the presence of silane compared to that in the absence of silane

Table 2. Cont.

Authors, Year	Study Design	Type of Adhesion Technique (Type, Time, Clinical Application)	Type of Porcelain	Sample Size (n)	Test Group	Control Group	Bracket Type	Intervention Test	Results	Conclusions
Mehmeti et al., 2017 [59]	In vitro	Phosphoric acid 120 s, composite resin-based bonding system, T light cured 40 s using light-emitting diode.	All-zirconium ceramic	20	n = 10–metallic bracket; n = 10–ceramic polycrystalline bracket.	NR	Metallic and ceramic polycrystalline	SBST	Force necessary to debond metallic brackets (sum of 10 tests = 70,797 N) of the zirconium crowns were higher than those of ceramic brackets (sum of 10 tests = 59,770 N), with a significant difference.	Metallic brackets compared with ceramic polycrystalline brackets, seem to create stronger adhesion with all-zirconium surfaces due to their better base surface design or retention mode. Also, ceramic brackets show higher fragility during debonding.
Yassaei et al., 2013 [60]	In vitro	G1: 9.6% HF; G2, 3 and 4: Er:YAG lasers of 1.6, 2, and 3.2 W.	Porcelain	100	Four groups: G1: n = 25–HF; G2: n = 25–Er:YAG lasers of 1.6; G3: n = 25–Er:YAG lasers of 2; G4: n = 25–Er:YAG lasers of 3.2	NR	Metallic	SBST	The mean shear bond strength in the laser group with power of 1.6 W (7.88 MPa) was more than that of the HF (7.4 MPa), 2-W power (7.52 MPa), and 3.2-W power (7.45 MPa) groups, but this difference was not statistically significant.	Er:YAG laser can be a suitable method for bonding of orthodontic brackets to porcelain surfaces.
Gardiner et al., 2019 [5]	In vitro	Hydrofluoric acid etch	Zirconia; lithium disilicate (IPS e.max); lithium silicate infused with zirconia (CELTRA DUO)	60	Zirconia (n = 20): 9.6%HF+silane (n = 10), silane (n = 10); IPS e.max (n = 20): 9.5% HF+silane (n = 10), silane (n = 10); CELTRA DUO (n = 20): 9.6%HF + silane (n = 10), silane (n = 10).	Enamel (n = 10): 35% PA etch	Metallic	SBST	SBST of the lithium silicate infused with zirconia groups were significantly less than the chemically pre-treated lithium disilicate group, however both materials, when chemical pre-treatment protocol was used, were not statistically different than the enamel control.	Orthodontic bonding to lithium silicate infused with zirconia yielded a weaker bond strength than bonding to traditional lithium disilicate, however, when the surface was pre-treated with hydrofluoric acid etch it provides a bond strength that is within an acceptable clinical range.

Table 2. Cont.

Authors, Year	Study Design	Type of Adhesion Technique (Type, Time, Clinical Application)	Type of Porcelain	Sample Size (n)	Test Group	Control Group	Bracket Type	Intervention Test	Results	Conclusions
Golshah et al., 2018 [4]	In vitro	10% HF acid 2 min and the following bonding protocols: G1: Transbond XT bonding agent cured 10 s; G2: silane plus Transbond XT bonding agent cured 10 s; G3: silane plus universal adhesive (G-Premio bond) cured 10 s; G4: universal adhesive cured 10 s.	Glazed feldspathic porcelain	40	G1: Transbond XT bonding agent (n = 10); G2: silane plus Transbond XT bonding agent (n = 10); G3: silane plus universal adhesive (G-Premio bond) (n = 10); G4: universal adhesive (n = 10).	NR	Metallic	SBST	The highest and the lowest SBST values were noted in groups silane plus universal adhesive (17.06 ± 2.58 MPa) and universal adhesive (9.85 ± 4.76 MPa), respectively. Type of adhesive had no significant effect on SBST ($p = 0.611$). However, the effect of application of silane on SBST was significant ($p = 0.000$). Groups subjected to the application of silane showed higher SBST values than others.	Universal adhesive and Transbond XT were not significantly different in SBST. However, application of silane significantly increased the bond strength.
Hosseini et al., 2013 [61]	In vitro	0.75, 1, 1.25, 1.5- and 2-W neodymium-doped yttrium aluminum garnet (Nd:YAG) laser 10 s; hydrofluoric acid 9.6% 4 min	Glazed porcelain	72	n = 12-HF; n = 12-0.75-Nd:YAG laser; n = 12-1-Nd:YAG laser; n = 12-1.25-Nd:YAG laser; n = 12-1.5-Nd:YAG laser; n = 12-2-Nd:YAG laser.	NR	Metallic	SBST	The mean ± SD of the shear bond strength in the laser group 0.75, 1, 1.25, 1.5, and 2 W and HF group was 2.2 ± 0.9, 4.2 ± 1.1, 4.9 ± 2.4, 7 ± 1.7, 9.6 ± 2.7, and 9.4 ± 2.5, respectively. Together with the increased power of laser, the mean shear bond strength was increased continuously and no significant differences were found between the HF group and the laser groups with power of 1.5 or 2 W	1.5 and 2 W powers of Nd:YAG laser can be used as an alternative method for porcelain etching.
Naseh et al., 2018 [10]	In vitro	9.6% hydrofluoric acid and divided into two groups: silane, air-dried. Transbond XT primer light-cured; Assure Plus, air-dried.	Feldspathic; lithium disilicate	40	n = 10-feldspathic with Assure Plus; n = 10-IPS E-max with Assure Plus	n = 10-feldspathic with silane+Transbond; n = 10-IPS E-max with silane+Transbond.	Metallic	SBST	Bracket bond to lithium disilicate by Assure Plus was significantly stronger than that to Feldspathic porcelain ($p = 0.041$).	Assure Plus provided high bond strength between ceramic and brackets and minimized damage to lithium disilicate ceramic during debonding. Assure Plus is recommended for use in orthodontic treatment of adults with ceramic restorations.

Table 2. Cont.

Authors, Year	Study Design	Type of Adhesion Technique (Type, Time, Clinical Application)	Type of Porcelain	Sample Size (n)	Test Group	Control Group	Bracket Type	Intervention Test	Results	Conclusions
Cevik et al., 2018 [17]	In vitro	G1: 37% phosphoric acid 4 min; G2: 9.6% hydrofluoric acid 3 min; G3: grinding with diamond burs 20 μm with a high-speed handpiece 30s in wet conditions; G4: Nd:YAG laser 15 Hz 1 W 30 s with pulse duration range was 300 μs; G5: Airborne-particle abrasion 50 μm alumina (Al_2O_3) particles 2.5 bars of pressure 10 s at a direction perpendicular to the surface with the distance of 10 mm.	Feldspathic porcelain	60	G1: 37% phosphoric acid (n = 10); G2: 9.4% hydrofluoric acid (n = 10); G3: grinding with diamond burs (n = 10); G4: Nd:YAG laser (n = 10); G5: Airborne-particle abrasion (n = 10).	Without surface treatment (n = 10).	Ceramic	SBST	Using G5 specimens resulted in the highest shear bond strength value of 8.58 MPa for feldspathic porcelain. However, the other specimens showed lower values: G3 (6.51 MPa), G4 (3.37 MPa), G2 (2.71 MPa), G1 (1.17 MPa), and control group (0.93 MPa).	Airborne-particle abrasion and grinding can be used as surface treatment techniques on the porcelain surface for a durable bond strength. Hydrofluoric acid and phosphoric acid etching methods were not convenient as surface treatment methods for the feldspathic porcelain.
Juntavee et al., 2018 [7]	In vitro	Er-YAG laser power 200 mJ, 10 W, 20 Hz, 10 s-pulse length for 20 s; Etching with 9.5% HF acid gel 5 s (E5) or 15 s (E15).	Machined ceramic specimens: Empress® CAD, and e.max® CAD; Ceramic veneering metal (d.Sign® porcelain (1.27 mm thickness) over d.Sign® 10 metal (0.23 mm thickness)).	45	n = 15-Er-YAG laser; n = 15-HF 5 s; n = 15-HF 15 s.	NR	Ceramic	SBST	Significant differences in bond strength among groups were found related to surface treatment ($p < 0.05$), but not significant difference upon type of ceramics ($p > 0.05$). E15 provided higher bond strength than Er-YAG laser and E5 ($p < 0.05$).	Bond strength was affected by surface treatment. Both Er-YAG laser and E15 treated surface provided higher bond strength than E5. Considering possibly inducing defect on ceramic surface, Er-YAG laser seems to provide better favorable surface preparation than others. Treated ceramic surface with Er-YAG prior to bracket bonding is recommended.

Table 2. Cont.

Authors, Year	Study Design	Type of Adhesion Technique (Type, Time, Clinical Application)	Type of Porcelain	Sample Size (n)	Test Group	Control Group	Bracket Type	Intervention Test	Results	Conclusions
Sabuncuoglu et al., 2016 [62]	In vitro	G1: Cylindrical diamond bur rotate at 40,000 rpm 3 s; G2: 37% Orthophosphoric acid 2 min; G3: 9,6% HF 2 min; G4: SB with 50 μm aluminum oxide at 60 psi for 3 s at a distance of 10 mm; G5: SB+HF; G6: Nd:YAG laser wavelength 1064nm (300 μm fiber), 2 W power and frequency of 10 Hz for 10 s in a pulse mode (100 μs) using a sweeping motion at approximately 2 mm distance; G7: Er:YAG laser 2 W, 10 Hz, 10 s, 2 mm.	Feldspathic	70	G1: Diamond bur (n = 10); G2: Orthophosphoric acid (n = 10); G3: Hydrofluoric acid (n = 10); G4: Sandblasted with aluminum oxide (n = 10); G5: SB+HF (n = 10); G6: Nd:YAG laser (n = 10); G7: Er:YAG laser (n = 10).	NR	NR	SBST	The highest SBST values were observed for SB + HF, with no significant difference between SB+HF and HF. SBST values for Diamond bur were significantly lower than those of all other groups tested.	Diamond bur alone is unable to sufficiently etch porcelain surfaces for bracket bonding. SB+HF results in a significantly higher shear-bond strength than HF or SB alone. Nd:YAG or Er:YAG laser was found to be more effective and less time-consuming than both HF acid and SB.
Aksakalli et al., 2015 [63]	Ex vivo	G1: SB with alumina particles 50 μm, at 65-70 psi, 10 s, 10 mm (SB); G2: 9,6% HF 4 min; G3: Er: YAG irradiation from 1 mm distance, 2 W, 10 Hz, 200 mJ, 100-μs pulse length, energy density of 25.31 J/cm² for 10 s.	Porcelain laminate veneer	39	G1: SB (n = 13); G2: HF (n = 13); G3: Er:YAG (n = 13).	NR	NR	SBST	The highest shear bond strength values were obtained with group HF (10.8 ± 3.8 MPa) and group ER (9.3 ±1.5 MPa), whereas group SB revealed the lowest values. The sandblasting method did not demonstrate any ideal bond strength values; however, the 9.6% hydrofluoric acid etching and Er: YAG laser did.	The Er: YAG laser can be selected for bonding brackets to porcelain surfaces with acceptable bond strength and minimal surface damage as compared to the other methods.

Table 2. Cont.

Authors, Year	Study Design	Type of Adhesion Technique (Type, Time, Clinical Application)	Type of Porcelain	Sample Size (n)	Test Group	Control Group	Bracket Type	Intervention Test	Results	Conclusions
Lestrade et al., 2021 [64]	In vitro/Ex vivo	G1: Bond enhancer (Assure, Reliance, IL, USA); G2: Green stone at 25,000 rpm; G3: Diamond bur at 25,000 rpm; G4: SB 25 μm aluminum oxide particles, distance 10 mm, 10 s; SB with Rocatec (3 M ESPE, MN, USA) 100 μm aluminum oxide particles treated with silicon dioxide.	Lithium disilicate	70	G1: Porc-Etch, 9.6% HF, Porcelain Conditioner, silane, bond enhancer (Assure, Reliance, IL, USA) (n = 10); G2: green stone (n = 10); G3: diamond burr (n = 10); G4: SB (n = 10); G5: SB with Rocatec (n = 10).	n = 10–HF + silane; n = 10–teeth with 37% phosphoric acid + self-etching + primer + adhesive.	Metallic	SBST	No significant differences were found in SBST values, with the exception of surface roughening with a green stone prior to HF and silane treatment. This protocol yielded slightly higher bond strength which was statistically significant	The present in-vitro study found that SBST values for ceramic pretreatment all fell within an acceptable clinical range and similar to the bond strength of enamel. No significant differences were found in the SBST values, with the exception of roughening with a green stone prior to HF and silane treatment, which yielded slightly higher bond strength.
Poosti et al., 2012 [65]	In vitro	Tungstem carbide burrs; 9.6% Hydrofluoric acid 4 min; Er:YAG; Neodymium-doped yttrium aluminum garnet laser (Nd: YAG) 10 s.	Glazed porcelain	100	G1: tungsten carbide burs (n = 20); G2: tungsten carbide burs + 9.6% hydrofluoric acid (n = 20); G3: 0.8-W Nd:YAG laser (n = 20); G4: 2W Er:YAG laser (n = 20); G5: 3-W Er:YAG laser (n = 20).	NR	Metallic	SBST	Although Tukey's test showed SBST in tungsten carbide burs+ 9.6% hydrofluoric acid and Nd:YAG laser were significantly higher than the other groups, they did not differ with each other significantly ($p > 0.05$). The results revealed that SBST of 9.6% hydroflouric acid and Nd:YAG Laser was in an acceptable range for orthodontic treatment.	Nd:YAG laser was shown to be an acceptable substitute for hydrofluoric acid while Er:YAG laser with the mentioned power and duration was not a suitable option.
AlShahrani et al., 2019 [66]	In vitro	G1: 9.6% Hydrofluoric acid+ S 60 s; G2: Er,Cr:YSGG laser 2 mm, 4.5 W, 30 Hz, 60 s; G3: Fractional carbon dioxide (CO_2) laser 10 W, 200 Hz, 3 mm, 60s, pulse duration 1.75 ms; G4: SB Al_2O_3 10 mm, 2.8 MPa, 20 s; G5: Monobond etch & prime, Ivoclar Vivadent, Schaan, Liechtenstein.	Lithium disilicate	50	G2: Er,Cr:YSGG laser+ S (n = 10); G3: CO_2 laser + S (n = 10); G4: SB (n = 10); G5: Self-Etch Glass Ceramic Primer (n = 10).	G1: HF+ S (n = 10).	Metallic and ceramic polycrystalline	SBST	The highest SBST values were presented by HF + S (21.08 ± 1.06). The lowest SBST values were displayed by Al_2O_3 (12.61 ± 0.45). SBST of samples conditioned with self-etch glass ceramic primer showed significant difference amongst all experimental groups (16.76 ± 0.81).	Lithium disilicate ceramics photosensitized with CO_2, and Er,Cr:YSGG has a potential to be recommended in clinical settings alternate to HF+S when bonded to metallic bracket.

Table 2. Cont.

Authors, Year	Study Design	Type of Adhesion Technique (Type, Time, Clinical Application)	Type of Porcelain	Sample Size (n)	Test Group	Control Group	Bracket Type	Intervention Test	Results	Conclusions
May et al., 2015 [67]	In vitro	10% HF 20 s; aluminum oxide blasting 15 s, pressure at 80 psi, 5 mm; 35% phosphoric acid 30 s; CoJet blasting; S.	Eris ceramic; d. Sign ceramic	120	n = 60–Eris Ceramic; n = 15 -10% HF; n = 15–10% HF + S; n = 15 -aluminum oxide blasting + 35% phosphoric acid + S; n = 15 -CoJet blasting + 35% phosphoric acid + S); n = 60–d.Sign Ceramic; n = 15 -10% HF; n = 15-10% HF + S; n = 15 -aluminum oxide blasting + 35% phosphoric acid + S; n = 15 -CoJet blasting + 35% phosphoric acid + S).	NR	Metallic	SBST	There were statistically significant differences among the ceramics ($p = 0.01$) and surface treatments ($p = 0.0001$), but it did not show interaction among them ($p = 0.14$).	The tested ceramics performed similarly in terms of bond strength; the use of S after HF was responsible for the increase of bond strength values; HF+ S, as well as aluminum oxide +phosphoric acid+S provided significantly higher bond strength values to metallic brackets; the CoJet system did not result in significantly higher values than those observed for aluminum oxide blasting, becoming similar to the groups treated with HF without S; aluminum oxide blasting followed by phosphoric acid etching and S presented results similar to the treatment with HF + S.
Alqerban, 2021 [68]	In vitro	G2: S; G3: HF 9.5% 60 s; G4: SB 50 um Al$_2$O$_3$, 1 mm, 2.8 atm, 15 s; G5: Self-etch ceramic primer (Monobond etch & prime, Ivoclar Vivadent, Schaan, Liechtenstein) (SECP) 60 s; G6: Er,Cr:YSGG laser 4.5 W, 30 Hz, 1 mm.	Lithium disilicate	90	G2: S 30 s (n = 15); G3: HF + UB + S 30 s (n = 15); G4: SB (n = 15); G5: SECP (n = 15); G6: Er,Cr:YSGG laser + S 20s (n = 15).	G1: HF + S 20s (n = 15).	Metallic	SBST	The highest SBST values were observed in HF+ UB + S (18.21 ± 1.241) and the lowest SBST values IN S only (5.21 ± 0.23). Specimens surface conditioned with HF+ S (17.85 ± 1.25), HF+ UB + S (18.21 ± 1.241) and Er,Cr:YSGG laser+ S (17.09 ± 1.114) unveiled comparable SBST values ($p > 0.05$).	Lithium disilicate conditioned with Er,Cr:YSGG laser has a potential to be used in clinical settings alternate to HF.

Table 2. Cont.

Authors, Year	Study Design	Type of Adhesion Technique (Type, Time, Clinical Application)	Type of Porcelain	Sample Size (n)	Test Group	Control Group	Bracket Type	Intervention Test	Results	Conclusions
Elsaka, 2016 [69]	In vitro	9% HF 1 min; 37% H_3PO_4 1 min; Diamond ceramic grinding bur (VOCO, Cuxhaven, Germany) 6000–10,000 rpm; Silica coating using Cojet system (CJ).	Vita Enamic (VE) CAD/CAM hybrid ceramic	240	n = 120-ceramic bracket (n = 30-HF; n = 30-H_3PO_4; n = 30-diamond ceramic grinding bur; n = 30—J). n = 120-metal bracket (n = 30-HF; n = 30-H_3PO_4; n = 30-diamond ceramic grinding bur; n = 30—J).	NR	Ceramic and metal brackets	SBST	SBST was significantly affected by the type of bracket and by type of treatment ($p < 0.001$). Specimens treated with CJ presented with significantly higher SBST compared to other groups ($p < 0.05$). Improvements in SBST values (MPa) were found in the following order: CJ	HF	Bur [H_3PO_4. Ceramic bracket showed higher SBST compared to metal bracket.	Surface treatment of VE CAD/CAM hybrid ceramic with silica coating enhanced the adhesion with ceramic and metal brackets. Ceramic bracket provided higher bond strength com-pared to metal bracket.
Falkensammer et al., 2012 [70]	In vitro	5% HF 60/30 s, 9.6% buffered HF 9.6%, 60/30 s; SB Al_2O_3/SiO_2 particles.	Metal- and all-ceramic veneering; feldspathic; leucite; leucite-free; fluorapatite.	960	The four types of ceramic were allocated to each of the six conditioning groups, resulting in 24 subgroups of 40 brackets each.	NR	NR	SBST	HF 5% or SB resulted in significantly ($p < 0.001$) higher bond strengths (mean values: 34.11 and 32.86 MPa, respectively) than with HF 9.6% (mean value: 12.49 MPa). Etching time or SB particles had no influence on bond strength.	Different conditioning procedures have an effect on ceramic microstructures and bracket adhesion. High SBST (29.74–36.80 MPa) were found for all ceramic surfaces when HF 5% or SB, indicating a higher risk of ceramic fracture. The HF 9.6% appeared to have a minor conditioning effect, resulting in a lower SBST (9.34–15.92 MPa), but fewer ceramic fractures. A short etching time (30 s) was as effective as standard etching (60 s). SB SiO_2 showed no advantage as compared with SB Al_2O_3.

Table 2. Cont.

Authors, Year	Study Design	Type of Adhesion Technique (Type, Time, Clinical Application)	Type of Porcelain	Sample Size (n)	Test Group	Control Group	Bracket Type	Intervention Test	Results	Conclusions
Kim et al., 2017 [71]	In vitro	SB Al_2O_3 and CO (Colet TM); S: Zirconia Prime Plus (ZPP) and SBU.	Zirconia	120	n = 10–Al_2O_3 + S–T; n = 10–Al_2O_3 + S–N; n = 10–Al_2O_3 + ZPF–T; n = 10–Al_2O_3 + ZPF–N; n = 10–Al_2O_3 + SBU–T; n = 10–Al_2O_3 + SBU–N; n = 10–CO + S–T; n = 10–CO + S–N; n = 10–CO + ZPP–T; n = 10–CO + ZPP–N; n = 10–CO + SBU–T; n = 10–CO + SBU–N.	NR	Metallic	SBST	CO-SBU had the highest bond strength after T. CO-S significantly higher SBST than Al_2O_3–S. CO-ZPP lower bond strength than Al_2O_3-ZPP before thermocycling, but the SBST increased after T.	CO-SBU showed the highest shear bond strength. Sandblasting with either AL or CO improved the mechanical bonding by increasing the surface area, and all primer groups showed clinically acceptable increase of SBST for orthodontic treatment.
Alaqeel, 2020 [72]	In vitro	Heat-treatment	Lithium disilicate glass-ceramic	120	n = 60-heat treated specimens (n = 15-neutralized, bonded with resin based cement; n = 15-neutralized, bonded with water based cement; n = 15-non-neutralized, bonded with resin based cement; n = 15-non-neutralized, bonded with water based cement).	n = 60-non-heat treated specimens (n = 15-neutralized, bonded with resin based cement; n = 15-neutralized, bonded with water based cement; n = 15-non-neutralized, bonded with resin based cement; n = 15-non-neutralized, bonded with water based cement).	NR	SBST	The heat-treated showed statistically significant higher bond strength in all the sub- groups, and the acid-neutralized samples showed higher bond strength using both types of cement; however, the increase was statistically significant only in resin-based cement-bonded samples. Resin-based cement-bonded samples showed higher bond strength than water-based cement-bonded samples.	Pre-etching heat treatment and post-etching acid neutralization of the cementing surface of lithium disilicate glass-ceramic significantly improve the initial bond strength to orthodontic brackets.

Table 2. Cont.

Authors, Year	Study Design	Type of Adhesion Technique (Type, Time, Clinical Application)	Type of Porcelain	Sample Size (n)	Test Group	Control Group	Bracket Type	Intervention Test	Results	Conclusions
Guida et al., 2019 [73]	In vitro	10%, HF 60s; S 3 min; HF + S; MDP—The adhesive system (Ambar, FGM, Joinville, Brazil—primer and adhesive combined in one bottle) containing MDP (10-methacryloyloxydecyl dihydrogen phosphate) applied in two layers. The first drop of adhesive was vigorously brushed on the bonding surface for 10 s, air-thinned before the second layer of adhesive was applied for 10 s, air-thinned, and light cured for 10 s.	Lithium disilicate-based glass-ceramic.	240	n = 20-BM-HF; n = 20-BM-S; n = 20-BM-HF + S; n = 20-BM-MDP; n = 20-BCp-HF; n = 20-BCp-S; n = 20-BCp-HF + S; n = 20-BCp-MDP; n = 20-BCm-HF; n = 20-BCm-S; n = 20-BCm-HF + S; n = 20-BCm-MDP.	BM—Stainless steel, metal bracket (Abzil, 3M Brazil, São Jose do Rio Preto, SP, Brazil) with a traditional mesh for mechanical retention	Metallic (BM) and ceramic brackets (monocrystalline (BCm) and polycrystalline (BCp).	SBST	BCm with HFS or HF showed the highest median σ values, 10.5 MPa and 8.5 MPa respectively. In contrast, the BCp with MDP showed the lowest median σ value (0.8 MPa), which was not statistically different from other MDP-treated groups.	The failure mode was governed by the glass-ceramic surface treatment, not by the bracket type. Quantitative (σ values) and qualitative (fracture mode) data suggested a minimum of 5 MPa for brackets bonded to glass-ceramic, which is the lower critical limit bond strength for a comprehensive orthodontic treatment.
Martalia et al., 2020 [74]	In vitro	9% HF; Silane Ultradent; Ortho Solo bonding and Grengloo; adhesive bracket; Single Bond Universal 3 M ESPE.	Porcelain veneers	28	n = 7–9% HF 90 s, aquades 5 s, air spray 5 s, Silane, air spray 60 s, Ortho Solo, Grenglo adhesive, light-curing for 20 s; n = 7–9% HF 90 s, aquades 5 s, air spray 5 s, Single Bond, light-curing 10 s, Grenglo adhesive, light-curing for 20 s; n = 7–9% HF 90 s, aquades 5 s, air spray 5 s, Ortho Solo, Grenglo adhesive, light-curing for 20 s.	n = 7–Single Bond, light-curing 10 s, apply Grenglo adhesive to bracket mess and the last step do light-curing for 20 s.	Metallic	SBST	The shear bond strengths between groups were significantly different ($p < 0.05$). The greatest bracket shear bond strength and lowest porcelain surface roughness were found in hydrofluoric acid, silane, bonding, and adhesive.	Silane applied separately from bonding and acid has great shear bond strength and low porcelain surface roughness.
Jivanescu et al., 2014 [75]	In vitro	Relyx U200 dual cure resin cement; Bluglloo light cure composite	Porcelain-fused-to-metal	16	n = 8-Relyx U200 dual cure resin cement; n = 8-Bluglloo light cure composite.	NR	Metallic	TBST	No statistically significant differences among the two cements in terms of tensile bond strength.	Both dental materials may be recommended for orthodontic bracket bonding to ceramic surfaces, with equally successful results. However, further testing on an increased number of specimens may be considered for more accurate data.

Table 2. Cont.

Authors, Year	Study Design	Type of Adhesion Technique (Type, Time, Clinical Application)	Type of Porcelain	Sample Size (n)	Test Group	Control Group	Bracket Type	Intervention Test	Results	Conclusions
Park et al., 2013 [76]	In vitro	37% Phosphoric acid 1 min, wash, dry with electric light 5 min, light curing 40 s, Transbond 37 °C of water bath for 24 h. Laser irradiation-Er:YAG laser 140 μm of the wave length and 20% of air water ratio, 20 Hz per second, 2 W, 1 mm distance, 20 s irradiation, dry 5 s, Transbond 40 s enlightening 37 °C of water bath for 24 h.	Zirconia and Ceramic	150	n = 10-Metal with phosphoric acid n = 10-Metal with laser acid; n = 10-Metal with laser + phosphoric acid n = 10-Ceramic with phosphoric acid; n = 10-Ceramic with laser acid; n = 10-Ceramic with laser + phosphoric acid; n = 10-Zirconia with phosphoric acid; n = 10-Zirconia with laser acid; n = 10-Zirconia with aser + phosphoric acid.	n = 10-Tooth with Phosphoric acid; n = 10-Tooth with Laser acid; n = 10-Tooth with Laser + phosphoric acid.	NR	SBST	Changed as the most in ceramic in laser irradiation. Bonding strength according to the etching method was the most in laser irradiation and acid etching in ceramic and in zirconia.	Ceramic crown with acid treatment was recommended because of relatively high in bonding strength.
Hellak et al., 2016 [77]	In vitro/Ex vivo	Self-etching no-mix adhesives (iBond™ and Scotchbond™); Total etch system Transbond XT™.	Glass-ceramic veneering (IPS e.maxTM Press, IPS e-max ZirCAD for inLabTM was used as high-strength zirconia and VITAblocsTM Mark II, C2II4 for CERECTM/inLab (VITA Zahnfabrik, Bad Sackingen, Germany) was used as a monochromatic feldspathic ceramic.	270	n = 240 divided into eight restorative surface groups (n = 30), of which Glass-ceramic veneering (n = 90) and all of the surfaces were divided into three subgroups with different adhesives (n = 10).	n = 30-Human enamel with Transbond XT primer; n = 30-Human enamel with iBond. n = 30-Human enamel with Scotchbond Universal	Metallic	SBST	Significant differences in SBST were found between the control group and experimental groups.	Transbond XT showed the highest SBST on human enamel. Scotchbond Universal on average provides the best bonding on all other types of surface (metal, composite, and porcelain), with no need for additional primers. It might therefore be helpful for simplifying bonding in orthodontic procedures on restorative materials in patients.

207

Table 2. Cont.

Authors, Year	Study Design	Type of Adhesion Technique (Type, Time, Clinical Application)	Type of Porcelain	Sample Size (n)	Test Group	Control Group	Bracket Type	Intervention Test	Results	Conclusions
Lee et al., 2015 [32]	In vitro	G1: SB 50 µm, 5 s at pressure of 40 psi, 5 mm; G2: 9% HF acid 4 min; G3: porcelain primer (PP) thin coat; G4: zirconia primer (ZP) thin coat.	Zirconia	40	G1: nonglazed zirconia treated with SB + ZP (n = 10); G2: glazed zirconia treated with SB + etching + ZP (n = 10); G3: glazed zirconia treated with SB + etching + PP (n = 10); G4: glazed zirconia treated with SB + etching + ZP + PP (n = 10).	NR	Metallic	SBST	Group G2 showed significantly lower shear bond strength than did the other groups. No statistically significant differences were found among groups G1, G3, and G4.	Porcelain primer is the more appropriate choice for bonding a metal bracket to the surface of a full-contour glazed zirconia crown with resin cement.

ACPS—3-acryloxypropyltrimethoxysilane; Al2O3—aluminium oxide; ANOVA—one-way analysis of variance; APA—Air-particle abrasion; ARI—adhesive Remnant Index; AST—adhesion strength test; atm—standard atmosphere; BCm—monocrystalline brackets; BCp—polycrystalline brackets; BIS-EMA—bisphenol A diglycidyl methacrylate ethoxylated; BIS-GMA—bisphenol A-glycidyl methacrylate; BM—metallic brackets; BTSE—bis-1,2-(triethoxysilyl) ethane; CB—ceramic brackets; Cj—Colet system; CO—Colet TM; CO2—carbon dioxide; CSBS—cyclic shear bond strength; DB—deglazing using diamond bur; df—degrees of freedom; E15—hydrofluoric acid 15s; E5—hydrofluoric acid 5s; Er: CrYSGG—erbium, chromium:yttrium-scandium-gallium-garnet; Er:YAG—Erbium:yttrium-aluminum-garnet; FC—feldspathic ceramic; G—group; H3PO4—orthophosphoric acid; HF—hydrofluoric acid; Hz—hertz; IP—IPS e.max CAD; LDC—lithium di silicate; Led—light-emitting diode; LU—lava ultimate; MB—methylene blue; MDP–10-methacryloyloxydecyl dihydrogen phosphate; MEP—monobond etch & prime; MIC—aluminum oxide microetching; min—minute(s); mj—millijoule; mm—millimeter; MPa—megapascal pressure unit; mz—Monolithic zirconium oxide ceramic; Nd:YAG—neodymium-doped yttrium aluminium garnet; np—no-primer; NR—not reported; p—p-value; PA—phosphoric acid; PDT—photodynamic therapy; PFM—porcelain fused to metal; PP—porcelain primer; psi—pounds of force per square inch of area; rpm—revolutions per minute; s—second(s); S—silane; S@SB2—adper single bond 2; S@SBU—silane + single bond universal; SB—sandblasting; SB2—single bond 2; SBST—shear bond strength test; SBU—single bond universal; sd—standard deviation; SECP—monobond etch and prime; SiO2—silicon dioxide; sp—short pulse; ssp—super short pulse; T—thermocycled; TBST—tensile bond strength test; TEGDMA—triethylene glycol dimethacrylate; TS—tribochemical silica coating UB—ultrasonic bath; UDMA—bisphenol A-glycidyldimethacrylate and urethane dimethacrylate; VE—Vita Enamic; VM—VITA Mark II; ZP—zirconia primer; ZPP—zirconia prime plus.

Study	Structured summary	Scientific background and rationale	Objectives and/or hypotheses	Intervention of each group	Outcomes definition	Sample size determination	Allocation sequence generation	Allocation concealment mechanism	Implementation	Blinding	Statistical methods	Outcomes and estimation	Limitations	Funding information	Protocol (if available)
Alqerban, 2019	Y	Y	Y	Y	Y	N	N	N	N	N	Y	N	N	Y	N
Goldshah et al., 2018	Y	Y	Y	Y	Y	Y	Y	N	N	N	Y	N	Y	Y	N
Mirhashemi et al., 2018	Y	Y	Y	Y	Y	N	N	N	N	N	Y	N	Y	N	N
Hellak et al., 2016	Y	Y	Y	Y	Y	N	N	N	N	N	Y	N	Y	Y	N
Lestrade et al., 2016	Y	Y	Y	Y	Y	N	N	N	N	N	Y	N	N	N	N
Mehmeti et al., 2017	N	Y	Y	N	N	N	N	N	N	N	Y	N	Y	Y	N
Cevik et al., 2017	Y	Y	Y	Y	Y	N	N	N	N	N	Y	Y	N	Y	N
Martalia et al., 2020	Y	Y	Y	Y	Y	Y	N	N	N	N	Y	N	N	N	Y
Sabuncuoglu et al., 2016	Y	Y	Y	Y	Y	N	N	N	N	N	Y	N	Y	N	N
Falkensammer et al., 2012	Y	Y	Y	Y	N	N	N	N	N	N	Y	N	N	N	N
AlShahrani et al., 2019	Y	Y	Y	N	Y	N	N	N	N	N	Y	N	N	N	N
Kim et al., 2017	Y	Y	Y	Y	Y	N	N	N	N	N	Y	N	Y	Y	N
Jivanescu et al., 2014	N	Y	N	N	Y	N	N	N	N	N	Y	N	N	N	N
Lee et al., 2015	Y	Y	Y	Y	Y	N	N	N	N	N	Y	N	N	N	N
Juntavee et al., 2018	Y	Y	Y	Y	N	N	N	N	N	N	Y	Y	N	Y	N
Park et al., 2013	Y	N	N	N	Y	N	N	N	N	N	Y	N	N	N	N
Guida et al., 2019	Y	Y	Y	Y	Y	N	N	N	N	N	Y	N	N	Y	N
Poosti et al., 2012	Y	Y	Y	Y	N	N	N	N	N	N	Y	N	Y	N	N
Hosseini et al., 2013	Y	Y	Y	Y	N	N	N	N	N	N	N	N	N	N	N
May et al., 2015	Y	Y	Y	Y	Y	N	N	N	N	N	Y	N	N	N	N
Naseh et al., 2018	Y	Y	Y	Y	Y	Y	N	N	N	N	Y	N	N	Y	N
Gardiner et al., 2019	Y	Y	Y	Y	Y	N	N	N	N	N	Y	Y	Y	Y	N
Alaqeel, 2020	Y	Y	Y	Y	N	N	N	N	N	N	Y	N	Y	Y	N
Aksakalli et al., 2014	Y	Y	Y	Y	N	N	N	N	N	N	Y	N	Y	N	N
Elsaka et al., 2015	Y	Y	Y	Y	Y	N	N	N	N	N	Y	N	Y	Y	N
Yassaei et al., 2013	Y	Y	Y	N	Y	N	N	N	N	N	Y	N	N	N	N
Tahmasbi et al., 2019	Y	Y	Y	Y	Y	N	N	N	N	N	Y	N	Y	Y	N
Costa et al., 2012	Y	Y	Y	Y	Y	N	N	N	N	N	Y	N	N	N	N
Kurt et al., 2019	Y	Y	Y	Y	Y	N	N	N	N	N	Y	N	N	N	N
Dalaie et al., 2016	Y	Y	Y	N	Y	Y	N	N	N	N	Y	Y	N	N	N
Ramos et al., 2012	Y	Y	Y	Y	Y	N	N	N	N	N	Y	N	N	N	N
Juntavee et al., 2020	Y	Y	Y	Y	N	N	N	N	N	N	Y	N	N	Y	Y
Stella et al., 2015	Y	Y	Y	Y	Y	N	N	N	N	N	N	Y	N	N	N
Abdelnaby, 2011	Y	Y	Y	Y	Y	N	N	N	N	N	Y	N	N	N	N
Kaygisiz et al., 2015	Y	Y	Y	Y	N	N	N	N	N	N	Y	N	Y	Y	N
Dilber et al., 2016	Y	Y	Y	Y	Y	N	N	N	N	N	Y	N	Y	N	N
Cevik et al., 2016	Y	Y	Y	Y	N	N	N	N	N	N	Y	N	N	Y	N
Epperson et al., 2017	Y	Y	Y	Y	Y	N	N	N	N	N	Y	N	Y	N	N
Mehmeti et al., 2019	Y	Y	Y	N	Y	N	N	N	N	N	Y	N	Y	Y	N
Baeshen, 2021	Y	Y	Y	Y	Y	N	N	N	N	N	Y	N	Y	Y	N
Ihsan et al., 2019	Y	Y	Y	Y	N	N	N	N	N	N	Y	N	N	Y	N
Saraç et al., 2011	Y	Y	Y	Y	Y	Y	N	N	N	N	Y	N	N	N	N
Al-Hity et al., 2012	Y	Y	N	Y	N	N	N	N	N	N	Y	N	N	N	N
Recen et al., 2021	Y	Y	Y	Y	N	N	N	N	N	N	Y	Y	N	Y	N
Durgesh et al., 2016	Y	Y	Y	Y	N	N	N	N	N	N	Y	N	N	N	N
Durgesh et al., 2020	Y	Y	Y	Y	N	N	N	N	N	N	N	N	N	N	N
García-Sanz et al., 2019	Y	Y	Y	Y	N	N	N	N	N	N	Y	N	Y	Y	N
Mohammed et al, 2019	Y	Y	N	N	Y	N	N	N	N	N	Y	N	N	Y	N
Mehmeti et al., 2018	Y	Y	N	Y	N	N	N	N	N	N	Y	N	Y	Y	N
Bavbek et al., 2014	Y	Y	Y	Y	N	N	N	N	N	N	Y	Y	N	N	N
Asiry et al., 2018	Y	Y	Y	Y	N	N	N	N	N	N	Y	N	N	Y	N
Ghozy et al., 2020	Y	Y	Y	Y	N	N	N	N	N	N	Y	N	N	Y	N
Lee et al., 2015	Y	Y	N	Y	N	N	N	N	N	N	Y	N	N	N	N
Erdur et al., 2015	Y	Y	Y	Y	Y	N	N	N	N	N	Y	N	N	N	N
Mehta et al., 2016	Y	Y	Y	Y	N	N	N	N	N	N	Y	Y	Y	Y	N
Miersch et al., 2019	Y	Y	Y	N	Y	Y	Y	N	N	N	Y	Y	Y	Y	N
Girish et al., 2012	Y	Y	Y	Y	N	N	N	N	N	N	Y	N	N	Y	N
Topcuoglu et al., 2013	Y	Y	Y	Y	N	N	N	N	N	N	Y	N	N	Y	N
Najafi et al., 2014	Y	Y	Y	Y	N	N	N	N	N	N	Y	N	N	Y	N
Akpinar et al., 2015	Y	Y	Y	Y	N	N	N	N	N	N	Y	N	N	N	N
Gonçalves et al., 2011	Y	N	N	N	N	N	N	N	N	N	Y	N	N	N	N
Alavi et al., 2020	Y	Y	Y	Y	N	N	N	N	N	N	Y	N	Y	Y	N
Ahrari et al., 2012	Y	Y	N	Y	N	N	N	N	N	N	Y	N	N	N	N
Mirhashemi et al., 2018	Y	Y	Y	Y	N	N	N	N	N	N	Y	Y	Y	Y	N
Franz et al., 2019	Y	Y	N	Y	N	N	N	N	N	N	Y	Y	Y	Y	Y
Hsu et al., 2015	Y	Y	Y	N	Y	N	N	N	N	N	Y	N	Y	N	N
Xu et al., 2018	Y	Y	Y	Y	N	N	N	N	N	N	Y	N	N	Y	N
Yu et al., 2021	Y	Y	Y	Y	N	N	N	N	N	N	Y	N	N	N	N
Zhang et al., 2016	Y	Y	Y	Y	N	N	N	N	N	N	Y	N	N	Y	N
Sandoval et al., 2020	Y	Y	N	Y	N	N	N	N	N	N	Y	N	N	N	N
Asiry et al., 2018	Y	Y	Y	Y	N	N	N	N	N	N	Y	N	N	Y	N

Figure 2. Y—yes; N—no. Risk of bias of the included studies.

Only two studies not reported a structured abstract, calculation of the sample size [59,75] or scientific background and rationale [38,76]. Regarding the randomization process, only two studies reported these items [4,23,47]. All studies not reported researcher blinding to the interventions. Y—yes; N—no. Only a few studies reported the estimated size of outcomes [5,7,27,30,46]. No studies reported information relative to the protocol domain, except for three [15,43,74].

3.2. Meta-Analysis

For the quantitative analysis, only studies that used metallic brackets adhered to felspathic ceramics and lithium disilicate were selected. These studies were pooled regarding the main surface treatment used, although different protocols (concentrations, applications times, energies ...) were used. Studies that presented other bracket types presented highly heterogeneous methodologies, making impossible its comparison. Also, regarding the other ceramic types, it was not possible to find studies with similar methodologies to be compared.

The meta-analysis regarding the feldspathic ceramics (Figure 3) presents the lower adhesion values for the treatments with fine bur (T1) and orthophosphoric acid (T3), without statistically significant differences between them, but significantly lower than all other treatments ($p < 0.001$). With increased adhesion values the sandblasting technique alone (T2), presents statistically significant differences ($p < 0.001$) for all groups, including the sandblasting + hydrofluoric acid group (T6), although less significant ($p < 0.05$). The group that uses LASER (T5) for surface preparation presents the following highest adhesion value with statistically significant differences ($p < 0.001$) T1, T2, T3, T4 and T7 groups and $p < 0.05$ to T5 group. The highest adhesion values were found in the LASER with hydrofluoric acid (T7) or hydrofluoric acid alone (T4) groups, without statistically significant differences between them, but being significantly higher than the others ($p < 0.001$).

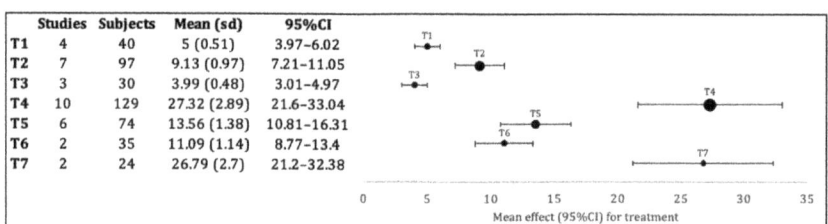

Figure 3. Forest plot of brackets adhesion to feldspathic ceramics with diverse superficial treatments. T1: Fine bur group; T2: Sandblasting (Al_2O_3) group; T3: orthophosphoric acid group; T4: hydrofluoric acid group; T5: LASER group; T6: Sandblasting (Al_2O_3) with hydrofluoric acid group; T7: LASER with hydrofluoric acid group. For each surface treatment, the number of studies included, the totality of samples evaluated, mean and standard deviation (SD), and 95% confidence intervals are described. Adhesion values are presented in MPa.

The meta-analysis that evaluates lithium disilicate ceramics (Figure 4) presents the statistically significant lowest adhesion values for the orthophosphoric acid (T3) group ($p < 0.001$). Still with low adhesion values, but higher than the previous ones, we find the fine bur group (T1), with statistically significant differences regarding all the other groups ($p < 0.001$). With increased adhesion values, we have the sandblasting technique (T2) and the hydrofluoric acid alone (T4) groups, without statistically significant differences between them, but with statistically significant differences ($p < 0.001$) with all other groups. The highest adhesion values are found in the LASER alone group (T5), with statistically significant differences from all other groups ($p < 0.001$).

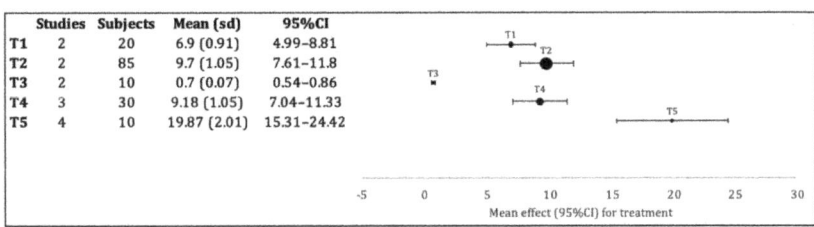

Figure 4. Forest plot of the evaluation of brackets adhesion to lithium disilicate ceramic with diverse superficial treatments. T1: Fine bur group; T2: Sandblasting (Al_2O_3) group; T3: orthophosphoric acid group; T4: hydrofluoric acid group; T5: LASER group. For each surface treatment, the number of studies included, the totality of samples evaluated, mean and standard deviation (SD), and 95% confidence intervals are described. Adhesion values are presented in MPa.

For the two ceramic types evaluated in the meta-analysis, the surface presenting the lowest results is the orthophosphoric acid, with adhesion values close to 0 MPa, such as 3.99 MPa ± 0.48 for felspathic ceramics and 0.7 MPa ± 0.07 for lithium disilicate. These low adhesion results are also observed in surface treatments using only fine drill wear, with 5 MPa ± 0.51 and 6.9 MPa ± 0.91; and sandblasting with 9.13 MPa ± 0.97 and 9.7 MPa ± 1.05 for feldspathic ceramics and lithium disilicate respectively.

The treatment with the highest values for lithium disilicate ceramics is the LASER treatment with 19.87 MPa ± 2.01, while for feldspathic ceramics it is the LASER treatment with hydrofluoric acid with 26.79 MPa ± 2.7 and the treatment with hydrofluoric acid alone with 27.32 MPa ± 2.89.

When comparing the same surface treatments on the two types of ceramics, substantially different adhesion values are obtained, as an example of hydrofluoric acid with such different performances as 27.32 MPa ± 2.89 for feldspathic and 9.18 MPa ± 1.05 for disilicate. The LASER treatment also presents some differences when we compare feldspathic ceramics with lithium disilicate with 13.56 MPa ± 1.38 and 19.87 MPa ± 2.01, respectively.

4. Discussion

The main purpose of this review was to identify the most efficient and reliable bonding protocol for orthodontic brackets to ceramic surfaces. As this is a complex and sensitive process it is essential to determine the best protocol to achieve the best results [2,4,10,12].

The last systematic review regarding this topic was published in 2014. This previous paper, that solely included in vitro studies, concluded that the best protocol would be etching with 9.6% hydrofluoric acid for 60 s, rinsing for 30 s, air-drying, and finally applying the silane [78]. With new articles emerging in recent years a new systematic review is warranted. Since we included papers published from 2011, all recent literature was scrutinized and included if relevant.

As previously stated, to ensure an acceptable shear bond strength (SBS) capable of resisting not only chewing but also forces induced by orthodontic appliances, optimal ceramic surface conditioning techniques are necessary. The present results revealed that the most studied conditioning methods include 37%/37.5% orthophosphoric acid, 4%/9%/9.5%/9.6%/10% hydrofluoric acid, silane application, sandblasting/air abrasion with aluminum oxide, diamond bur roughening, single bond universal adhesive and the use of different types of LASER, such as Er:YAG laser, CO_2 laser, Er:CrYSGG laser, Nd:YAG laser, Cr:YSGG laser, FS laser.

4.1. Design and Bracket Material

The included studies present several different combinations of ceramic surface conditioning techniques to understand which one achieves a better SBS value. Some studies prove that although the ceramic surface conditioning method is the most important factor in achieving acceptable clinical values for SBS, it is not exclusive. Factors such as the material and design of the bracket, type of ceramic surface, and etch time also affect SBS. Mehmeti et al. states that the bracket type used significantly affects the SBS value and is a valid clinical concern [57]. On the other hand, Guida et al. showed that the failure rate is closely related to the glass-ceramic surface conditioning and that the bracket type is inconsequential [73]. According to Mehmeti et al., metallic brackets seemingly provide stronger adhesion with all-zirconium surfaces when compared to ceramic polycrystalline brackets, which can be attributed to their improved base surface design [59]. However, this is opposed to the findings of Al-Hity et al. which revealed that bonding strength of ceramic brackets on porcelain significantly exceeds that of metal brackets [19]. Different testing protocols and materials used can explain the contradictory results, since these two factors have a profound impact on the obtained results.

4.2. Orthophosphoric Acid, Fine Burr and Sandblasting

In our systematic analysis, the lowest adhesion values were verified with orthophosphoric acid, fine burr, and with slightly higher values, sandblasting treatments. Although these treatments created microroughness that could improve adhesion, their use alone presented unsatisfactory results. According to three authors (Mohammed et al., Mehta et al. and Girish et al.), the sandblasting method in association with the application of silane reaches the maximum SBS, while the use of 37% orthophosphoric acid has the lowest SBST and is deemed unsuitable for bonding ceramic brackets [21,27,31]. In this situation, we can attribute the good SBS scores to the use of silane, which alone presents high bond strength forces.

Other studies, regarding surface roughening revealed that the use of sandblasting or diamond burs along with the application of hydrofluoric acid significantly improved bond strength [52]. Sandblasting with SiO_2 was shown to have no advantage when compared to sandblasting with AL_2O_3 [70].

4.3. Hydrofluoric Acid

The etching process partially dissolves the ceramic matrix, increasing the surface area by creating microchannels, this allows for the penetration of resin cement, thus providing finer conditions for increased bond strength.

However, since the available brands of porcelain have dissimilar particle sizes and crystalline structure, different outcomes are to be expected when testing various ceramic surfaces and brands. The heterogeneity of the reviewed studies can be attributed to structural differences in porcelain surfaces (besides the brackets' base designs), which may result in higher or lower bond strength. As example, a paper by Kurt et al. published in 2019, reported that the highest SBS value was found in feldspathic ceramics previously treated with hydrofluoric acid [24]; however, Saraç et al. demonstrated that for any conditioning method, leucite-reinforced ceramic, in general, showed a higher SBS when compared to feldspathic and fluoroapatite ceramics [47].

As stated above, the etching agent HF increases the available surface area for adhesion. Higher HF concentrations promote more ceramic dissolution, which may be linked to higher bond strength values [79]. Such results support the use of HF as surface treatments when bonding ceramic restorations [80]. This can explain the results obtained in the feldspathic ceramics group, where the HF groups (alone or in combination with a laser) presented higher adhesion values. However, the HF promoted significantly lower adhesion values in the disilicate lithium group. Lithium silicate is more susceptible to HF action than feldspathic. HF concentrations above 5% used for more than 20 s significantly influence the characteristics of the material, promoting a decrease in the material strength [81]. Additionally, higher HF concentrations can also result in worse adhesion, as shown in an in vitro study by Pérez et al. [82].

The use of HF also produces insoluble fluorosilicate salts that remain on the material's surface (if not removed by other methods, such as ultrasonic cleaning), which can affect the adhesion [83]. Also, the overall reduced number of studies included for this material and the different experimental methodologies used can affect the observed results. Taken together, such factors and differences in the material composition regarding feldsphatic ceramics can explain the obtained values for the disilicate lithium group.

Also, the acid etching time was inconsistent as different studies used different methodologies. According to Falkensammer et al. this factor is not preponderant for achieving SBS, according to their study an etching time of 30 s was as effective as standard conditioning (60 s) [70]. However, Costa et al. revealed that an etching time of 60 s significantly improved the SBS of brackets to feldspathic ceramic surfaces [34].

4.4. Silane

The use of silane improves the bond strength of brackets to ceramic surfaces [23,67]. Silane forms chemical bonds with both organic and inorganic surfaces, resulting in a stronger connection between surfaces. Furthermore, Zhang et al. reported that HF acid etching followed by silane was the best suited method for bonding on silica based ceramics and, according to Tahmasbi et al. SBS of bracket to porcelain mainly relies on the use of silane rather than the type of adhesive chosen [9,25].

4.5. Adhesive System

The chosen adhesive protocol will influence the bond strength of brackets to ceramic surfaces. According to the results of the studies reviewed, ceramic surfaces treated with blasting aluminum oxide followed by Single Bond Universal™ application had an improved SBS and caused less cohesive damage to the ceramic [51].

4.6. LASER

Recent publications studied alternatives that involve irradiating the ceramic surface with different laser types. The bond strength obtained through the combination of Er:YAG laser and HF acid on the ceramic surface may be sufficient for bonding brackets [28]. Also, according to Cevik et al. hydrofluoric acid and phosphoric acid etching methods were not suitable as surface treatment methods for feldspathic porcelains [17]. Contrarily, other studies revealed that the Er:YAG laser with the recommended settings (intensity and duration) is not a suitable alternative to the application of HF, however the laser Nd: YAG has been shown more promising results [30,65].

The results of this systematic review indicated that laser irradiation and/or HF-etching are the two surface treatments that allow greater resin-ceramic bonding. Laser irradiation emits a wavelength which is absorbed by ceramic materials, creating microretentions which improve resin-ceramic bonding [84]. Feitosa et al. compared 5 types of surface treatment and have found that Er:YAG laser promotes higher surface roughness, producing an improvement in the tensile strength. Regarding laser application time, these authors suggested times greater than 5 s, since some regions on the laser-treated surface had a similar morphologic appearance to the control group [85]. An article published in 2013 compared fractional CO_2 laser with different intensities with hydrofluoric acid, showing that 10 and 15 W laser were higher shear bond strength than HF-etching with better results in deglazed specimens [29]. More recently, Mirhashemi et al. suggested that laser combined with HF promotes higher shear bond strength than laser groups only [30].

In lithium disilicate ceramic crowns, the results revealed that irradiation with different types of lasers can be effective in obtaining an adequate SBS. Conditioning with Er,Cr:YSGG and CO_2 laser has the potential to be used in clinical settings alternative to HF+S when bonding to metallic brackets [66]. However, contrary to the previously mentioned statements, the study by Alavi et al. concluded that neither CO_2 nor Nd:YAG lasers resulted in adequate surface changes for bonding ceramic brackets when compared to conditioned samples with HF [16]. This is also confirmed by Mirhashemi et al. who demonstrated that although conditioning with Er:CrYSGG met SBS requirements for orthodontic brackets, the SBS must be improved through refinement of the irradiation details [30]. Regarding zirconia crowns, FS laser at 200 mW and 60 μm is ideal treatment for conditioning, producing good SBS while also having a more sustainable energy consumption [53].

Importantly, no studies regarding the combined use of HF with laser (T7) included lithium disilicate ceramics, so we cannot ascertain if high bond values similar to the ones observed in the feldspathic ceramics could be obtained, or if the ceramic type is a decisive factor, like for the HF treatment.

Due to the lack of homogeneity in methodology within the currently available literature investigating the bond strength of orthodontic brackets to ceramic surfaces, the present review results present some limitations. To overcome this, calibrated studies analyzing the same parameters using the same protocols should be performed, hence providing stronger evidence. Further research focusing on surface changes, the architecture of the bracket base and the type of the adhesive resin should be performed.

5. Conclusions

Surface treatment protocols cannot be universal for all ceramic and/or all bracket types. Based on our results, we can conclude that for felspathic ceramics, the surface treatment which provides the best adhesion values is the use of hydrofluoric acid alone or concomitantly with LASER. For lithium disilicate ceramics, the treatment with the best results is the use of LASER alone, although combination with HF was not evaluated.

Lower bond strengths were observed in the orthophosphoric acid and fine burr groups. Further high-quality studies with similar methodologies regarding the ceramic type, surface protocol, surface changes, the architecture of the bracket base and the type of the adhesive resin are required.

Author Contributions: Conceptualization, A.B.P. and I.F.; Methodology, F.M.; Software, C.M.M.; validation, C.N., R.T. and M.R.; Formal analysis, B.O. and F.P.; Investigation, F.V.; Resources, I.F. and C.M.M.; data curation, B.O. and E.C.; Writing—original draft preparation, A.B.P.; Writing—review and editing, F.M. and M.R.; visualization, C.N., R.T., F.P.; Supervision, F.V. and E.C.; Project administration, F.V.; Funding acquisition, E.C. All authors have read and agreed to the published version of the manuscript.

Funding: This research received no external funding.

Institutional Review Board Statement: Not applicable.

Informed Consent Statement: Not applicable.

Data Availability Statement: The data presented in this study are available on request from the corresponding author.

Conflicts of Interest: The authors declare no conflict of interest.

References

1. Alzainal, A.H.; Majud, A.S.; Al-Ani, A.M.; Mageet, A.O. Orthodontic Bonding: Review of the Literature. *Int. J. Dent.* **2020**, *2020*, 8874909. [CrossRef] [PubMed]
2. González-Serrano, C.; Phark, J.-H.; Fuentes, M.V.; Albaladejo, A.; Sánchez-Monescillo, A.; Duarte, S.; Ceballos, L. Effect of a single-component ceramic conditioner on shear bond strength of precoated brackets to different CAD/CAM materials. *Clin. Oral Investig.* **2021**, *25*, 1953–1965. [CrossRef] [PubMed]
3. Lopes, G.V.; Correr-Sobrinho, L.; Correr, A.B.; de Godoi, A.P.T.; Vedovello, S.A.S.; de Menezes, C.C. Light Activation and Thermocycling Methods on the Shear Bond Strength of Brackets Bonded to Porcelain Surfaces. *Braz. Dent. J.* **2020**, *31*, 52–56. [CrossRef]
4. Golshah, A.; Mohamadi, N.; Rahimi, F.; Pouyanfar, H.; Tabaii, E.; Imani, M. Shear Bond Strength of Metal Brackets to Porcelain Using a Universal Adhesive. *Med. Arch.* **2018**, *72*, 425. [CrossRef] [PubMed]
5. Gardiner, R.; Ballard, R.; Yu, Q.; Kee, E.; Xu, X.; Armbruster, P. Shear bond strength of orthodontic brackets bonded to a new all-ceramic crown composed of lithium silicate infused with zirconia: An in vitro comparative study. *Int. Orthod.* **2019**, *17*, 726–732. [CrossRef]
6. Durgesh, B.H.; Alhijji, S.; Hashem, M.I.; Al Kheraif, A.A.; Durgesh, P.; Elsharawy, M.; Vallittu, P.K. Influence of tooth brushing on adhesion strength of orthodontic brackets bonded to porcelain. *Biomed. Mater. Eng.* **2016**, *27*, 365–374. [CrossRef]

7. Juntavee, N.; Juntavee, A.; Wongnara, K.; Klomklorm, P.; Khechonnan, R. Shear bond strength of ceramic bracket bonded to different surface-treated ceramic materials. *J. Clin. Exp. Dent.* **2018**, *10*, e1167–e1176. [CrossRef]
8. Mehmeti, B.; Kelmendi, J.; Iiljazi-Shahiqi, D.; Azizi, B.; Jakovljevic, S.; Haliti, F.; Anić-Milošević, S. Comparison of Shear Bond Strength Orthodontic Brackets Bonded to Zirconia and Lithium Disilicate Crowns. *Acta Stomatol. Croat.* **2019**, *53*, 17–27. [CrossRef]
9. Tahmasbi, S.; Shiri, A.; Badiee, M. Shear bond strength of orthodontic brackets to porcelain surface using universal adhesive compared to conventional method. *Dent. Res. J. (Isfahan.)* **2020**, *17*, 19. [CrossRef]
10. Naseh, R.; Afshari, M.; Shafiei, F.; Rahnamoon, N. Shear bond strength of metal brackets to ceramic surfaces using a universal bonding resin. *J. Clin. Exp. Dent.* **2018**, *10*, e739-45. [CrossRef]
11. Pinho, M.; Manso, M.C.; Almeida, R.F.; Martin, C.; Carvalho, Ó.; Henriques, B.; Silva, F.; Pinhão Ferreira, A.; Souza, J.C.M. Bond Strength of Metallic or Ceramic Orthodontic Brackets to Enamel, Acrylic, or Porcelain Surfaces. *Materials* **2020**, *13*, 5197. [CrossRef] [PubMed]
12. Kaya, Y.; Unalan Degirmenci, B.; Degirmenci, A. Comparison of the Shear Bond Strength of Metal Orthodontic Brackets Bonded to Long-term Water-aged and Fresh Porcelain and Composite Surfaces. *Turkish J. Orthod.* **2019**, *32*, 28–33. [CrossRef] [PubMed]
13. Ghozy, E.A.; Shamaa, M.S.; El-Bialy, A.A. In vitro testing of shear bond strength of orthodontic brackets bonded to different novel CAD/CAM ceramics. *J. Dent. Res. Dent. Clin. Dent. Prospects* **2020**, *14*, 239–243. [CrossRef] [PubMed]
14. Kara, M.; Demir, O.; Dogru, M. Bond Strength of Metal and Ceramic Brackets on Resin Nanoceramic Material With Different Surface Treatments. *Turkish J. Orthod.* **2020**, *33*, 115–122. [CrossRef] [PubMed]
15. Juntavee, P.; Kumchai, H.; Juntavee, N.; Nathanson, D. Effect of Ceramic Surface Treatment and Adhesive Systems on Bond Strength of Metallic Brackets. *Int. J. Dent.* **2020**, *2020*, 7286528. [CrossRef] [PubMed]
16. Alavi, S.; Samie, S.; Raji, S.A.H. Comparison of lithium disilicate–reinforced glass ceramic surface treatment with hydrofluoric acid, Nd:YAG, and CO2 lasers on shear bond strength of metal brackets. *Clin. Oral Investig.* **2021**, *25*, 2659–2666. [CrossRef]
17. Cevik, P.; Eraslan, O.; Eser, K.; Tekeli, S. Shear bond strength of ceramic brackets to surface-treated feldspathic porcelain after thermocycling. *Int. J. Artif. Organs* **2018**, *41*, 160–167. [CrossRef]
18. Faggion, C.M. Guidelines for Reporting Pre-clinical In Vitro Studies on Dental Materials. *J. Evid. Based Dent. Pract.* **2012**, *12*, 182–189. [CrossRef]
19. Al-Hity, R.; Gustin, M.-P.; Bridel, N.; Morgon, L.; Grosgogeat, B. In vitro orthodontic bracket bonding to porcelain. *Eur. J. Orthod.* **2012**, *34*, 505–511. [CrossRef]
20. Durgesh, B.H. Experimental silane primer and grit blasting distance in orthodontic bonding of zirconia surfaces. *Ceram.-Silikaty* **2020**, *64*, 469–477. [CrossRef]
21. Mohammed, M.A.; Bhuminathan, S. A Comparative Evaluation of Shear Bond Strength of Orthodontic Brackets Bonded to Porcelain Fused Metal Crowns Treated with Different Surface Conditioning Techniques—An Invitro Study. *Indian J. Public Health Res. Dev.* **2019**, *10*, 2416. [CrossRef]
22. Dilber, E.; Aglarcı, C.; Akın, M.; Özcan, M. Adhesion of metal brackets to glassy matrix and hybrid CAD/CAM materials after different physico-chemical surface conditioning. *J. Adhes. Sci. Technol.* **2016**, *30*, 1700–1709. [CrossRef]
23. Miersch, S.; König, A.; Mehlhorn, S.; Fuchs, F.; Hahnel, S.; Rauch, A. Adhesive luting of orthodontic devices to silica-based ceramic crowns—Comparison of shear bond strength and surface properties. *Clin. Oral Investig.* **2020**, *24*, 3009–3016. [CrossRef] [PubMed]
24. Kurt, İ.; Çehreli, Z.C.; Özçırpıcı, A.A.; Şar, Ç. Biomechanical evaluation between orthodontic attachment and three different materials after various surface treatments: A three-dimensional optical profilometry analysis. *Angle Orthod.* **2019**, *89*, 742–750. [CrossRef] [PubMed]
25. Zhang, Z.; Qian, Y.; Yang, Y.; Feng, Q.; Shen, G. Bond strength of metal brackets bonded to a silica-based ceramic with light-cured adhesive. *J. Orofac. Orthop./Fortschritte der Kieferorthopädie* **2016**, *77*, 366–372. [CrossRef]
26. Recen, D.; Yıldırım, B.; Othman, E.; Çömlekoğlu, M.E.; Aras, I. Bond strength of metal brackets to feldspathic ceramic treated with different surface conditioning methods: An in vitro study. *Eur. Oral Res.* **2021**, *55*, 1–7. [CrossRef] [PubMed]
27. Mehta, A.S.; Evans, C.A.; Viana, G.; Bedran-Russo, A.; Galang-Boquiren, M.T.S. Bonding of Metal Orthodontic Attachments to Sandblasted Porcelain and Zirconia Surfaces. *Biomed Res. Int.* **2016**, *2016*, 5762785. [CrossRef]
28. Xu, Z.; Li, J.; Fan, X.; Huang, X. Bonding Strength of Orthodontic Brackets on Porcelain Surfaces Etched by Er:YAG Laser. *Photomed. Laser Surg.* **2018**, *36*, 601–607. [CrossRef]
29. Ahrari, F.; Heravi, F.; Hosseini, M. CO_2 laser conditioning of porcelain surfaces for bonding metal orthodontic brackets. *Lasers Med. Sci.* **2013**, *28*, 1091–1097. [CrossRef]
30. Mirhashemi, A.; Chiniforush, N.; Jadidi, H.; Sharifi, N. Comparative study of the effect of Er:YAG and Er;Cr:YSGG lasers on porcelain: Etching for the bonding of orthodontic brackets. *Lasers Med. Sci.* **2018**, *33*, 1997–2005. [CrossRef]
31. Girish, P.; Dinesh, U.; Bhat, C.R.; Shetty, P.C. Comparison of Shear Bond Strength of Metal Brackets Bonded to Porcelain Surface using Different Surface Conditioning Methods: An in vitro Study. *J. Contemp. Dent. Pract.* **2012**, *13*, 487–493. [CrossRef]
32. Lee, J.-Y.; Kim, J.-S.; Hwang, C.-J. Comparison of shear bond strength of orthodontic brackets using various zirconia primers. *Korean J. Orthod.* **2015**, *45*, 164. [CrossRef]
33. Ihsan, S.S.A.; Mohammed, S.A. Comparison of Shear Bond Strength of Orthodontic Buccal Tube Bonded to Zirconia Crown after Using Two Different (10-MDP)- Containing Adhesive Systems. *Int. J. Med. Res. Health Sci.* **2019**, *8*, 69–78.

34. Costa, A.R.; Correr, A.B.; Puppin-Rontani, R.M.; Vedovello, S.A.; Valdrighi, H.C.; Correr-Sobrinho, L.; Vedovello Filho, M. Effect of bonding material, etching time and silane on the bond strength of metallic orthodontic brackets to ceramic. *Braz. Dent. J.* **2012**, *23*, 223–227. [CrossRef]
35. Dalaie, K.; Mirfasihi, A.; Eskandarion, S.; Kabiri, S. Effect of bracket base design on shear bond strength to feldspathic porcelain. *Eur. J. Dent.* **2016**, *10*, 351–355. [CrossRef]
36. Kaygisiz, E.; Egilmez, F.; Ergun, G.; Yuksel, S.; Cekic-Nagas, I. Effect of different surface treatments on bond strength of recycled brackets to feldspathic porcelain. *J. Adhes. Sci. Technol.* **2016**, *30*, 45–55. [CrossRef]
37. Topcuoglu, T.; Oksayan, R.; Topcuoglu, S.; Coskun, M.E.; Isman, N.E. Effect of Er:YAG Laser Pulse Duration on Shear Bond Strength of Metal Brackets Bonded to a Porcelain Surface. *Photomed. Laser Surg.* **2013**, *31*, 240–246. [CrossRef]
38. Gonçalves, P.R.A.; de Moraes, R.R.; Costa, A.R.; Correr, A.B.; Nouer, P.R.A.; Sinhoreti, M.A.C.; Correr-Sobrinho, L. Effect of etching time and light source on the bond strength of metallic brackets to ceramic. *Braz. Dent. J.* **2011**, *22*, 245–248. [CrossRef] [PubMed]
39. Akpinar, Y.Z.; Irgin, C.; Yavuz, T.; Aslan, M.A.; Kilic, H.S.; Usumez, A. Effect of Femtosecond Laser Treatment on the Shear Bond Strength of a Metal Bracket to Prepared Porcelain Surface. *Photomed. Laser Surg.* **2015**, *33*, 206–212. [CrossRef] [PubMed]
40. Asiry, M.A.; Alshahrani, I.; Hameed, M.S.; Durgesh, B.H. Effect of Surface Conditioning Protocols and Finishing on Bonding Orthodontic Brackets to Ceramics. *J. Biomater. Tissue Eng.* **2018**, *8*, 591–596. [CrossRef]
41. Erdur, E.A.; Basciftci, F.A. Effect of Ti:sapphire laser on shear bond strength of orthodontic brackets to ceramic surfaces. *Lasers Surg. Med.* **2015**, *47*, 512–519. [CrossRef]
42. Asiry, M.A.; AlShahrani, I.; Alaqeel, S.M.; Durgesh, B.H.; Ramakrishnaiah, R. Effect of two-step and one-step surface conditioning of glass ceramic on adhesion strength of orthodontic bracket and effect of thermo-cycling on adhesion strength. *J. Mech. Behav. Biomed. Mater.* **2018**, *84*, 22–27. [CrossRef]
43. Franz, A.; Raabe, M.; Lilaj, B.; Dauti, R.; Moritz, A.; Müßig, D.; Cvikl, B. Effect of two different primers on the shear bond strength of metallic brackets to zirconia ceramic. *BMC Oral Health* **2019**, *19*, 51. [CrossRef]
44. Yu, J.; Zhang, Z.; Yang, H.; Wang, Y.; Muhetaer, A.; Lei, J.; Huang, C. Effect of universal adhesive and silane pretreatment on bond durability of metal brackets to dental glass ceramics. *Eur. J. Oral Sci.* **2021**, *129*, e12772. [CrossRef]
45. Abdelnaby, Y.L. Effects of cyclic loading on the bond strength of metal orthodontic brackets bonded to a porcelain surface using different conditioning protocols. *Angle Orthod.* **2011**, *81*, 1064–1069. [CrossRef]
46. Cevik, P.; Karacam, N.; Eraslan, O.; Sari, Z. Effects of different surface treatments on shear bond strength between ceramic systems and metal brackets. *J. Adhes. Sci. Technol.* **2017**, *31*, 1105–1115. [CrossRef]
47. Sarac, Y.S.; Kulunk, T.; Elekdag-Turk, S.; Sarac, D.; Turk, T. Effects of surface-conditioning methods on shear bond strength of brackets bonded to different all-ceramic materials. *Eur. J. Orthod.* **2011**, *33*, 667–672. [CrossRef] [PubMed]
48. Hsu, H.-M.; Chang, C.-J.; Liu, J.-K. Effects of Various Acid-Silane Surface Treatments on Bond Strength of Metal Brackets to Porcelain Crowns. *J. Med. Biol. Eng.* **2015**, *35*, 375–380. [CrossRef]
49. Durgesh, B.H.; Alhijji, S.; Hashem, M.I.; Kheraif, A.A.; Malash, A.M.; Divakar, D.D.; Shahrani, O.A.; Asmari, M.A.; Matinlinna, J.P. Evaluation of an Experimental Silane Primer System in Promoting Adhesion Between Orthodontic Bracket and Ceramic. *J. Biomater. Tissue Eng.* **2016**, *6*, 239–245. [CrossRef]
50. Bavbek, N.C.; Roulet, J.-F.; Ozcan, M. Evaluation of microshear bond strength of orthodontic resin cement to monolithic zirconium oxide as a function of surface conditioning method. *J. Adhes. Dent.* **2014**, *16*, 473–480. [CrossRef]
51. Lima Sandoval, P.C.; Ratto Tempestini Horliana, A.C.; Calabró Calheiros, F.; de Moura-Netto, C.; Gonçalves, F.; Antunes Santos, A.M.; Volpi Mello-Moura, A.C. Evaluation of shear strength in metallic brackets bonded to ceramic surface. *Chirurgia (Bucur)* **2020**, *33*, 18–23. [CrossRef]
52. Zarif Najafi, H.; Oshagh, M.; Torkan, S.; Yousefipour, B.; Salehi, R. Evaluation of the Effect of Four Surface Conditioning Methods on the Shear Bond Strength of Metal Bracket to Porcelain Surface. *Photomed. Laser Surg.* **2014**, *32*, 694–699. [CrossRef]
53. García-Sanz, V.; Paredes-Gallardo, V.; Bellot-Arcís, C.; Martínez-León, L.; Torres-Mendieta, R.; Montero, J.; Albaladejo, A. Femtosecond laser settings for optimal bracket bonding to zirconia. *Lasers Med. Sci.* **2019**, *34*, 297–304. [CrossRef]
54. Stella, J.P.F.; Oliveira, A.B.; Nojima, L.I.; Marquezan, M. Four chemical methods of porcelain conditioning and their influence over bond strength and surface integrity. *Dental Press J. Orthod.* **2015**, *20*, 51–56. [CrossRef]
55. Epperson, M.; Vazirani, N.; Armbruster, P.C.; Kee, E.L.; Xu, X.; Ballard, R.W. Hybrid crowns—Bonding protocols and shear bond strength. *Australas. Orthod. J.* **2021**, *33*, 40–47. [CrossRef]
56. Ramos, T.; Lenza, M.; Reges, R.; Freitas, G. Influence of ceramic surface treatment on shear bond strength of ceramic brackets. *Indian. J. Dent. Res.* **2012**, *23*, 789. [CrossRef]
57. Mehmeti, B.; Haliti, F.; Azizi, B.; Kelmendi, J.; Shahiqi, D.I.; Jakovljevic, S.; Milosevic, S.A. Influence of different orthodontic brackets and chemical preparations of ceramic crowns on shear bond strength. *Australas. Med. J.* **2018**, *11*, 107–112. [CrossRef]
58. Baeshen, H.A. Influence of photodynamic therapy and different conventional methods on conditioning of lithium di silicate ceramics bonded to metallic brackets: An assessment of bond strength. *Photodiagnosis Photodyn. Ther.* **2021**, *34*, 102210. [CrossRef] [PubMed]
59. Blerim, M.; Azizi, B.; Kelmendi, J.; Iljazi-Shahiqi, D.; Alar, Ž.; Anić-Milošević, S. Shear Bond Strength of Orthodontic Brackets Bonded to Zirconium Crowns. *Acta Stomatol. Croat.* **2017**, *51*, 99–105. [CrossRef]

60. Yassaei, S.; Moradi, F.; Aghili, H.; Lotfi Kamran, M.H. Shear bond strength of orthodontic brackets bonded to porcelain following etching with Er:YAG laser versus hydrofluoric acid. *Orthod. Art Pract. Dentofac. Enhanc.* **2013**, *14*, e82–e87. [CrossRef] [PubMed]
61. Hosseini, M.H.; Sobouti, F.; Etemadi, A.; Chiniforush, N.; Ayoub Bouraima, S. Scanning Electron Microscope Comparative Evaluation of Feldspathic Porcelain Surfaces under Irradiation by Different Powers of Neodymium-Doped Yttrium Aluminium Garnet (Nd:YAG) Laser. *J. lasers. Med. Sci.* **2013**, *4*, 75–78.
62. Alakuş Sabuncuoğlu, F.; Ertürk, E. Shear bond strength of brackets bonded to porcelain surface: In vitro study. *J. Istanbul. Univ. Fac. Dent.* **2016**, *50*, 9–18. [CrossRef] [PubMed]
63. Aksakalli, S.; Ileri, Z.; Yavuz, T.; Malkoc, M.A.; Ozturk, N. Porcelain laminate veneer conditioning for orthodontic bonding: SEM-EDX analysis. *Lasers Med. Sci.* **2015**, *30*, 1829–1834. [CrossRef]
64. Lestrade, A.M.; Ballard, R.W.; Xu, X.; Yu, Q.; Kee, E.L.; Armbruster, P.C. Porcelain surface conditioning protocols and shear bond strength of orthodontic brackets. *Australas. Orthod. J.* **2021**, *32*, 18–22. [CrossRef]
65. Poosti, M.; Jahanbin, A.; Mahdavi, P.; Mehrnoush, S. Porcelain conditioning with Nd:YAG and Er:YAG laser for bracket bonding in orthodontics. *Lasers Med. Sci.* **2012**, *27*, 321–324. [CrossRef]
66. AlShahrani, I.; Kamran, M.A.; Almoammar, S.; Alhaizaey, A. Photosensitization of lithium di-silicate ceramic by Er, Cr: YSGG and fractional carbon dioxide laser bonded to orthodontic bracket. *Photodiagnosis Photodyn. Ther.* **2019**, *28*, 273–276. [CrossRef]
67. May, N.B.; Araújo, É.; Vieira, L.C.C. Shear bond strength of ceramic brackets after different pre-treatments in porcelain surface. *Brazilian J. Oral Sci.* **2015**, *14*, 31–35. [CrossRef]
68. Alqerban, A. Lithium di silicate ceramic surface treated with Er,Cr:YSGG and other conditioning regimes bonded to orthodontic bracket. *Saudi Dent. J.* **2021**, *33*, 188–193. [CrossRef]
69. Elsaka, S.E. Influence of surface treatments on bond strength of metal and ceramic brackets to a novel CAD/CAM hybrid ceramic material. *Odontology* **2016**, *104*, 68–76. [CrossRef]
70. Falkensammer, F.; Freudenthaler, J.; Pseiner, B.; Bantleon, H.P. Influence of surface conditioning on ceramic microstructure and bracket adhesion. *Eur. J. Orthod.* **2012**, *34*, 498–504. [CrossRef]
71. Kim, J.; Park, C.; Lee, J.-S.; Ahn, J.; Lee, Y. The Effect of Various Types of Mechanical and Chemical Preconditioning on the Shear Bond Strength of Orthodontic Brackets on Zirconia Restorations. *Scanning* **2017**, *2017*, 6243179. [CrossRef]
72. Alaqeel, S.M. The effect of heat treatment and surface neutralization on bond strength of orthodontic brackets to lithium disilicate glass-ceramic. *J. Mech. Behav. Biomed. Mater.* **2020**, *103*, 103605. [CrossRef]
73. Di Guida, L.A.; Benetti, P.; Corazza, P.H.; Della Bona, A. The critical bond strength of orthodontic brackets bonded to dental glass–ceramics. *Clin. Oral Investig.* **2019**, *23*, 4345–4353. [CrossRef] [PubMed]
74. Martalia, C.; Anggitia, C.; Hamid, T.; Sjamsudin, J. The comparison of shear bond strength of metal orthodontics bracket to porcelain surface using silane and single bond: An in vitro study. *J. Int. Oral Health* **2020**, *12*, 470. [CrossRef]
75. Jivanescu, A.; Bratu, D.C.; Zaharia, R.; Marsavina, L. Tensile Bond Strength Evaluation of Two Adhesive Cements Used for Bonding Orthodontic Metal Brackets to Porcelain Fused-to-metal Crowns. *Mater. Plast.* **2014**, *51*, 465–467.
76. Park, K.-S.; Kim, N.-J.; Lee, C.-J.; Park, J.-H. Study on the Shear Bond Strength of Orthodontic Bracket according to the Type of Artificial Tooth Crown and Etching Method. *Int. J. Clin. Prev. Dent.* **2013**, *9*, 71–78.
77. Hellak, A.; Ebeling, J.; Schauseil, M.; Stein, S.; Roggendorf, M.; Korbmacher-Steiner, H. Shear Bond Strength of Three Orthodontic Bonding Systems on Enamel and Restorative Materials. *Biomed Res. Int.* **2016**, *2016*, 6307107. [CrossRef]
78. Grewal Bach, G.K.; Torrealba, Y.; Lagravère, M.O. Orthodontic bonding to porcelain: A systematic review. *Angle Orthod.* **2014**, *84*, 555–560. [CrossRef]
79. Garboza, C.S.; Berger, S.B.; Guiraldo, R.D.; Fugolin, A.P.P.; Gonini-Júnior, A.; Moura, S.K.; Lopes, M.B. Influence of Surface Treatments and Adhesive Systems on Lithium Disilicate Microshear Bond Strength. *Braz. Dent. J.* **2016**, *27*, 458–462. [CrossRef] [PubMed]
80. da Cunha, P.F.J.S.; Tavares, J.G.; Spohr, A.M.; Bellan, M.C.; Bueno, C.H.; Cardoso, L.I. Examining the effects of acid etching duration on the bond strength between two CAD/CAM materials and one composite resin. *Odontology* **2021**. [CrossRef]
81. May, M.M.; Fraga, S.; May, L.G. Effect of milling, fitting adjustments, and hydrofluoric acid etching on the strength and roughness of CAD-CAM glass-ceramics: A systematic review and meta-analysis. *J. Prosthet. Dent.* **2021**, in press. [CrossRef] [PubMed]
82. Caparroso Pérez, C.; Latorre Correa, F.; Arroyave Hoyos, L.J.; Grajales Gaviria, C.A.; Medina Piedrahita, V.M. In vitro evaluation of the effect of hydrofluoric acid concentration and application time on adhesion to lithium disilicate. *Rev. Fac. Odontol. Univ. Antioq.* **2014**, *26*, 62–75.
83. dos Santos, D.; Bitencourt, S.; da Silva, E.; Matos, A.; Benez, G.; Rangel, E.; Pesqueira, A.; Barão, V.; Goiato, M. Bond strength of lithium disilicate after cleaning methods of the remaining hydrofluoric acid. *J. Clin. Exp. Dent.* **2020**, *12*, e103–e107. [CrossRef]
84. Zeidan, L.C.; Esteves, C.M.; Oliveira, J.A.; Brugnera, A.; Cassoni, A.; Rodrigues, J.A. Effect of different power settings of Er,Cr:YSGG laser before or after tribosilicatization on the microshear bond strength between zirconia and two types of cements. *Lasers Med. Sci.* **2018**, *33*, 233–240. [CrossRef] [PubMed]
85. Feitosa, F.A.; de Araújo, R.M.; Tay, F.R.; Niu, L.; Pucci, C.R. Effect of high-power-laser with and without graphite coating on bonding of resin cement to lithium disilicate ceramic. *Sci. Rep.* **2017**, *7*, 17422. [CrossRef] [PubMed]

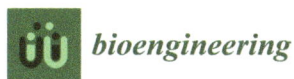 *bioengineering*

Systematic Review

The Biological Effects of 3D Resins Used in Orthodontics: A Systematic Review

Inês Francisco [1,*], Anabela Baptista Paula [1,2,3,4,5], Madalena Ribeiro [1], Filipa Marques [1], Raquel Travassos [1], Catarina Nunes [1], Flávia Pereira [1], Carlos Miguel Marto [2,3,4,5,6], Eunice Carrilho [2,3,4,5] and Francisco Vale [1]

[1] Faculty of Medicine, Institute of Orthodontics, University of Coimbra, 3004-531 Coimbra, Portugal; anabelabppaula@sapo.pt (A.B.P.); madalenaprata@hotmail.com (M.R.); filipa.p.s.marques@gmail.com (F.M.); raqueltravassos.91@gmail.com (R.T.); mcal9497@hotmail.com (C.N.); fppereira_@hotmail.com (F.P.); fvale@fmed.uc.pt (F.V.)
[2] Faculty of Medicine, Institute of Integrated Clinical Practice, University of Coimbra, 3004-531 Coimbra, Portugal; cmiguel.marto@uc.pt (C.M.M.); eunicecarrilho@gmail.com (E.C.)
[3] Faculty of Medicine, Area of Environment Genetics and Oncobiology (CIMAGO), Coimbra Institute for Clinical and Biomedical Research (iCBR), University of Coimbra, 3004-531 Coimbra, Portugal
[4] Centre for Innovative Biomedicine and Biotechnology (CIBB), University of Coimbra, 3004-531 Coimbra, Portugal
[5] Clinical Academic Center of Coimbra (CACC), 3004-531 Coimbra, Portugal
[6] Faculty of Medicine, Institute of Experimental Pathology, University of Coimbra, 3004-531 Coimbra, Portugal
* Correspondence: ines70.francisco@gmail.com

Abstract: Three-dimensional (3D) resin medical-dental devices have been increasingly used in recent years after the emergence of digital technologies. In Orthodontics, therapies with aligners have gained popularity, mainly due to the aggressive promotion policies developed by the industry. However, their systemic effects are largely unknown, with few studies evaluating the systemic toxicity of these materials. The release of bisphenol A and other residual monomers have cytotoxic, genotoxic, and estrogenic effects. This systematic review aims to analyze the release of toxic substances from 3D resins used in Orthodontics and their toxic systemic effects systematically. The PICO question asked was, "Does the use of 3D resins in orthodontic devices induce cytotoxic effects or changes in estrogen levels?". The search was carried out in several databases and according to PRISMA guidelines. In vitro, in vivo, and clinical studies were included. The in vitro studies' risk of bias was assessed using the guidelines for the reporting of pre-clinical studies on dental materials by Faggion Jr. For the in vivo studies, the SYRCLE risk of bias tool was used, and for the clinical studies, the Cochrane tool. A total of 400 articles retrieved from the databases were initially scrutinized. Fourteen articles were included for qualitative analysis. The risk of bias was considered medium to high. Cytotoxic effects or estrogen levels cannot be confirmed based on the limited preliminary evidence given by in vitro studies. Evidence of the release of bisphenol A and other monomers from 3D resin devices, either in vitro or clinical studies, remains ambiguous. The few robust results in the current literature demonstrate the absolute need for further studies, especially given the possible implications for the young patient's fertility, which constitutes one of the largest groups of patients using these orthodontic devices.

Keywords: aligner; cytotoxicity; estrogenicity; invisalign; monomer; retainer; 3D resin

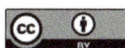

1. Introduction

Clear aligner systems have been around for many years in the Orthodontic practice; however, in recent years, the rapid development in this area led to the creation of large production facilities, increasing their availability to the population. With the launch of the Tooth Positioner (TP Orthodontics) in the mid-20th century, which allowed for only slight orthodontic movements, many advances were made within clear aligner systems to allow for more complex tooth movements and occlusal corrections [1–3]. Moreover, since Align Technology's FDA approval in 1998, the popularity of orthodontic aligners within the general public has risen, creating a market demand and increasing the number of companies that offer these services [2,4–6].

These systems improved throughout the years and also retained some advantages compared to conventional orthodontic treatment. As orthodontists treat an increasingly older population, there is a rise in aesthetic concerns, favoring the use of these systems [1,2]. Another advantage is that the clear aligner systems were noted by Cardoso et al. [7] to be less painful when compared to the conventional bracket system. Reduced chair time and fewer emergencies are also listed as advantages, and treatment time seems to decrease compared to conventional systems, albeit only in mild to moderate and non-extraction cases [8,9]. Regarding oral hygiene, there is no consensual standpoint as some authors describe similar outcomes in aligner and conventional bracket patients, and others observe better hygiene and less plaque build-up in aligner patients and fewer enamel lesions as a result [3–6,8].

Although some of the clear aligner systems may seem to replace conventional appliances completely, these systems also present some drawbacks compared to their older counterparts [1]. Some studies indicate that clear aligner systems are less effective in controlling anterior buccolingual inclination and rotation movements in rounder teeth, and some difficulties may also be experienced to establish ideal occlusal contacts. As mentioned above, although general treatment time is decreased, in extraction cases, it is increased when compared to conventional systems [1,4,5,8,9]. As recently as 2020, concerns about the toxicity of clear aligners rose depending on their fabrication method. Studies revealed that the plastics used in clear aligner systems might have adverse effects on the activity and viability of the gingival cells and severe reproductive toxicity in an in vitro environment, highlighting potential future risks of their use in humans [10,11].

These devices are made using thermoformed, which is usually made with polyurethane with an integrated elastomer, or 3D printed plastics through different processes. Each of these manufacturing techniques presents its own set of advantages and handicaps. For example, the thermoformed method produces aligners with an irregular thickness which can create difficulties within the treatment itself. This approach is also associated with increased cytotoxicity, which is most likely due to the heating process required during the fabrication process [3,10]. As for the 3D printed plastics, these are thought to be less unsustainable and cheaper in the long run. The 3D printed plastics manufacturing method uses computer-aided design and computer-aided manufacturing technology (CAD/CAM) through additive methods (adding layers successively), subtractive methods (grinding or milling of industrially prefabricated materials), or through liquid materials (e.g., stereolithography). Although they are usually fabricated with highly cytotoxic materials such as polymethyl methacrylate (PMMA), the curing process seems to reduce this incidence but not eliminate it completely [2,3,12,13]. However, these findings are not consensual. Post processing procedures of these devices (e.g., polishing) or their sterilization (e.g., autoclaving or gamma irradiation) can also remove the uncured monomer. However, these procedures can lead to a decrease in mechanical strength. Incomplete conversion of monomers into polymers, with a marked decrease in the degree of conversion, can enhance the release of monomers, namely methyl methacrylate (MMA), triethylene glycol dimethacrylate (TEGDMA), 2-hydroxyethyl methacrylate (HEMA), and bisphenol A glycidyl methacrylate (Bis-GMA) [14,15]. These monomers can induce local negative effects such as cytotoxicity and mutagenicity, and systemic ones such as teratogenicity and estrogenicity [16–18]. Degradation and metabolization of these monomers can cause irreversible damage to cellular DNA. Other authors demonstrated the induction of glutathione sequestration and an increase in oxidative stress [19,20]. These phenomena can lead to changes in the cell cycle and eventually cell death by apoptosis [21–23]. Rogers et al. [11] reported severe reproductive toxicity after exposing murine oocytes to the materials used in clear aligner manufacturing regardless of their ISO-certification of biocompatibility or marketing ploys. On the opposite side, Eliades et al. [10] found no cytotoxicity from aligners (Invisalign) after soaking them in a saline solution for two months in a glass container set at 37 °C. These are both stand-alone research projects that have not been replicated, making it impossible for comparisons.

The purpose of this review is to assess the release of toxic substances from 3D resins used in Orthodontics and their toxic systemic effects.

2. Materials and Methods

This systematic review was registered in PROSPERO with the ID 282126 number and was drawn up following the Preferring Items for Systematic and Meta-Analyses and Meta-Analyses (PRISMA) guidelines. The Population, Intervention, Comparison, and Outcome (PICO) question asked was "Does the use of 3D resins in orthodontic devices induce cytotoxic effects or changes in estrogen levels?".

The literature search was carried out in several databases such as PubMed (www.ncbi.nlm.nih.gov/pubmed), Cochrane Library (www.cochranelibrary.com), Scopus (www.scopus.com), Web of Science Core Collection (webofknowledge.com/WOS), and EMBASE (www.embase.com).

The last search was performed on 1 September 2021, and the language filter was applied: English, Portuguese, and Spanish. The search formula for the PubMed database was: ("3D resins" OR "3D print *" OR "invisalign" OR "Suresmile" OR "essix" OR "aligners" OR "thermoplastic aligner" OR "vacuum-formed retainer" OR "clear aligner" OR "orthodontic aligners") AND ("bisphenol-A" OR "BPA" OR "monomer" OR "release" OR "ethoxylated bisphenol A-dimethacrylate" OR "Bis-EMA" OR "urethane dimethacrylate" OR "UDMA" OR "triethylene glycol dimethacrylate" OR "TEGDMA" OR "polyethylene glycol diacrylate" OR "PEGDA") AND ("estrogenicity" OR estrogen OR "toxicity"[Subheading] OR toxicity[Text Word] OR "cytotoxicity"). Similar search formulas were used for the remaining databases. The references of the included studies were searched for additional relevant studies.

Three independent reviewers scrutinized the studies by title and abstract. Potential eligible studies were selected in accordance with the defined inclusion criteria: in vitro, in vivo, ex vivo, and clinical studies; and studies evaluating the release monomers from 3D resins such as 3D printed or thermoformed orthodontic devices. Studies that only presented a chemical analysis of the aligners or considerations about the synthesis of the polymers that constitute them were excluded. Studies describing fixed orthodontic retainers with composite resins were also excluded. Two external elements were consulted in case of doubt or in the absence of consensus.

After the eligibility process, the articles were divided into categories according to the study type: in vitro, in vivo, or clinical. For each, the following information was extracted: author and date, study design, fabrication technique, resin composition, cell line type, sample size, test group, exposure time, assay type, results, and main conclusions. In addition, for the in vivo and clinical studies, the intervention group (time of use), study measure, and the outcome data were also recorded.

The in vitro studies' risk of bias was assessed using the guidelines for the reporting of pre-clinical studies on dental materials by Faggion Jr. [24]. For the in vivo studies, the Systematic Review Centre for Laboratory animal Experimentation (SYRCLE) risk of bias tool was used. For the clinical studies, the Cochrane tool was used.

3. Results

The search, scrutiny, and eligibility processes are described in Figure 1. The initial search resulted in 400 articles, to which five papers identified in cross-references were added. After removing the duplicates, 283 articles remained. These were scrutinized by title and abstract, resulting in 24 papers. Finally, 19 studies were read in full, and fourteen articles were included in the qualitative assessment, from which several data were analyzed, and the study of bias was carried out. The disparity of methodologies and different types of aligners/splints did not allow a quantitative analysis, so a meta-analysis was not carried out.

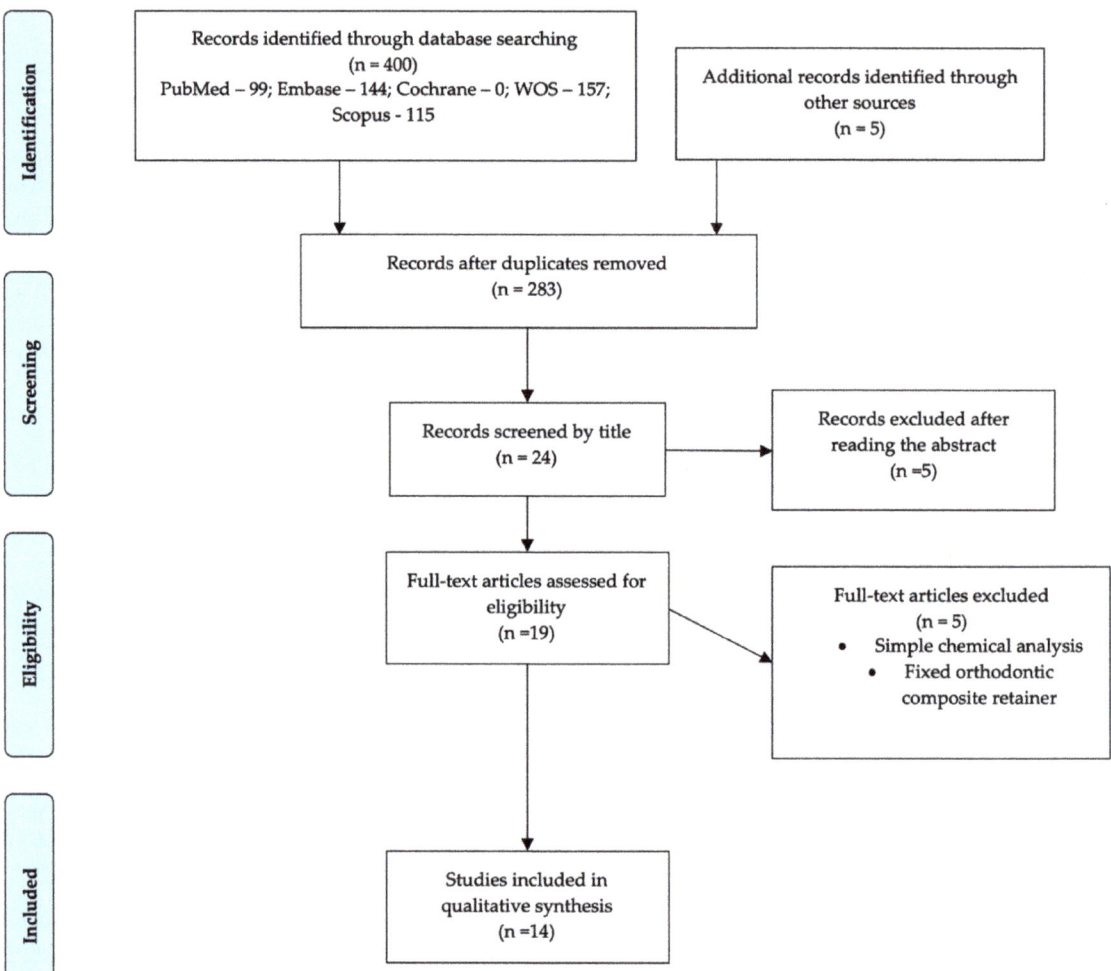

Figure 1. Flow Diagram of the eligibility of publication scrutiny according to PRISMA guidelines.

3.1. Cytotoxicity Evaluation

Of the 14 studies included in the qualitative analysis, one was a clinical study (RCT), one was an in vivo model, and the remaining 12 were in vitro studies. To assess cytotoxicity in vitro studies, those using cell lines, cell cultures, or a chemical analysis of extracts were included [10,11,25–34]. This evaluation was carried out through several assays, namely, the MTT assay, XTT assay, morphology, mass spectroscopy, gas chromatography, among others.

With the in vivo studies, the evaluation of cytotoxicity was carried out through the investigation of chemical and metallic elements in blood samples after exposure to aligners [35]. Similarly, in the included RCT, BPA levels in saliva samples from individuals exposed to aligners were assessed [36].

3.1.1. In Vitro Studies

The materials used in the included studies are thermoformable resins, either printed on 3D devices or made with cold acrylics manually (Table 1). The methodology of in vitro studies is very diverse. Some studies only chemically assess the release of monomers into the medium through the extracts technique [10,25,26,28–30,32–34]. Most use these enriched media to assess their effect on cell culture through indirect contact assays. The cell lines used are mostly fibroblasts [10,27,32,33], progenitor cells such as oocytes, or estrogen sensitive cell lines [10,11,30]. Other studies also mechanically assess structural changes in aligners or retainers. Most studies report the release of monomers, especially bisphenol A (BPA), from all the devices. In some of them, these values are below the levels considered toxic. Thermoformable devices have lower monomer release values than those 3D printed, and devices made manually with heat polymerization. Another study by Alifui et al. states that only resinous materials, whether thermoformable or 3D printed, with authorization to be used for medical devices, should be recommended [34].

3.1.2. In Vivo Studies

The animal study included in the systematic review evaluated some metals' levels after using aligners or retainers in Wistar rats (Table 2). The evaluation was carried out using blood samples after several times of use. This study concluded an increase in metal levels, mainly with retainers, but they are not considered toxic. Furthermore, there is a decrease in these elements' levels after 2 weeks. Although conducted in an animal model, this study makes an extrapolation to the levels in humans, supporting that its clinical use is safe [35].

3.1.3. Clinical Studies

As mentioned above, only one clinical study evaluated the monomers' release after retainer placement (Table 3) [36]. This analysis measured BPA levels in the patients' saliva before placement and after 1 day, 1 week, and 1 month. All retainer types show increased levels of BPA, but only thermoformable retainers (VFRs) show statistically significant increases. Hawley retainers, either thermal or chemical polymerize, are the most recommended for clinical use.

3.2. Risk of Bias

The quality assessment of the in vitro and in vivo studies is summarized in Figures 2 and 3, respectively. Concerning in vitro studies, only one study [30] reported the process of allocation sequence generation. All in vitro studies did not describe the mechanism used to implement the random allocation sequence, how researchers were blinded after assignment to the intervention, and where the full trial protocol can be accessed. All studies stated objectives and/or hypotheses except for two [11,34]. Regarding the in vivo study, half of the items evaluated were not presented (allocation concealment, random housing, caregiver and/or researcher blinding, random outcome assessment, and outcome assessor blinding) [35].

The included RCT was considered to have a high risk of bias due to deviations from the randomization process and intended interventions (Figure 4) [36].

Table 1. Summary of parameters and results from in vitro included studies.

Authors, Year	Study Design	Fabrication Technique	Resin Composition	Cell Line	Sample Size (n)	Test Group	Time	Assay Type	Results	Conclusions
Eliades T. et al., 2009 [10]	Extract Technique	Thermoformed	Invisalign appliances	Cytotoxicity Human gingival fibroblasts; Estrogenicity MCF-7: Estrogen-sensitive MDA-MB-231 human breast adenocarcinoma—estrogen-insensitive.	3 sets of aligners; n = 6 (96 aligner eluents per group).	Test group: invisalign at 5%, 10%, 20%; Control group: Vehicle at 5%, 10%, 20%.	2 months	Cytotoxicity (by modification of the MTT assay); Estrogenicity (assays involved 2 cell lines: MCF-7 and MDA-MB-231).	Cytotoxicity (optical density of human gingival fibroblasts); Estrogenicity was assessed by the proliferation of MCF-7 and MDA-MB-231.	No cytotoxicity or estrogenic activity of Invisalign appliances was documented in this in vitro assay.
Kurzmann C. et al., 2017 [27]	Direct and indirect contact	Resins for Stereolithographic 3D-Printed	Clear resin (FLGPCL02), Dental SG resin (FLDGOR01)	L929 cell line, Human gingiva fibroblasts	n = 96-well culture plates	Test group: Clear (exposed to printed Clear resin) and Dental SG (exposed to Dental SG resin); Control group: W/O (untreated control).	24 h	Macroscopic and scanning electron microscopy.	When exposed to the materials, the cellular activity of L929 cells and gingival fibroblasts was observed.	The impact of Clear and Dental SG resins depends on the processing stage of the material.
Rogers H. et al., 2021 [11]	Ex vivo + in vitro (direct and indirect)	3D-printed using Form 2 SLA printers	Dental SG (DSG-FLDGOR01, Lot Nos. XN232N05, XK244N01, XK242N01, XK25N01, XH084N05) and Dental LT Clear (DLT-FLDLCL01, Lot Nos. XK484N02, XH043N02, XK29N02).	Mouse oocytes	n = 540	Test group: DSG and DLT wells; Control group: polystyrene control.	168 h	Mass spectroscopy	Exposure to DSG and DLT was proved to induce rapid mammalian oocyte degeneration in vitro.	The use of two 3DP resins revealed severe reproductive toxicity.
Kessler A. et al., 2020 [28]	Extract technique	3D-printed using Rapidshape D20 II (RS), Solflex 350 (SF), Form2 (Form).	3Delta Guide (UDMA, TMPTA, TPO); Freeprint Splint (Acrylated resin, Aliphatic urethane acrylate, TPGDA, THMA, TPO); Fotodent Guide (BIS-EMA, Acrylresin, HEMA, HPMA, Monoester with 1,2-Propandiol, TPO); Nextdent SG (Methacrylic oligomers, Phosphine oxide); V-printed SG (BIS-EMA, UDMA, TPO).	Chemical analysis: Eluted in methanol and water for 3 days.	n = 4	Not reported	3 days	Finnigan Trace GC ultra gas chromatograph connected to a DSQ mass spectrometer.	The elution in methanol (total of twelve) and water (total of four) detected the release of substances.	The material and the printing device have a significant influence on the release of monomers from 3D-printed surgical guides.

Table 1. Cont.

Authors, Year	Study Design	Fabrication Technique	Resin Composition	Cell Line	Sample Size (n)	Test Group	Time	Assay Type	Results	Conclusions
Kotyk M. et al., 2014 [29]	Extract technique	Thermoformed	Biocryl Essix (prethermoformed and thermoformed); Biocryl Retainer (prethermoformed and thermoformed); Dentsply Raintree Essix (prethermoformed), Dentsply Essix (thermoformed), Invisalign aligner (unused and used).	Chemical analysis: Eluted in artificial saliva; Bisphenol-A (BPA) leached from orthodontic materials.	n = 8 retainer materials, cut into pieces of an unspecified number.	Not reported	2 weeks	Gas chromatography/mass spectroscopy (GC-MS).	In the first 3 days of artificial saliva immersion, BPA leaching was observed.	- BPA was found to leach from thermoformed Biocryl acrylic resin retainer material; - BPA was below the reference dose for daily intake; - evidence suggests the patient BPA exposure should be minimized or even eliminated.
Naqbi A. et al., 2018 [30]	Indirect contact (extract technique)	Thermoformed	Vivera retainers (from the manufacturer and after retrieved from patients).	Estrogen-sensitive MCF-7 Estrogen-insensitive MDA-MB-231.	n = 12 (6 or each of the two groups; 48 aligner eluents per group).	Test group: retainers sterilized with gamma-irradiation, retainers sterilized with autoclaving; Control group: retainers not subjected to any sterilization mode.	14 days	Cytotoxicity and Estrogenicity.	No significant proliferation of MCF-7, and MDA-MB-231 cells were induced by the three samples.	- Vivera retainers did not seem to exhibit cytotoxicity or estrogenic activity; - Vivera retainers can be used as part-time removable oral appliances following the manufacturer's instructions.
Schuster S. et al., 2004 [31]	Mechanical test	Thermoformed	Invisalign appliances	Mechanical analysis	n = 10 samples of aligners before intraoral placement and after retrieval; n = 12 samples of same aligners after placement intraorally for 22hours for 2 weeks.	Not reported	2 weeks	Reflection microscopy, FTIR, scanning electron microscopy, Vickers hardness, Gas chromatography-mass spectroscopy (GC-MS).	Retrieved Invisalign appliance shows a morphological variation (Reflection microscopy, FTIR, scanning electron microscopy, Vickers hardness). Substance leaching (GC-MS): no residual monomers or oxidative byproducts were detected.	No definitive consensus on the reactivity and biological properties can be established.

Table 1. *Cont.*

Authors, Year	Study Design	Fabrication Technique	Resin Composition	Cell Line	Sample Size (n)	Test Group	Time	Assay Type	Results	Conclusions
Xu Y. et al., 2021 [32]	Mechanical test Direct contact test + extract test	Stereolithographically (SLA) printed	Dental LT Clear resin (UDMA, HEMA, EGDMA, HPA)	L929 mouse fibroblasts	n = 12	Not reported	Mechanical test—12 h Direct and indirect—12 h, 24 h, 72 h	Flexural strength test Scanning electron microscopy Metabolic activity.	No alterations were detected on the samples for less than 1 h. When post-rising prolonged to 12 h could be observed surface fissures.	The removal of cytotoxic methacrylate monomers by post rinsing could be achieved in 5 min. Further extending the post-rinsing time did not improve the cytocompatibility but rather reduced the flexural strength of the SLA-printed acrylic. - If the 3D printed material is mistakenly post-rinsed overnight(12 h), the resulting surface defects and strength reduction may not be acceptable.
Wedekind L. et al., 2021 [33]	Indirect contact	Additive manufacturing (3D-printing; SHERAprint-ortho plus); Subtractive manufacturing (SHERAeco-disc PM20); Conventional manufacturing (SHERAORTHOMER).	Polymethyl methacrylate (PMMA) (THFMA, BDDMA, TPGDA).	Human gingival fibroblasts	Not reported	Each sample eluted with water and methanol	24 h and 72 h	GC/MS analysis XTT based cell viability assay.	With the solvent methanol, the released components exceeded the cytotoxic concentrations; In water eluates, only THFMA was determined from SHERAprint-ortho plus in concentrations of non-cytotoxic levels.	With the solvent methanol, released components from the investigated splint materials exceeded cytotoxic concentrations in HGFs calculated for a worst-case scenario in splint size. In the water eluates, only the methacrylate THFMA could be determined from SHERAprint-ortho plus in concentrations below cytotoxic levels in HGFs. Therefore, in the physiological (water/saliva) situation, a health risk is of minor relevance.

Table 1. *Cont.*

Authors, Year	Study Design	Fabrication Technique	Resin Composition	Cell Line	Sample Size (n)	Test Group	Time	Assay Type	Results	Conclusions
Alifui-Segbaya F. et al., 2018 [34]	Indirect contact (extract technique)	EnvisionTec's digital processing (DLP) and Formlab's reverse stereolithography (SL) systems	E-Denture (ED), E-Guard (EG), Dental SG (DSG) methacrylates.	Zebrafish embryo model	n = 10	- E-Denture (ED); - E-Guard (EG); - Dental SG (DSG) methacrylates; - control.	96 h and 120 h	FTIR spectroscopy	Biocompatibility was influenced by physicochemical characteristics of materials.	- Despite the twofold increase in DC (%) for nTx EG, it was unsafe in zebrafish bioassays; hence there is a limited correlation between conversion rate and biological performance. - The study concludes that it is preferable to use approved materials, apposite manufacturing parameters, and post-processing techniques that together ensure optimal results for medical devices.
Kopperud H. et al., 2011 [25]	Extract technique	Heat-cure (Orthocryl). Light-cured (Triad VLC), Thermoplastic (Biocryl C, Essix A+, Essix Embrace) resins.	Methyl methacrylate (MMA), acetonitrile, ammonium acetate, 2,4-dinitro-phenylhydrazine (DNPH), distilled water, 2-hydroxyethyl methacrylate (2-HEMA), methanol and UDMA.	Chemical analysis: Eluted in formaldehyde	n = 5	Not reported	10 days	Gas chromatography/mass spectroscopy (GC-MS) and liquid chromatography/mass spectrometry.	Leaching methacrylate monomers from prefabricated thermoplastic plates are lower than those from powder-and-liquid-based material and from paste material.	Orthodontic prefabricated thermoplastic plates should be preferred.
Nakano H. et al., 2019 [26]	Indirect contact	3D-printed	Acrylic-epoxy hybrid light-curing resins	Not reported	n = 8	Okamoto Chemicals (3D-1M: 1); NextDent (Ortho Clear); ISO20795-2	24 h and 72 h	Cellular toxicity LDH-test Cell Viability WST1 test Mechanical experiments Stereolithography.	Have successfully developed a 3D biocompatible resin, without cellular toxicity but with not yet ideal mechanical properties.	Achieved a biocompatible 3D-printed resin that releases no toxic materials to humans or the environment.

Table 2. Summary of parameters and results from in vivo included studies.

Authors, Year	Study Design	Sample Size (n)	Test Groups	Fabrication Technique	Resin Composition	Outcome Time	Study Measure Outcome	Results	Conclusions
Chen S. et al., 2016 [35]	In vivo	Mini-screw implant + thermoplastic sample Wistar (n = 80).	Test group of aligner (n = 30); Test group of retainer (n = 30); Control group (n = 10); Blank group (n = 10).	Thermoformed	- Invisalign Smart Track aligners; - Erkodur retainers.	T1: 28 days; T2: 56 days; T3: 112 days.	0.5 mL blood samples (rat orital vein); Inductively coupled plasma mass spectrometry (ICP-MS).	- Al, Ti, V, Cr, Fe, Co, Ni, Cu, Zn were detected in polymeric retainers; - Al, Ni, Zn, Sn were detected in polymeric aligners.	- The metal elements in polymeric materials evaluated in blood did not exceed toxic values; - The identified element levels decrease after 2 weeks.

Table 3. Summary of parameters and results from clinical included studies.

Authors, Year	Study Design	Sample Size (n, Sex)	Control Group	Intervention Group (Time of Use)	Fabrication Technique	Resin Composition	Outcome Time (Hours)	Study Measure Outcome	Results	Conclusions
Raghavan A. et al., 2017 [36]	RCT	n = 45: G1(n = 15); G2(n = 15); G3(n = 15. Sex: not reported	Not reported	T0: before placement; T1: 1h after placement; T2: 7 days after placement; T3: 30 days after placement.	G1: Biostar vacuum thermoforming system (VFR); G2: Hawley retainer Heat cure method; G3: Hawley retainer Chemical cure method (in both arches).	G1: Essix ACE Plastic Vacuum-formed retainers (VFRs); G2: DPI Heat Cure Hawley retainers (compression molding technique); G3: DPI Cold Cure chemical cure ("sprinkle" on technique).	180 saliva samples T0: Group 1—0.00001 ± 0.0001, Group 2—0.00006 ± 0.00004, Group 3—0.00009 ± 0.00006; T1: Group 1—1.20236 ± 0.35643, Group 2—0.00091 ± 0.00081, Group 3—0.06031 ± 0.02550; T2: Group 1—2.38420 ± 1.79714, Group 2—0.00045 ± 0.00008, Group 3—0.00363 ± 0.00050; T3: Group 1—0.020396 ± 0.08709, Group 2—0.00067 ± 0.001410, Group 3—0.00934 ± 0.00237.	BPA levels in the saliva	BPA levels: G1: T1 > T0 (+1.20 ppm); T2 > T1 (+1.18 ppm); T3 < T2 (−2.18 ppm); G2 and G3: T1 > T0; T2 < T3; T3 > T2.	- Increases BPA levels in saliva in all groups after placement of the retainers; - BPA levels were found to be larger in VFRs, followed by Hawley retainers by chemical cure, and finally Hawley retainers by heat cure; - VFRs increase BPA levels after placement to 1 week but decrease after 1 month; - Hawleys retainers (heat and chemical) decrease after placement to 1 week but increase after 1 month.

Study		Structured summary	Scientific background and rationale	Objectives and/or hypotheses	Intervention of each group	Outcomes definition	Sample size determination	Allocation sequence generation	Allocation concealment mechanism	Implementation	Blinding	Statistical methods	Outcomes and estimation	Limitations	Funding information	Protocol (if available)
Al Naqbi et al., 2018		Y	Y	Y	Y	Y	N	Y	N	N	N	Y	N	N	N	N
Kotyk et al., 2014		Y	Y	Y	Y	Y	N	N	N	N	N	N	N	N	N	N
Kessler et al., 2020		Y	Y	Y	Y	N	N	N	N	N	N	Y	N	N	N	N
Eliades et al., 2009		Y	Y	Y	Y	Y	N	N	N	N	N	Y	N	Y	N	N
Kopperud et al., 2010		Y	Y	Y	Y	Y	N	N	N	N	N	Y	Y	N	Y	N
Nakano et al., 2019		Y	Y	Y	Y	N	N	N	N	N	N	N	N	Y	N	N
Schuster et al., 2004		Y	Y	Y	Y	Y	N	N	N	N	N	N	N	Y	N	N
Wedekind et al., 2021		Y	Y	Y	Y	Y	N	N	N	N	N	Y	N	N	Y	N
Xu et al., 2021		Y	Y	Y	Y	Y	N	N	N	N	N	Y	Y	N	N	N
Kurzmann et al., 2017		Y	Y	Y	Y	Y	N	N	N	N	N	Y	N	Y	Y	N
Rogers et al., 2021		Y	Y	N	Y	Y	N	N	N	N	N	Y	N	N	N	N
Alifui-Segbaya et al., 2018		Y	Y	N	Y	Y	N	N	N	N	N	Y	N	N	Y	N

Y-Yes; N-No

Figure 2. Risk of bias of the in vitro studies.

Study	Domain	
Cheng et al., 2016	Sequence generation	U
	Baseline characteristics	Y
	Allocation concealment	N
	Random housing	N
	Caregiver and/or researcher blinding	N
	Random outcome assessment	N
	Outcome assessor blinding	N
	Incomplete outcome data	U
	Selective outcome reporting	Y
	Other sources	Y

U-unclear; Y-Yes; N-No

Figure 3. Risk of bias of the in vivo study.

Study	Domain	
Raghavan et al., 2017	Bias arising from the randomization process	H
	Bias due to deviations from the intended interventions	H
	Bias due to missing outcome data	L
	Bias in the measurement of the outcome	SC
	Bias in selection of the reported result	SC
	Overall bias	H

H-High; L-Low; SC- Some concerns

Figure 4. Risk of bias of the RCT study.

4. Discussion

The present systematic review is set to appraise the release of toxic substances from 3D resins used in Orthodontics and its toxic systemic effects [11,13].

The development of 3D printing and advancements made in biocompatible resin materials propelled an expeditious evolution in several areas of Medicine. Nonetheless, the cytotoxic potential of 3D printed products is yet to be comprehensively researched as there is currently scarce information on this subject, and publications do not seem to reach consensual conclusions [37]. According to Eliades et al. [10], when assessing Invisalign's cytotoxicity and estrogenicity, there were no discerning results regarding these biological effects. These results are confirmed by Iliadi et al. [37] in their systematic review of clinical and in vitro research of thermoplastic materials used in clear aligner systems, which did not report there were proven cytotoxic or estrogenic effects associated with these devices. These results agree with the findings of this systematic review. However, the qualitative report of the included studies did not allow for the establishment of a definitive consensus on the reactivity and biological properties of the clear aligners. The disparity between the results of the included studies can be explained by the methodological differences across the studies, namely the absence of sample randomization, intervention protocols, and follow-up times (varying from 24 h to 2 months).

Kurzmann et al. [27] studied the biocompatibility and the response of the oral soft tissues to 3D printed resins. This study was set out to reveal whether 3D printed resins such as Clear Resin and Dental SG resin have an impact on human gingival fibroblasts at different processing stages. It was later concluded that the effect depends on the processing stage; in a liquid stage, the clear resin was shown to be more impactful in cell activity when compared to Dental SG resin. The in vitro study by Kopperud et al. [25] analyzed leachable monomers, additives, and degradation products from three different kinds of materials (heat-cured resin, light-cure resin, and thermoplastic) and concluded that thermoplastic materials are the least leachable out of the three.

Presently, there are concerns regarding environmental pollution promoted by the excessive use of plastics and how this affects most, if not all, ecosystems, and, in turn, how these man-made disruptions affect human health. Over time, plastic can degrade, generating micro- or nanoparticles, which leads to a plastic additives release and the absorption of environmental chemicals. This breakdown means that humans and other animals are constantly exposed to these particles through their own food or water sources, possibly causing endocrine disruption and other issues associated with plastic toxicity [38–40]. In addition, with the increased use of these systems and a varying number of aligners per patient, there is a rising sustainability concern, as the materials used in their fabrication are non-recyclable. Rogers et al. [11] evaluated the cytotoxic potential of 3D printed dental resins using mouse oocytes in vivo. The tested resins were Dental SG resins (DSG) and Dental LT Clear (DLT), classified as biocompatible for medical use and currently used in dental surgical guides and oral retainers. This publication concluded that although these resins are considered biocompatible, they exhibit reproductive toxicity in mouse oocytes after direct and indirect exposure.

The articles that were included in this paper have inherent limitations. With reviews such as these, one must always account for bias risks, as different methodologies were used, assessment criteria, and accessibility to the literature. For instance, some studies compare the conventional bracket system with clear aligners with no consideration for the severity of the malocclusion nor patient cooperation, which can lead to uneven results when such studies are replicated, which is not possible many times, fueling the current replication crisis we face as investigators in a scientific field [5,9]. Furthermore, the aging of clear aligners in the oral cavity is not equal to in vitro conditions since the intra-oral environment can expose the aligners to various heat shocks, as from the ingestion of hot drinks. The oral cavity also has an alkaline environment that might promote BPA release [10]. However, identifying BPA release in clinical studies is a complex evaluation, as it requires ethical considerations.

It should also be considered that most patients using aligners are in their reproductive years. Although most of the studies report that the monomers' release is below the toxic level, these systems require a constant change of trays, thus exposing the same individual to additive sources of BPA regularly [31].

Given the lack of literature on this subject, it is necessary to conduct further studies with similar methods focusing on the same aligner manufacturing processes and resin composition to achieve more homogeneous results, matching protocols and setting evaluation timings. Most articles published are based on in vitro studies, and despite their scientific contribution, in vivo and mainly clinical studies are required since there is increasing utilization of these systems. While further studies are not available, the orthodontists must act with caution, using the aligners for simple cases that require short treatment periods or only in non-fertile ages. In addition, orthodontists should advise patients not to ingest hot foods and instruct them on how to correctly care for the aligners to avoid the release of cytotoxic monomers.

5. Conclusions

Within the scope of this review, it was noted that studies evaluating the biological effects of 3D resins in orthodontics are mostly conducted in vitro. Although mixed results are described, 3D printed aligners may present higher levels of cytotoxicity and genotoxicity when compared to thermoplastic resins, particularly those that have not been subjected to a final surface treatment. As such, clinical studies analyzing saliva, blood, or even urine samples must be carried out in the future to determine the levels of monomers released in humans upon the use of these devices.

Author Contributions: Conceptualization, A.B.P. and I.F.; methodology, C.M.M. and E.C.; acquisition of data, R.T., C.N. and F.P.; software, C.M.M.; validation, C.N., R.T. and M.R.; formal analysis, F.P.; investigation, F.V.; resources, I.F. and C.M.M.; data curation, E.C.; writing—original draft preparation, A.B.P., F.M. and M.R.; writing—review and editing, A.B.P., I.F., C.M.M., F.V., F.M. and M.R.; visualization, C.N., R.T. and F.P.; supervision, F.V. and E.C.; project administration, F.V.; funding acquisition, E.C. All authors have read and agreed to the published version of the manuscript.

Funding: This research received no external funding.

Institutional Review Board Statement: Not Applicable.

Informed Consent Statement: Not Applicable.

Data Availability Statement: The data presented in this study are available on request from the corresponding author.

Conflicts of Interest: The authors declare no conflict of interest.

References

1. Kassam, S.K.; Stoops, F.R. Are clear aligners as effective as conventional fixed appliances? *Evid. Based Dent.* **2020**, *21*, 30–31. [CrossRef]
2. Weir, T. Clear aligners in orthodontic treatment. *Aust. Dent. J.* **2017**, *62*, 58–62. [CrossRef] [PubMed]
3. Maspero, C.; Tartaglia, G.M. 3D Printing of Clear Orthodontic Aligners: Where We Are and Where We Are Going. *Materials* **2020**, *13*, 5204. [CrossRef]
4. Borda, A.F.; Garfinkle, J.S.; Covell, D.A.; Wang, M.; Doyle, L.; Sedgley, C.M. Outcome assessment of orthodontic clear aligner vs fixed appliance treatment in a teenage population with mild malocclusions. *Angle Orthod.* **2020**, *90*, 485–490. [CrossRef]
5. Zheng, M.; Liu, R.; Ni, Z.; Yu, Z. Efficiency, effectiveness and treatment stability of clear aligners: A systematic review and meta-analysis. *Orthod. Orthod. Res.* **2017**, *20*, 127–133. [CrossRef] [PubMed]
6. Tamer, I.; Oztas, E.; Marsan, G. Orthodontic Treatment with Clear Aligners and The Scientific Reality Behind Their Marketing: A Literature Review. *Turkish J. Orthod.* **2019**, *32*, 241–246. [CrossRef] [PubMed]
7. Cardoso, P.C.; Espinosa, D.G.; Mecenas, P.; Flores-Mir, C.; Normando, D. Pain level between clear aligners and fixed appliances: A systematic review. *Prog. Orthod.* **2020**, *21*, 3. [CrossRef] [PubMed]
8. Ke, Y.; Zhu, Y.; Zhu, M. A comparison of treatment effectiveness between clear aligner and fixed appliance therapies. *BMC Oral Health* **2019**, *19*, 24. [CrossRef]

9. Rossini, G.; Parrini, S.; Castroflorio, T.; Deregibus, A.; Debernardi, C.L. Efficacy of clear aligners in controlling orthodontic tooth movement: A systematic review. *Angle Orthod.* **2015**, *85*, 881–889. [CrossRef]
10. Eliades, T.; Pratsinis, H.; Athanasiou, A.E.; Eliades, G.; Kletsas, D. Cytotoxicity and estrogenicity of Invisalign appliances. *Am. J. Orthod. Dentofac. Orthop.* **2009**, *136*, 100–103. [CrossRef] [PubMed]
11. Rogers, H.B.; Zhou, L.T.; Kusuhara, A.; Zaniker, E.; Shafaie, S.; Owen, B.C.; Duncan, F.E.; Woodruff, T.K. Dental resins used in 3D printing technologies release ovo-toxic leachates. *Chemosphere* **2021**, *270*, 129003. [CrossRef] [PubMed]
12. Tartaglia, G.M.; Mapelli, A.; Maspero, C.; Santaniello, T.; Serafin, M.; Farronato, M.; Caprioglio, A. Direct 3D Printing of Clear Orthodontic Aligners: Current State and Future Possibilities. *Materials* **2021**, *14*, 1799. [CrossRef]
13. Park, J.-H.; Lee, H.; Kim, J.-W.; Kim, J.-H. Cytocompatibility of 3D printed dental materials for temporary restorations on fibroblasts. *BMC Oral Health* **2020**, *20*, 157. [CrossRef] [PubMed]
14. Saeed, F.; Muhammad, N.; Khan, A.S.; Sharif, F.; Rahim, A.; Ahmad, P.; Irfan, M. Prosthodontics dental materials: From conventional to unconventional. *Mater. Sci. Eng. C* **2020**, *106*, 110167. [CrossRef]
15. Ali, U.; Karim, K.J.B.A.; Buang, N.A. A Review of the Properties and Applications of Poly (Methyl Methacrylate) (PMMA). *Polym. Rev.* **2015**, *55*, 678–705. [CrossRef]
16. Aretxabaleta, M.; Xepapadeas, A.B.; Poets, C.F.; Koos, B.; Spintzyk, S. Comparison of additive and subtractive CAD/CAM materials for their potential use as Tübingen Palatal Plate: An in-vitro study on flexural strength. *Addit. Manuf.* **2021**, *37*, 101693. [CrossRef]
17. Shin, J.-W.; Kim, J.-E.; Choi, Y.-J.; Shin, S.-H.; Nam, N.-E.; Shim, J.-S.; Lee, K.-W. Evaluation of the Color Stability of 3D-Printed Crown and Bridge Materials against Various Sources of Discoloration: An In Vitro Study. *Materials* **2020**, *13*, 5359. [CrossRef]
18. Li, P.; Schille, C.; Schweizer, E.; Kimmerle-Müller, E.; Rupp, F.; Heiss, A.; Legner, C.; Klotz, U.E.; Geis-Gerstorfer, J.; Scheideler, L. Selection of extraction medium influences cytotoxicity of dental alloys and its alloys. *Acta Biomater.* **2019**, *98*, 235–245. [CrossRef]
19. Atalayin, C.; Armagan, G.; Konyalioglu, S.; Kemaloglu, H.; Tezel, H.; Ergücü, Z.; Keser, A.; Dagci, T.; Önal, B. The protective effect of resveratrol against dentin bonding agents-induced cytotoxicity. *Dent. Mater. J.* **2015**, *34*, 766–773. [CrossRef]
20. Engelmann, J.; Leyhausen, G.; Leibfritz, D.; Geurtsen, W. Effect of TEGDMA on the intracellular glutathione concentration of human gingival fibroblasts. *J. Biomed. Mater. Res.* **2002**, *63*, 746–751. [CrossRef]
21. Schweikl, H.; Spagnuolo, G.; Schmalz, G. Genetic and Cellular Toxicology of Dental Resin Monomers. *J. Dent. Res.* **2006**, *85*, 870–877. [CrossRef]
22. Sancar, A.; Lindsey-Boltz, L.A.; Ünsal-Kaçmaz, K.; Linn, S. Molecular Mechanisms of Mammalian DNA Repair and the DNA Damage Checkpoints. *Annu. Rev. Biochem.* **2004**, *73*, 39–85. [CrossRef] [PubMed]
23. Samuelsen, J.T.; Dahl, J.E.; Karlsson, S.; Morisbak, E.; Becher, R. Apoptosis induced by the monomers HEMA and TEGDMA involves formation of ROS and differential activation of the MAP-kinases p38, JNK and ERK. *Dent. Mater.* **2007**, *23*, 34–39. [CrossRef]
24. Faggion, C.M. Guidelines for Reporting Pre-clinical In Vitro Studies on Dental Materials. *J. Evid. Based Dent. Pract.* **2012**, *12*, 182–189. [CrossRef] [PubMed]
25. Kopperud, H.M.; Kleven, I.S.; Wellendorf, H. Identification and quantification of leachable substances from polymer-based orthodontic base-plate materials. *Eur. J. Orthod.* **2011**, *33*, 26–31. [CrossRef]
26. Nakano, H.; Kato, R.; Kakami, C.; Okamoto, H.; Mamada, K.; Maki, K. Development of Biocompatible Resins for 3D Printing of Direct Aligners. *J. Photopolym. Sci. Technol.* **2019**, *32*, 209–216. [CrossRef]
27. Kurzmann, C.; Janjić, K.; Shokoohi-Tabrizi, H.; Edelmayer, M.; Pensch, M.; Moritz, A.; Agis, H. Evaluation of Resins for Stereolithographic 3D-Printed Surgical Guides: The Response of L929 Cells and Human Gingival Fibroblasts. *Biomed. Res. Int.* **2017**, *2017*, 4057612. [CrossRef] [PubMed]
28. Kessler, A.; Reichl, F.-X.; Folwaczny, M.; Högg, C. Monomer release from surgical guide resins manufactured with different 3D printing devices. *Dent. Mater.* **2020**, *36*, 1486–1492. [CrossRef] [PubMed]
29. Kotyk, M.W.; Wiltshire, W.A. An investigation into bisphenol-A leaching from orthodontic materials. *Angle Orthod.* **2014**, *84*, 516–520. [CrossRef]
30. Al Naqbi, S.R.; Pratsinis, H.; Kletsas, D.; Eliades, T.; Athanasiou, A.E. In Vitro Assessment of Cytotoxicity and Estrogenicity of Vivera® Retainers. *J. Contemp. Dent. Pract.* **2018**, *19*, 1163–1168. [CrossRef]
31. Schuster, S.; Eliades, G.; Zinelis, S.; Eliades, T.; Bradley, T.G. Structural conformation and leaching from in vitro aged and retrieved Invisalign appliances. *Am. J. Orthod. Dentofac. Orthop.* **2004**, *126*, 725–728. [CrossRef] [PubMed]
32. Xu, Y.; Xepapadeas, A.B.; Koos, B.; Geis-Gerstorfer, J.; Li, P.; Spintzyk, S. Effect of post-rinsing time on the mechanical strength and cytotoxicity of a 3D printed orthodontic splint material. *Dent. Mater.* **2021**, *37*, e314–e327. [CrossRef] [PubMed]
33. Wedekind, L.; Güth, J.-F.; Schweiger, J.; Kollmuss, M.; Reichl, F.-X.; Edelhoff, D.; Högg, C. Elution behavior of a 3D-printed, milled and conventional resin-based occlusal splint material. *Dent. Mater.* **2021**, *37*, 701–710. [CrossRef]
34. Alifui-Segbaya, F.; Bowman, J.; White, A.R.; Varma, S.; Lieschke, G.J.; George, R. Toxicological assessment of additively manufactured methacrylates for medical devices in dentistry. *Acta Biomater.* **2018**, *78*, 64–77. [CrossRef]
35. Chen, S.; Li, S.; Fang, D.; Bai, Y. Quantification of metal trace elements in orthodontic polymeric aligners and retainers by inductively coupled plasma mass spectrometry (ICP-MS). *Int. J. Clin. Exp. Med.* **2016**, *9*, 16273–16282.

36. Raghavan, A.S.; Pottipalli Sathyanarayana, H.; Kailasam, V.; Padmanabhan, S. Comparative evaluation of salivary bisphenol A levels in patients wearing vacuum-formed and Hawley retainers: An in-vivo study. *Am. J. Orthod. Dentofac. Orthop.* **2017**, *151*, 471–476. [CrossRef]
37. Iliadi, A.; Koletsi, D.; Papageorgiou, S.N.; Eliades, T. Safety Considerations for Thermoplastic-Type Appliances Used as Orthodontic Aligners or Retainers. A Systematic Review and Meta-Analysis of Clinical and In-Vitro Research. *Materials* **2020**, *13*, 1843. [CrossRef]
38. Huang, D.; Xu, Y.; Lei, F.; Yu, X.; Ouyang, Z.; Chen, Y.; Jia, H.; Guo, X. Degradation of polyethylene plastic in soil and effects on microbial community composition. *J. Hazard. Mater.* **2021**, *416*, 126173. [CrossRef] [PubMed]
39. Viera, J.S.C.; Marques, M.R.C.; Nazareth, M.C.; Jimenez, P.C.; Sanz-Lázaro, C.; Castro, Í.B. Are biodegradable plastics an environmental rip off? *J. Hazard. Mater.* **2021**, *416*, 125957. [CrossRef]
40. Jiang, B.; Kauffman, A.E.; Li, L.; McFee, W.; Cai, B.; Weinstein, J.; Lead, J.R.; Chatterjee, S.; Scott, G.I.; Xiao, S. Health impacts of environmental contamination of micro- and nanoplastics: A review. *Environ. Health Prev. Med.* **2020**, *25*, 29. [CrossRef] [PubMed]

MDPI
St. Alban-Anlage 66
4052 Basel
Switzerland
Tel. +41 61 683 77 34
Fax +41 61 302 89 18
www.mdpi.com

Bioengineering Editorial Office
E-mail: bioengineering@mdpi.com
www.mdpi.com/journal/bioengineering

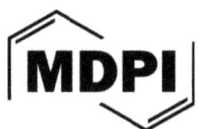